Communication and the care of people with dementia

John Killick
Kate Allan

Open University Press
Buckingham • Philadelphia

Open University Press
Celtic Court
22 Balmoor
Buckingham
MK18 1XW

email: enquiries@openup.co.uk
world wide web: www.openup.co.uk

and
325 Chestnut Street
Philadelphia, PA 19106, USA

First published 2001

A catalogue record of this book is available from the British Library

ISBN 0 335 20774 X (pb)   0 335 20775 8 (hb)

Library of Congress Cataloging-in-Publication Data
Killick, John, 1936–
    Communication and the care of people with dementia / John Killick, Kate Allan.
        p.   cm.
    Includes bibliographical references and index.
    ISBN 0–335–20775–8 — ISBN 0–335–20774–X (pbk.)
    1. Dementia. 2. Dementia—Patients—Care. 3. Interpersonal communication.
    I. Allan, Kate, 1965– II. Title.

RC521.K55 2001
362.1'9683—dc21   2001021076

Typeset by Type Study, Scarborough
Printed in Great Britain by Biddles Limited, Guildford and Kings Lynn

We dedicate this book to the people with dementia and their relatives who have participated in and supported the work which forms its basis. Their generous sharing has allowed us the kinds of insights which have the potential to change minds and hearts in the ways we so desperately need.

Contents

Part 3: Themes

Part 4: Implications

Part 5: Integration

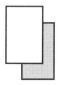

Acknowledgements

We would like to thank Professor Mary Marshall and our colleagues at the Dementia Services Development Centre at Stirling University and elsewhere for their support. There are others who have helped us with suggestions, criticisms, encouragement and technical assistance, all of which is much appreciated. These include Alastair Allan, Carole Archibald, Ailsa Cook, Bob Ferguson, Kate Foster and Faith Gibson.

Our appreciation goes to Westminster Health Care for sustained support of John as their writer in residence since 1992. They made it possible for him to undertake the learning process out of which this book was born.

Our families and friends have been endlessly forbearing during the time we have been working on the book, and we thank them for this.

We are grateful to the Linbury Trust for two grants which bought us time for writing.

Lastly we wish to acknowledge the following journals in which passages of the text have previously appeared: Psychologists Special Interest Group in Elderly People (PSIGE) newsletter, *Changes*, *Journal of Dementia Care*, *Mental Health Journal*, *Elderly Care* and *Signpost*.

Introduction

How much should the authors of a book know about the subject matter before setting out to write it? The idea of writing a book certainly could imply that it already exists somewhere, and only awaits transformation into physical reality. Perhaps it is so with some. This book has certainly not been like that. In many ways the process of bringing it into being has paralleled the experience of undertaking communication work with people with dementia, where it seems that the thoughts and ideas emerge only in the very process of talking and writing about them.

Our collaboration has taken the form of a series of extended and searching explorations of John's experiences. By the time we agreed to write the book together, he had spent five years working as a writer in residence with people with dementia. It had become clear to him early on in that period that important things were happening for people during the course of the work. It emerged only much later that important things were also happening to John. The next few years were spent (not exclusively) on a process of reflection on the nature, meaning and implications of the work. Prior to this John had proceeded largely intuitively, guided by a strong set of values, and developing new awareness and skills as he went, but not subjecting his experiences to conscious analysis.

Kate brought to this process a fascination with the subject, and a deep regard for the experience of the person with dementia. In keeping with her training and experience in psychology, she embarked on trying to achieve an understanding of what was actually going on in this kind of communication and relationship.

John endured a lot of cross-questioning in the course of our collaboration on this book. For example:

Why did you do that?
What did she do then?
How did you feel about it?
What do you think an observer would have made of that?
Would you do the same now?
What do you think that means?
How does that fit with what we think we already know?

It was often only while engaged in this process that we began to apprehend the complexity and subtlety of what had been going on, and there was a real sense of excitement in starting to give shape and expression to it. We hope that at least some of the quality of our enthusiasm comes across in the writing. Sometimes the sheer intricacy and shadowiness of what we have been exploring has felt daunting, even overwhelming. It seems that we are raising a whole lot of difficult and complicated subjects and then trying to string them all together into a coherent whole.

There are lots of maybes in the book. We really understand so little about dementia: what it is, how it affects people, and what are the best ways of thinking about it and responding to them. Quite often we found ourselves in the position of describing a set of circumstances, and then speculating on how they might be understood or interpreted. From here we have further speculated on the implications, and soon it feels as if we are sitting atop a set of interconnected limbs and we may wonder how we got there. Since we are all so early in the process of getting to grips with the meaning of dementia, we feel an attitude of tentativeness and openness should be the norm. You may find much that you disagree with us about, but if we have raised issues, prompted questions, excited curiosity and sometimes aroused passions then we will have achieved some success.

It will quickly become obvious that in the course of developing our argument we use a great many quotations – not only from people with dementia, but also from other writers in the dementia world and elsewhere – fiction, poetry and other areas of study. Our justification of this strategy is threefold: first, it is so often the case that another writer has made a point much more eloquently than we could ourselves; second (and this applies only if we have used their words fairly) the fact that someone else has said it reinforces our argument; and third, we believe strongly in the value of drawing on the thinking and experience of writers outwith the field of dementia care. It would also be fair to point out that sometimes finding the passage came first, and this then prompted us to develop a particular line of thinking. In this way we hope the book will be strengthened by its links with other subject areas and disciplines.

Throughout the book we have quoted extensively from the words of people with dementia in their conversations with John. In accordance with the principle of confidentiality we have done everything we can to seek permission to use these, from the individuals themselves, and often from their relatives as well. In all the texts names, places and certain other details have been changed in order to preserve anonymity. In addition to this, all of our chapter titles embody quotes from people with dementia. We have a very strong sense of responsibility in representing people's thoughts here, not only in terms of passing on messages which people clearly wanted others to be aware of, but also in protecting people who are in a vulnerable situation. It has been done in a spirit of respect, humility and the hope that their words and actions, which are so often powerful and vivid demonstrations of people's continued integrity and struggle, will help to improve the care of people with dementia everywhere. We therefore earnestly hope that no one will be offended or upset to recognize their words or those of a relative or friend. The book would be immeasurably the less without them, and its chances of making a difference much reduced.

We should briefly explain about the terminology we have used. Regarding the name of the condition itself, we refer to it simply as 'dementia'. We are aware in so doing that we are implying that there is just one thing called dementia, which of course is not true. However, it would quickly become unwieldy always to refer in the plural to what is probably a group of conditions which have features in common. We also wish to avoid referring to 'the dementias', which carries unfortunate overtones of people themselves being referred to as 'dementias'. We do not use the word 'disease' or 'illness' since this implies that dementia is purely a medical entity. Rather the more neutral term 'condition' is used, which being vaguer is more inclusive of the psychological and social aspects alongside the physical ones.

As regards talking about the person themselves, we reject the term 'sufferer', which is still the most common way of referring to the individual with the condition. It is too negative in tone, but even worse it defines the person entirely in terms of their having dementia. Instead we have used the phrase 'person with dementia' or 'people with dementia', and while this may be clumsy at times, it seems the clearest and most value-free description. We never describe a person as 'demented' since this again defines them in terms of the condition, and also implies that they have reached a qualitatively different state, perhaps even some kind of endpoint. (We should acknowledge that the terms 'sufferer' and 'demented' are used in some of the quotes employed.)

Since most of John's experience has been in nursing homes, much of the material quoted or discussed arises from that context. We appreciate, however, that there exists a great diversity in terms of the services used by people with dementia, including, increasingly, home-based support. Similarly most of his work has been with older people, though of course dementia affects people in their forties and fifties too. Whilst many of the issues raised will be common to both groups, some will differ.[1]

Although the material is complex we have tried to make the book as easy to use as possible. It is in five parts. The text is framed by two portraits, in their own words, of Alice and Jane, both of whom have dementia. The idea here is to present these individuals directly to the reader, to set the person with dementia centre stage. Alice raises all sorts of questions which we hope the book will go on to address, and Jane invites us to reflect on her words in the light of what has gone before.

In between come a series of chapters which can be broadly grouped into theoretical, practical and thematic categories. After the words of Alice, and a chapter on the idea of personhood in dementia, which provides the context and sets out the fundamental ideas and values of the book, Part 1 continues with material on the basics of communication. The four chapters in Part 2 constitute a guided tour of practical aspects of an interaction. The three chapters in Part 3 deal with larger themes which seem to have special significance. There could have been many more of these, but selectivity was necessary. Part 4 concentrates on implications of what has gone before for care practice, and also the ethical dimensions of the work. Because both of these subjects are all pervasive, we have given each a special role in the book. Sections on implications for care and ethical implications therefore appear at the end of most chapters.

Our starting points

We do not see ourselves as presenting a theory of dementia, nor indeed a theory of communication. We have not attempted to review the ideas of others. There is other work which does this, and it would simply have made this book too long. When relevant to our argument, however, we do refer to other authors and recommend work by them. But, of course, despite the lack of a coherent theory our arguments are based on a set of assumptions. Instead of delineating these, however, we have decided to identify some of the common beliefs about dementia which this book is setting out to challenge:

- that dementia is primarily a physical condition which leads to predictable deterioration in the person's cognitive, social and practical skills
- that what makes a human being a person is lost somewhere in the development of the condition
- that the ability to communicate, both verbally and nonverbally, is located within the individual, and steadily declines as the condition progresses
- that the individual has no meaningful inner life or awareness of what is happening to them
- that dementia undermines the need and capacity to maintain relationships or form new ones
- that all aspects of memory steadily deteriorate until the individual's existence is entirely unsupported by it
- that the individual progressively loses emotional coherence and control
- that dementia leads to a decline in all creative disposition and expression
- that other people are helpless to influence the progress of the condition, and that the result is always an experience of loss.

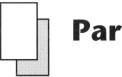 **Part 1:** Basics

1 Conversations with Alice: 'A far fetch'

Alice lives in a mental health unit in a nursing home in England. She is a short, dumpy woman in her mid-eighties. She has a shock of silvering hair, black bushy eyebrows and rather protruding blue eyes. Most of her days are spent walking around the unit attempting to engage other residents in conversations; her attitude in these exchanges is usually one of haughty impatience. Occasionally she sings 'Hee haw, hee haw' in raucous tones over and over in a manner which seems calculated to annoy. At other times she sleeps. There are days when she is too ill to talk at all.

Often, however, she appears deliberately to seek out John in order to unburden herself of ideas and feelings that she has been saving up. They have had over twenty extended conversations of this kind spread over as many weeks. His role is that of a befriender and listener as well as recorder, not that of a carer or clinician. His knowledge of her illness is minimal. He responds to her as a person. Their friendship is based on mutual trust. One day she says to him:

Anything you can tell people about how things are for me is important.

But at times she gets impatient with the process they are undertaking together. After working with John one day, and getting angry and upset with herself, she shouts to a member of staff:

Take this man away! I don't want to fill in any more of his questionnaires.

Underlying it all, however, there seems to be a sense of urgency in what she is doing. She says things like:

You're only coming in the nick of time. A lot of this has already faded.

Mostly she seems desperately to want to recall her life and times, and she approaches the task with positive resolve:

I don't think I'm going to forget this again. No, I think I'm going to manage it. Sort it out without a doubt.

At the same time she remembers that what she is embarked upon is, for her, a process fraught with difficulties:

It's a far fetch this writing of my life.

There is scope for humour and playfulness, however:

I must tell you the tale of my life, sir, but I don't want my tea to get cold.

This latter statement seems to carry a special significance when directed at John, which it has been on more than one occasion. She also enjoys saying things like:

Daniel in the Lion's Den
has slipped away by hissen.

These rhymes when occurring in the middle of prose conversations partake of the same enigmatic quality as many of her other utterances.

There are occasions when she realizes that willing the process cannot bring results:

I have the idea that too much fussing about memory makes it worse.

and:

It's so foolish to get yourself in a knot. Or to grieve about getting yourself into a knot.

Some memories come from very early in her life:

I had a younger sister, and when my mother asked her 'Do you remember father?' she said 'No, was he the poorly man in the bed?'

They may only last a few moments, or a sentence or two, as in:

I can hear my mother singing in the kitchen.

Sometimes a sense of fragmentation seems to be uppermost. The thought that everything is slipping away from her is very upsetting:

It's the terrific confusion of things that worries me more than anything else.

There appears to be an element of doubt about her own identity, as in:

This isn't my voice today. I've not heard myself sounding like this before. It isn't my cough either. It's a tomfool cough. And it belongs to Tom.

But despite this, she has a great need to try to make sense of what is happening to her:

I don't know why I came here. But I think it was for my health. You see, we know the Cause but cannot cope with the Effect.

She knows that she is not well, and perhaps believes that her problems might be hereditary:

I never expected to be in this silly condition. My grandmother would say quite frequently 'I do forget.' And now it has come to me.

Sometimes she rationalizes it, as in:

It's as the Lord made it that I have forgotten so many things. Just think if you carried all that around with you all your life!

Alice also speaks of her sense of loss regarding her intellectual powers:

The brilliance of my brain has slipped away when I wasn't looking.

And she gives expression to her need to understand what is going on:

After all, what is this lump of matter if you can't make sense of it?

She talks about her surroundings in a rather indirect way, as if she cannot bring herself to admit it is her own situation to which she is referring:

That's the Nursing Home over there, isn't it? Well I hope never to be there.

and:

There are lots of cars rolling up to that Nursing Home. Oh, I hope I don't have to go into one of those places.

She comments on features of the environment and the people in it:

The set-up here is very complicated. You have them howling around the place thinking it's straight forrard.

And:

We seem to be having rather a fussy do. The yowling has been enough to scare anyone's wits.

She appears to use an extended metaphor to talk about her experience of living in the home:

I'm suffering from monkey-puzzle. The monkey-puzzle is this place. The puzzle is: how do I cope with the monkeys?

Clearly the monkeys are despised authority figures, and they are linked to the 'peppering':

Well I've had my mouth nicely peppered this morning, not literally you understand.

'Peppering' appears to refer to being talked about behind one's back.

She has plenty to say on what seems to be the subject of her relationships with other residents:

The kids have told me straight. 'We don't like you.' I didn't like being told. But it's honest – I'm really pleased to know.

Sometimes Alice talks of being detained against her will:

As you well know I'm a prisoner here. My sister has stolen my life. Now I'm old and expected to dream my time away.

She seems to need to have a wider perspective on her situation:

I want a natural life where I can see my forebears and enjoy the fruits of my labours.

and:

I want to get to the point where it's a matter of course.

Alice's emotions range from the bleakest despair:

I'll end up dotty, I'm afraid they'll break me up for firewood. I'm good for nothing else.

to elation:

Oh, you know, we are cared for, aren't we? People try so hard to get us into a normal situation. It comes over me in a distinct feeling of joy.

Ultimately she seems aware of the power differential between herself and those who are in charge, and makes a rather stunning request of John:

Are you a person who could swing it for me with the authorities? I want you to ask them a question for me:
Would they please give me back my personality?

The purpose of this brief chapter has been to present a portrait of Alice in what were her current circumstances and state of mind as far as possible in her own words. The interpretations we have offered are provisional and subjective. Her style of speaking and the things she said were both absolutely distinctive and memorable, and also shared characteristics with those of other people John went on to meet, some of whom are quoted later in this book.

The last words must be Alice's own. This is a complete piece she dictated to John on his last visit. It illustrates many of the characteristics to which we have drawn attention. She responded to his questions about the phrasing she wanted. But once the text was finalized she showed no interest in either hearing it or viewing it.

I can't remember anything of today except the peppering of my tongue. Yes, my mouth was peppered again this morning. As an educated man, I thought perhaps you might be an expert in these matters. I believe it is all part of the monkey-puzzle.

These little monkeys have two legs, you know, and wear suits. These whiskers that are growing around the lower part of my face, I did think that they formed part of the category of the monkey-puzzle, just put there to irritate the newcomers. But what can't be cured must be endured. You wish the trouble was at Timbuktu, but if it can't be then it has to be here.

I've come to the conclusion that we should educate these monkeys. First of all, I should make it perfectly clear to them that there are certain things that are not done, even though I know that they are laughing their heads off behind my back.

This man who has just entered the room, is he to be trusted? Could he be one of the monkeys? No, I don't think so, he hasn't got the brain. But he doesn't seem very interested in us. Each morning he has his little sport. It doesn't involve me. Each day I watch it as an observer. I am thinking it might be a source of the peppering that is going on.

My sister definitely said to me 'Don't let them get you!' Talk about a monkey puzzle! Well I reckon they got me!'

If you said to me right now 'Would you like to give a present day outline of your life?' I wouldn't know. I'm here. I'm comfortable. But who put me here I wouldn't know. I never intended to be here. Yet it's familiar enough. And here's me whining away like some silly petted baby. Surely I must have been kidnapped to end up here long past my bedtime?

2 | **Personhood:** 'The truth is mine, not yours'

We start this chapter with an account of how John first encountered people with dementia in his work as a writer in residence. As well as being the beginning of the story of this book, this account seemed to us to be the best way of setting the scene for what is to follow.

For the previous year he had been writing the life histories of frail residents in nursing homes, and it had been agreed that he should try the same kind of approach with people with dementia. He knew nothing about the subject, however, and had never met anyone with the condition:

> The manager opened the door of the unit. As I entered he expressed the view that I would have little success in establishing any kind of communication with the residents, far less undertaking life history work with them. Then the door was locked behind me. I looked around the lounge and saw twenty to thirty people, some in chairs, others walking, but all displaying peculiar characteristics: strange repetitive movements, or making clumsy attempts to move furniture, or crying out or using unusual combinations of words. I was frightened, and remained so to a greater or lesser extent for two or three days. The reasons for this were various. People who behave strangely are upsetting, and even more so en masse. Part of this was simply fear of the unknown. I didn't understand what these people were saying or

doing, or the motivation behind their behaviour. I was afraid I might be harmed. Some of their physical characteristics and actions were repellent to me, and I worried that I might be 'contaminated' and become 'mad' myself.

All these feelings were entirely new for me. In every other environment I had encountered (for example prisons, hospices, schools), although I might not have understood everything that was going on, I grasped enough to allow me to feel comfortable. Here I understood nothing: my expectations of normality had been completely overturned. I couldn't reason with these people. I couldn't empathize with them. The most disturbing thing about all this was that it seemed to mean that ultimately I couldn't love them.

I was overcome by a feeling of immense helplessness. If you cannot exercise your humanity in ways which can help people, and they cannot give anything back to you, then no mutuality is possible. A basic part of being human is the belief that we all share something that is recognizable and communicable. In this situation, the inability to perceive any kind of similarity was compounded by a perception of their apparent lack of interest in me. My own selfhood was radically threatened by this experience.

A further factor which caused me distress was my appointed role. Other staff were there to carry out specific practical duties. They could escape into 'doing' from the awful existential truth that communication was impossible. My job, on the contrary, was to confront this reality head-on. I felt wholly inadequate. I was afraid to act in case I made an impossible situation worse. So I coped by cultivating invisibility in corners or taking to the staffroom to experience the relief of 'normal' encounters.

Despite finding these withdrawals necessary, I decided on the second day that if there was to be any kind of progress I must remain twenty-four hours a day on the unit. I hoped to become accustomed to the atmosphere, and to familiarize myself as fully as possible with the residents, and that through this my fear would lessen. This involved taking meals with them, and sleeping in their environment.

It was some time on the third day that I experienced a breakthrough. I had some real interactions with individuals, and these were positive in nature. One man approached me, took my hand and led me to a private place. He proceeded to confide some of his thoughts and feelings about the home to me. Another lady embarked on what was to become a series of encounters, and gave me permission to write down her words. In spite of very low initial expectations, here was clear evidence that communication was possible. It could not have been a more welcome discovery. With these developments I had an overwhelming sense of relief, and certainly no longer felt threatened by the residents. They had suddenly become people in my eyes, and I was filled with empathy for them. Of course they themselves hadn't changed at all. It was my perception which had profoundly altered.

This development enabled me to interpret their actions in different ways, and meaning suddenly blossomed. Instead of seeing their behaviours purely as symptoms of some terrible and mysterious disease, a kind of plague that had been visited upon them, I began to see many of the difficulties they experienced as closely related to problems of perception and of verbal expression. I found that they were often endearing traits. It became possible not only to recognize distinctive actions and mannerisms, but to perceive patterns and motivations underpinning them.

Relaxed at last, not uptight and wary, I became aware that people were reaching out to me, and also apparently offering friendship and consolation to another whom they perceived to be in the same situation as themselves. Once I got to this point I found that these people had more in common with human beings generally than I could possibly have imagined at first. Their humour, fellow-feeling, insightfulness and honesty were remarkable. This was a humbling experience, and accompanied by a great feeling of joy that my capacities could be fully used. This freed me to play a much fuller part in life on the unit. When someone couldn't remember something, I felt for them. When the words wouldn't come right, I found I could help. When someone took pleasure in something, I shared it.

By the end of the week I did not want to leave the unit. It was a wrench to be parted from so many friends with whom I had forged bonds of a unique kind.

All that took place in 1993; John has since worked with hundreds of people with dementia, sometimes writing down what they have to say and always reflecting upon any texts and the details of encounters. At first he deliberately read as little as possible about dementia as he was concerned that accumulating 'knowledge' and being exposed to the perspectives of others might interfere with the exploratory approach he was developing. After a couple of years, this need had subsided. He began to read about the subject, and has since talked to many interested people about his work and experiences.

In retrospect that week of initiation into the world of dementia can be viewed as a telescoping of the history of changes in attitudes during the 1990s towards dementia as a condition, and our responsibilities towards those who have it. Since it is important to understand about these changes, and the context of this book, let us attempt to tease out the parallels.

Making sense of the experience

At the beginning of the five days John saw dementia as a disease, a serious medical problem which had totally engulfed the person. Our western cultural inheritance disposes us strongly to understand differentness in medical terms, and as a result he would certainly have accepted an explanation like the following for what he saw:

> Alzheimer's Disease is a physical condition. The mental and emotional changes are a direct result of a set of catastrophic changes in the brain that lead to the death of the brain cells. The degeneration is irreversible.[1]

Reflecting our society's horror of the ageing process,[2] illness and disability, and eventual death, and given the fear and disgust that he felt initially, he might even have gone along with the description of the physical shell that was left behind as:

> this grotesque thing in the corner . . . an uncollected corpse.[3]

Those in the unit would certainly have been in danger of not being recognized as persons in the sense that it is normally understood.

As a writer John could see no place for himself in that environment, since communication appeared to be an impossibility. Again these were very much the attitudes commonly found at the beginning of the 1990s. In so far as the subject of communication was thought about at all, it was to chart what was perceived as the inevitable destruction of abilities, and the inexorable decline into incoherence and eventually silence and complete isolation. Blanket statements about the person being 'unable to communicate' were commonplace. The observed changes in the person's communicative skills were routinely attributed to core features of the dementia, and no acknowledgement was made of the role of psychological factors (for example, the impact of the person's own feelings about their difficulties, loss of confidence, and so on) and social influences (the attitudes and behaviour of others). This way of thinking reflected an understanding of the course of the condition always being uniformly progressive. Various 'stage theories' have been advanced,[4] but all are based on the expectation that the person's capacities and skills deteriorate in predictable and irreversible fashion.

If John's perceptions had not changed, he would have found himself contributing to what the psychologist Tom Kitwood (who is the main person associated with the changes in attitudes towards people with dementia) identified as the 'malignant social psychology' which surrounds people with the condition. The word 'malignant' here refers not to any kind of intentional maliciousness, but rather the social and interpersonal processes which inevitably follow from the categorization of human beings as no longer persons. Some examples will serve to illustrate:[5]

> Banishment – the person is either sent away or excluded, either physically, psychologically, or both – thus depriving them of sustaining human contact.

> Invalidation – the person's subjectivity, especially their feelings, is either denied, not acknowledged or dismissed as insignificant.

Labelling – the diagnostic category becomes the foundation for attempts to understand, and attempts to communicate with, the person.

Stigmatization – the person is treated as an outcast.

As a result of this treatment, the person with dementia was basically isolated – at best tended physically, but otherwise left to drift in their unknown and apparently unknowable world until they died. The fact that John had encountered these people in a group, and seen them as being essentially indistinguishable from one another, intensified his experience of alienation. This parallels society's attitudes towards older people generally, and the additional factors of illness and disability serve to consign them to an even more anonymous and irrelevant collective.

The change in John's attitudes and perceptions came when he began to make contact with people as individuals. What followed from this was a series of interactions which demonstrated that far from being part of an undifferentiated group, every person with dementia was unique and responded to a distinctive approach. What is more, they did not just absorb his attention but expressed a great range and depth of human qualities in return. He realized that instead of being isolated, these people desperately needed to continue in relationships despite the difficulties they encountered. Things that they said could be written down, and emerged as being of profound interest. Although at first people's words were the most salient aspect of their communication, later the nonverbal dimensions of encounters emerged as being highly significant, as did interactions which did not include words at all.

What lies at the heart of these observations and experiences is the idea of personhood. Are people with dementia truly persons, with all that that implies, or have they, through the progression of the condition, lost that which we feel to be essential? Many thinkers have defined personhood in terms of characteristics and abilities which are located within the individual, such as insight, rationality and memory.[6] These criteria appear to exclude people, such as those with dementia, who have difficulty in these areas. Kitwood's central thesis is that these ways of defining personhood are mistaken. Instead he proposed that it is:

a standing or status which is bestowed on one human being, by others, in the context of relationship and social being. It implies recognition, respect and trust.[7]

This is indeed exactly what John had experienced. It was through encountering people with dementia and finding ways to communicate with them that their personhood became a reality. By the end of that week John had already begun to perceive what his later experiences would reinforce: that people with dementia are truly persons and have a meaningful contribution to make to our shared humanity. The implications of such an idea are something we are all still in the process of discovering, and we explore further the concept of personhood later in this chapter.[8] But in order to appreciate this reality we must be prepared to recognize and challenge the values which go along with what the ethicist Stephen Post has called our 'hypercognitive culture' in which:

clarity of mind and economic productivity determine the value of a human life.[9]

It is difficult to overestimate the extent to which our culture and our thinking are organized around the idea that an intelligent human being is more valuable than one who is not considered to be such. Questions about who has the power to define the idea of intelligence, and what happens to those who do not qualify, rarely arise. We are hugely reluctant to recognize, nurture and celebrate other human qualities, and this serves to impoverish us all.

In the development of his ideas Kitwood argued forcefully that we need to undergo a fundamental shift of perspective away from seeing the person as being entirely overtaken by dementia, with all the emphasis on deficit and deterioration, and where essentially everything the person is and does is interpreted as being part of the condition. Instead the focus should be on the person, who they are, how they understand and experience their world, and what they need in order to maintain their sense of self.[10] Kitwood summarized this position with the simple yet revolutionary formulation:

PERSON with dementia
rather than
person with DEMENTIA

This way of conceptualizing dementia has been termed the 'psychosocial' model, which Kitwood saw as an expansion of the 'biomedical' model or 'standard paradigm', rather than an alternative to it. In other words, Kitwood accepted that there was a neurological basis for change in the individual, but emphasized the importance of its interaction with psychological and social factors. Since each individual is unique, the particular ways in which they are affected and the condition develops are similarly unique. As thinking in this area has progressed, however, some have raised the possibility that dementia is an entirely socially constructed condition with no physical basis at all.[11] The arguments continue, but in the meantime we need to proceed with an open mind, and an acceptance that dementia remains something of an unknown quantity. We have a long way to go in achieving a full understanding of its nature and consequences for the individual person.[12]

Having set out a model of dementia, the next step was to consider what it suggested in terms of practical responses. Kitwood developed the concept of what he called 'person-centred care', which was essentially a set of values and strategies to recognize, maintain and even enhance the personhood of the individual through all aspects of the care process. He made high claims for this approach:

> If personhood is to be maintained, it is essential that each individual be appreciated in his or her uniqueness. Where there is empathy without personal knowledge, care will be aimless and unfocused. Where there is personal knowledge without empathy, care will be detached and cold. But when empathy and personal knowledge are brought together, miracles can happen.[13]

For the next few years, the idea of person-centred care was widely taken up within the world of services. This happened despite the fact that neither Kitwood nor anyone else had done much to spell out exactly what was involved in providing such care. It is only very recently that some have begun to question the concept seriously, pointing out that we are very far off understanding and following through on the implications of personhood in the care of people with dementia. Among these is specialist nurse Tracy Packer, who says:

> Every week, shocked family carers, social workers and agency nursing staff in particular, describe incidents to me that would not be taking place so frequently if true person-centred care really was as widely implemented as we sometimes like to believe.[14]

Ian Morton, a specialist in dementia care who has a background in nursing, has devoted a whole book to tracing the origins of this approach.[15] He sees the American psychologist Carl Rogers with his client-centred therapy as under-pinning Kitwood's formulation and placing it within a historical context.[16] Alongside the development of Kitwood's ideas are other approaches which have played a part in altering attitudes to dementia. These include Naomi Feil's validation therapy,[17] Fiona Goudie and Graham Stokes's resolution therapy,[18] and Gary Prouty's pre-therapy.[19] What all these approaches have in common is their person-centred focus, and together they create a culture in which the person is acknowledged in all their individuality and complexity, and innovations of a humane kind can flourish.

The special role of communication

If it is true, as those we have cited maintain, that the quality we call person-hood is made real through relationships with others, then this is clearly where the crucial issues in the care of people with dementia lie. Further, central to the business of relationships is communication. We cannot be truly in relationship with others if we are not in communication with them.

This leads us to ask: what do we mean by the term 'communication'? While this is a fair question, in keeping with our approach in the book generally, we do not intend to make a specific attempt to pin this concept down. Our wish is that an open, inclusive approach be adopted, since we are still at an early stage in exploring the different forms communication can take and the possi-bilities it confers.

Before going on to explore the place of communication in the care of people with dementia, we need now to take more time to explore the role of communication in all of our lives. As with so many things, we do not appreciate our dependence on it until it is damaged or disrupted. How might this arise in relation to communication? It is certainly not necessary to have dementia to experience the consequences in terms of emotional distress, and even a disturbance in one's sense of self, through the withdrawal of normal communication. Being temporarily deaf because of an ear infection or unable to speak because of laryngitis provides a powerful illustration of how much our sense of things being normal relies on the capacity to communicate. This can also be demonstrated in social ways. The experience of being 'sent to Coventry' is normally associated with children, but it also happens in the adult world. Military cadet James Pelosi suffered severe physical and emotional consequences through being 'silenced' by his colleagues for an alleged misdemeanour.[20] The period of punishment went on for 19 months, and during this time no one in his company spoke to him or acknowledged him in any way. Despite being a particularly resilient character he lost 26 pounds in weight, and such were the psychological effects that when it was finally over, he said: 'It was just as if I was a person again.' It is no exaggeration, then, to say that communication is a basic human need, as John has elsewhere described it, it is a 'matter of the life and death of the mind'.[21] Perhaps we have yet properly to recognize that it is also a matter of the life and death of the body.

As we have seen, the traditional response has been very much to exclude those with dementia from the sphere of normal human communication, both in terms of ignoring what the person has to say and giving up any attempts to engage properly with them. Having come a long way in terms of recognition of the socially constructed nature of personhood, we are now in a position to wonder whether much of what we see when we encounter the individual – withdrawal, lack of competence – challenging behaviour and disturbed language and nonverbal expression, rather than being due to brain damage, is actually the result of the deprivation of opportunities for real communication. This has all the characteristics of the classic self-fulfilling prophecy. By labelling the individual and withdrawing them from normal interactions, we can precipitate the kinds of features and behaviours which we then consider evidence of the dementia. This in turn magnifies our own distorted responses, which triggers deeper distress and disorganization in the individual. And so it goes on.

Another crucially important facet of this interpersonal scenario is that of stigma. The sociologist Erving Goffman talks of those people who carry some form of stigma (whether it is physical disfigurement, a history of criminal behaviour or whatever) as being 'discredited', as having a 'spoiled identity' and lacking acceptance from others.[22] Once we have labelled someone in a negative way, the scene is set for the dynamics of stigma to set in, and again this often takes a circular form.

It is also important to recognize that our own deep-rooted fears of illness, deterioration and death strongly dispose us to avoid confronting the reality of the experience of people who have conditions like dementia. The assumption that communication is no longer possible is a convenient way of letting ourselves off this particular hook. To acknowledge that, underneath the dementia, the other person is much more similar to oneself than different, is to countenance the possibility that their difficulties may one day be our own or those of someone we love. These are deep waters.

The message arising from all of this is clear: we must devote much greater energy to supporting the individual in remaining in communication, and therefore relationship, with those around them. This is undoubtedly a challenge. Although we need to maintain an open mind on the question of what is socially induced as opposed to neurologically determined, it is undeniable that *something* is happening to people who develop dementia and this can make communication very difficult. In order to keep the channels open we must not only invest a lot of effort, but also be ready to challenge our own attitudes regarding, for example, what counts as communication, and our behaviour, for example by slowing down and taking more time to encourage, support and listen. As researcher Malcolm Goldsmith put it:

> We have to be willing to try and enter their 'world', with all its alternative boundaries and conventions, rather than expect them to respond to ours.[23]

Communication is an inherently mutual activity. By committing ourselves to the goal of true communication, we are also committing ourselves to being personally involved in what happens, we are engaging our own personhood in the enterprise. And it is an uncertain business. When we set out to establish a relationship with the individual, we can neither know what is going to happen, nor what it is going to mean. Real communication has the potential to make us aware of new problems, to challenge our ways of understanding people and their behaviour, and, at a very deep level, to change our own ways of seeing and experiencing our world. This is what a professor of social work, Faith Gibson, was recognizing when she posed the question 'Can we risk person-centred communication?' Having explored it from many different points of view, she concluded:

> We must employ whatever power we have in the world of dementia care for this purpose. We must use our present knowledge, our skills and feelings, to communicate. We are morally obliged to continue working in extending our limited understanding, developing our embryonic skills and taming our deep anxieties.[24]

Of course, as well as the risks, there are real rewards too. Entering into true communication and relationship with people with dementia not only has the potential to enhance the well-being of the individual and transform the experience of providing care for them, but also offers rich benefits in terms of personal and spiritual development to us too. This idea is central to the book.

Further facets of personhood

We shall now spend time exploring the nature and scope of the concept of personhood, since a greater understanding in this sphere will serve to inform and guide our efforts in the area of communication. Many of these are complex ideas, and they have a way of becoming slippery and intangible as soon as you start to think about them, but they are crucial and relevant to our subject. We do not present them in any particular order of priority, and they overlap and interlink in complicated ways.

Consciousness and self-consciousness

The phenomenon of consciousness is at the heart of being human, and our most intimate and significant experiences are inextricably linked with this quality. To put it in the simplest terms, consciousness is what makes us different from robots or computers, and probably all other animals. For example, the experience we call sadness is altered greatly by the fact that when we are sad, we can recognize and label the feeling, compare it with previous experiences of sadness, perhaps attribute it to a cause, and have expectations about how much longer it is likely to last. In short, we can have thoughts and feelings about having thoughts and feelings, and this is possible through the phenomenon of consciousness. Through this and the bewildering multiplicity of sensations, cognitions and emotions which go to make up our inner lives we develop a feeling of what it is like to be ourselves, ultimately a sense of self. As well as enabling us to adopt perspectives on specific states of mind or body, consciousness enables us to engage in reflection at the level of awareness of our overall circumstances, our state of health and well-being and its fragility, and ultimately to know that our time is limited, and that we will die.

At a further level, although we cannot have direct access to the consciousness of another person – we can never know directly about their joys or sufferings – the capacity for consciousness enables us to empathize and communicate with them, and this means that their experience becomes part of our own reality. The neurologist Antonio Damasio writes:

> Consciousness is, in effect, the key to a life examined, for better or for worse, our beginner's permit into knowing all about the hunger, the thirst, the sex, the tears, the laughter, the kicks, the punches, the flow of images we call thought, the feelings, the words, the stories, the beliefs, the music and the poetry, the happiness and the ecstasy. At its simplest and most basic level, consciousness lets us recognize an irresistible urge to stay alive and develop a concern for the self. At its most complex and elaborate level, consciousness helps us to develop a concern for other selves and improve the art of life.[25]

How do all these ideas relate to people with dementia? It seems safe to say that, as part of the belief that dementia destroys personhood, we have assumed that the individual's capacity for true consciousness is damaged or even obliterated, that there is no coherent sense of self and no real experience of subjectivity. If this kind of assumption does underpin our thinking in relation to people with dementia, it would be hard to overestimate its negative ramifications. It can only be through communication that we have a real opportunity to put these assumptions to the test.

The idea of the self

The word 'self' (and its variants – myself, yourself and so on) is used so frequently in our everyday thinking and conversations we give it no thought. But in using these words we are acknowledging that there is something to call a 'self' and that the idea is allied with what it is to be a person. The psychologist Rom Harré offers the following reflection on the nature of selfhood:

> the self, as the singularity we each feel ourselves to be, is not an entity. Rather it is a site, a site from which a person perceives the world and a place from which to act.[26]

As we discussed earlier, old ways of understanding dementia assumed that the condition is inherently destructive of selfhood. If we unpack this further we see that this can apply both to the destruction of whatever it is in a person that we call the 'self', and also to that person's sense of self, so that the person is assumed not only to be irretrievably lost to others, but also to themselves. And that this is all the more profound a loss for not being properly experienced as such – for if there is no self, there is no 'site' from which to experience loss, or anything else. The ethicist, Stephen Post, described dementia as

> an agonizing deterioration of the self . . . the very substratum of the self with respect to identity and coherence is on the path toward radical disintegration.[27]

While readily acknowledging that we do not fully understand the essential nature and workings of selfhood, we need to adopt a much more open attitude to questions about the preservation of selfhood in dementia than the one Post sets out here. This need arises both for practical purposes, so that we can address questions such as 'How should we behave in our dealings with people with dementia?' and for theoretical reasons 'How can we learn more about the nature of dementia and how it affects persons?'

Different selves

Whether or not you believe or feel yourself to have a kind of 'core' self which is the most fundamental part of you, our ordinary day-to-day experience is that of having a set of variants of the self or 'identities' that we call on at different times and in different situations. The self you experience at work or when going to a hospital appointment is probably different from the one you occupy when relaxing at home or when out with friends. The nature and extent of the variation in the experience and presentation of self is related to our attitudes and values, moods and feelings, our needs and motivations, the behaviour of others, and the characteristics and demands of a situation. This is a normal feature of our adaptability to the complexity and pressures of life.

Related to this is the fact that our convoluted social lives mean we have various roles in life, for example that of being a worker, mother, friend, neighbour, patient and so on.[28] The extent to which we see our own self being dominated by particular roles varies in accordance with personality, the attitudes of others and our life situation. A woman who has just become a mother may feel that her identity has suddenly become immersed in that role, whereas an older woman who has grandchildren who she sees only rarely is less likely to have a strong sense of herself in the role of a grandmother.

We need to consider questions about how the self and identity might relate to particular roles for people with dementia. Does the capacity to access and express different aspects of the self persist? Or is it that there is a narrowing down of the range? Perhaps over time people lose access to the various facets of their own self, meaning that they have a more restricted range of resources with which to cope with the demands of the situations in which they find themselves. For some people there may be a sense in which they are 'stuck' in the wrong version of the self, and this leads to apparent inappropriateness or incompetence. Our own responses to dementia may be as much to blame for this kind of disruption as anything inherent in the condition, and the very strangeness of the situations in which we force people with dementia to exist is likely to cause further disturbance to the workings of selfhood. This is what the psychologists Steven Sabat and Rom Harré are identifying in the following:

> Thus, if there is a loss of the capacity to present an appropriate self, in many cases the fundamental cause is to be found not in the neurofibrillary tangles and senile plaques in the brains of sufferers, but in the character of the social interactions and their interpretation that follow in the wake of the symptoms.[29]

We discuss the issue of roles in relation to people with dementia further in Chapter 12 on relationships.

Sometimes there can be very striking changes in the way a person with dementia appears to be experiencing themselves, and that is in connection with subjective age. We live in an age-conscious society, in which people are categorized and judged according to the number of years they have been alive. At the same time, the age we are and the age we feel are often very different. It is a fairly common observation that people with dementia seem sometimes to be convinced that they are much younger than they actually are, and speak and act from this point of view. What triggers such episodes and the exact nature of the experience is unknown, but it is certainly an interesting and perhaps very significant feature of the condition.

The possibility of helping people to explore and express their experience of selfhood, and of learning lessons about how we can help people to find the most constructive ways through this, can come about only through deep and genuine communication.

Stability and change

A further facet of the notion of self is that of its persistence over time. When we go to sleep at night we expect to wake up 'in' the same self the next morning, and when we make plans for a year or more ahead, we take it for granted that our dispositions and motivations will be similar then to how they are at present. When we look back in time, the feeling we have is of being the same self earlier in our lives, even if we can identify changes of various sorts. Although it is also true that when we meet someone we have not seen for years, we may remark 'She hasn't changed', as if it is somehow surprising that the passage of time and experience of life has not wrought more changes. Our world would be a very different and confusing place if people did not remain, in some core sense, constant throughout their lives.

That said, people do change in important ways, whether this is part of growing up or adult development and change. Sometimes change happens gradually and unconsciously, sometimes people deliberately set out to alter aspects of themselves. Events over which we have no control can also affect the self in a fundamental way. When a person is involved in an extreme event, such as a major accident or an act of violence, this can bring about sudden and radical change in what seem to be core aspects of self. And of course illness or accident can cause physical damage to the brain which has consequences for the nature of selfhood.

One of the most difficult and painful aspects of dementia is the perception that it can bring about changes in what seem to be defining aspects of the person. Until the 1990s it was assumed that this kind of change arose directly from brain damage. With a fuller understanding of psychological and social aspects of the condition, we are now able to recognize that such change could be as much the result of emotional and existential distress on the part of the person, and the effects of distorted and impoverished relationships with other people, as anything attributable to neurological change.

Sometimes changes occur in quite specific, maybe even limited, areas. Although there may be a loss of intellectual capacity, the person may remain recognizable in terms of their interpersonal or emotional style. A characteristic sense of humour may be retained, or a set of distinctive mannerisms or particular way of speaking. Or it may be that there are times when these features are absent, presumed lost, and then return for a while, restoring the sense of familiarity.

For other people, however, the kinds of changes the person is seen to undergo can be so radical that those around them might say that they are a different person altogether. Their personality or preferences may seem to have altered so significantly that it is no longer possible to predict what they might appreciate or enjoy. Aggressive impulses may appear in someone who was never known to lift a hand, or offensive language in an individual who previously demonstrated great restraint in that respect. Not all observed changes are negative. Some people seem to learn to enjoy new things or appreciate old things in a new way. Some relatives report on an enhanced emotional dimension to their relationships as if old and long-established barriers to affection have been broken down. Issues around the reality or perception of change in the self over time from the perspective of those around the individual are explored further in Chapter 12 on relationships.

But what is most interesting to us is the person's own perspective. With the recognition of retained personhood and the further possibilities that real communication confers, we are now in the position of being able to find out from the person themselves about their experience of change. This book is full of examples of what people say about this subject when given the opportunity.

Individuality and group membership

We all feel ourselves to be unique, different from others in many ways, obvious and subtle. Outward characteristics such as physical appearance, and the way we dress and adorn ourselves, are very visible examples of individuality, but our ways of thinking about things, beliefs and attitudes, quirks and foibles, likes and dislikes, and of course our individual history of experiences, and constellations of relationships, all go into making each one of us a one-off, unrepeatable person. Although we tend to see our individuality as something deriving from within us, a sense of individuality can be real only when it is acknowledged and upheld by others. People who have suffered the experience of incarceration in concentration camps, where active suppression and undermining of personal uniqueness is routine, attest to the socially constructed nature of a sense of individuality.

Alongside a feeling of being unique, as social beings we all need to have a sense of commonality with others, to seek membership of a group. We all define ourselves partly in terms of connections with other people, whether the link is predominantly cultural, emotional, professional, political or based in shared interest, activity or outlook. This need for connection with others is another important way in which personal identity is created and maintained, but it also means that we exist in a state of tension between being an individual and being a member of a group. Both confer benefits and make demands.

Although we now appreciate that recognition of each person's individuality is basic to good care, when a group of people with dementia is encountered for the first time it may seem, as in John's experience, that the similarities in the way people appear and conduct themselves are striking. No doubt some of this derives from the way we organize services for people with dementia. But with careful and sympathetic attention it does not take long for people to emerge as individuals with all their indefinable distinctiveness.

It seems safe to assume that people with dementia have a great need for us both to recognize and reflect their individuality and to affirm their need for relationships. Communication is the only way we can do this.

Self-image and self-esteem

Our self-image consists in the beliefs we hold about ourselves, and what we see as being our core and defining characteristics and values. For example, you may see yourself as being hardworking and tough-minded, and that these characteristics are more central to your identity than, say, your political views or your enjoyment of Indian food. These perceptions may be more or less in accordance with how others see you, but what is most important is that you believe them, and they influence how you make sense of situations, and how you respond to them. Also, like other aspects of the self, one's self-image is bound to change over time, but for most people certain aspects remain stable over long periods, perhaps a lifetime.

Intimately intertwined with our self-image is self-esteem – how positively or negatively, sympathetically or critically we regard ourselves. For personal well-being and an optimal level of functioning, we need to feel at ease with ourselves, and to have a sense of being a basically decent and competent person. Of course each individual will have their own ideas about what qualifies one in this regard. Self-esteem is a variable entity. Some days we feel more buoyant than others, and sometimes self-esteem is higher or lower for more sustained periods. Persistently low self-esteem is associated with a range of psychological difficulties, mental illnesses, physical maladies and destructive behaviours. It is a big factor in the quality of relationships.

Absolutely related to that of self-esteem is the notion of confidence. The ability to approach something with the expectation of success is just as important, perhaps more so, than the capacity to do it. For if we do not believe in ourselves, our skills and knowledge, however sophisticated, will remain unexercised. Self-belief or confidence rises and falls with self-esteem. A boost to self-esteem may give us the confidence to try something new, and success will, in turn, bolster our evaluation of ourselves. Conversely a blow to self-esteem is likely to damage confidence. We are increasingly recognizing that confidence is a major issue for people with dementia. So much of what happens to them constitutes an assault on this facet of their personhood it is hardly surprising that they give up doing things, which is then labelled by others as evidence of dementia leading to further confidence-damaging restrictions.

As a diverse group, people with dementia obviously come into the condition with a very wide range in terms of self-image and self-esteem, but because of our culture's negative attitudes towards ageing, illness and dementia in particular, the experiences the person has had in connection with their condition are likely to have constituted an assault on their self-esteem. There is also the fact that once a person has been identified as having dementia, it is almost as if they have lost the right to define their own identity. Dementia trumps everything else. In more specific terms, what we value most in ourselves will affect the experience of dementia. Someone who derived their self-esteem largely from taking care of others will construe their experience of dementia differently from someone whose identity was built more around the use of their intellectual abilities or practical skills.

One of the aims of in-depth communication specifically, and good dementia care generally, is to learn more about how the person sees themselves and therefore their world, and how they are affected by their experience of dementia. Issues of how their self-image and self-esteem can be maintained or even enhanced can then be addressed, it is hoped with the result of helping them to re-establish confidence in a whole range of ways. These themes are developed throughout the book, but we give particular consideration to how we make sense of our experiences in Chapter 6.

Personality

Personality can be thought of as the set of psychological characteristics and dispositions that makes each of us a unique, recognizable and, up to a point, predictable human being. The concept of personality underpins a large range of different aspects of what goes into making up a human being – what interests, excites or moves us, how we relate to others, and how we filter and organize the complexity that spins around us into a meaningful whole. Personality characteristics are evident in very young infants, and through the miracle of human development unfold and find expression right through the lifespan.

In dementia, personality change is often identified as one of the prominent features, and usually as a problematic one, as when a gentle person becomes aggressive or someone who has been restrained becomes 'disinhibited'. Our understanding of the relationship between the self and personality, and what happens in the context of dementia is very shallow and almost entirely problem focused. We need much more openness in this regard. Again we have to think about the distinction between change which is organic in nature and that which derives from psychological and interpersonal pressures, the person's ways of coping and the quality of their relationships. There is also the possibility of positive change in the context of dementia, something which can pave the way for enhanced relationships and greater enjoyment of various aspects of living.

The physical self

We all inhabit a body which serves as the physical manifestation of the self. The relationship between the body and the self is typically complex. Sometimes we are inclined to think of our bodies as being somehow separate from the more essential self. In his examination of the metaphors we employ in understanding our bodies, and in particular the experience of pain, physician and thinker Jonathan Miller says:

> Our body is not, in short, something we have, it is a large part of what we actually are: it is by and through our bodies that we recognise existence in

the world, and it is only by being able to move in and act upon the world that we can distinguish it from ourselves.[30]

Our experience of our body is affected both by our own feelings about it (whether, for example, it works well, or gives us pain, or we like or dislike its appearance), and also others' reactions to it. It is a fact that people's characters and intentions are judged according to their appearance.[31] Our society places a high premium on bodies taking a certain form, and exercises deep prejudice against the reality of the ageing body, and bodies which are affected by illness and disability. For many the sense of separateness of self and body seems to magnify with age, resulting in an increasing feeling of alienation from the physical. Here is the feminist Barbara Macdonald on this subject:

> My hands are large and the backs of my hands begin to show the brown spots of aging. Sometimes lately, holding my arms up reading in bed or lying with my arms clasped around my lover's neck, I see my arm with the skin hanging loosely from the forearm and cannot really believe that it is my own. It seems disconnected from me; it is someone else's, it is the arm of an old woman. It is the arm of such old women as I myself have seen, sitting on benches in the sun with their hands folded in their laps; old women I have turned away from. I wonder now, how and when these arms came to be my own – arms I cannot turn away from.[32]

Presumably these realities are no less powerful for people with dementia. As well as confronting change in the psychological and cognitive domain, they are also faced with changes in their physical self and capacities, including those that are associated with general ageing, those directly connected with dementia, and also those which are a result of other conditions. Pain may be a major factor affecting the person's day-to-day experience. But alongside the physical aspects, their own and others' attitudes towards the body may constitute as much of a handicap as its actual characteristics. It is quite commonly observed that people begin to fail to recognize themselves at all, perhaps remaining convinced that they are much younger than they actually are. This may be a more extreme expression of the kind of feelings Barbara Macdonald describes, but it may be complicated and compounded by other forms of identity disturbance which accompany dementia or arise as a response to our bewilderment and fear of the condition.

Another crucial aspect of the physical self relates to sensory change and loss. Our relationship with the world of things and people is mediated entirely by the senses, and later life is often a time when changes begin to occur in this sphere. We understand little about how our capacity to perceive the world around us is related to experience of the self, but we should certainly not underestimate the impact of sensory change on this. The academic John Hull writes of his experience of blindness:

To what extent is loss of the image of the face connected with loss of the image of the self? Is this one of the reasons why I often feel I am a mere spirit, a ghost, a memory? Other people have become disembodied voices, speaking out of nowhere, going into nowhere. Am I not like this too, now that I have lost my body?[33]

More specifically, we know almost nothing about the experience of those who have long-established sensory disability before the onset of dementia.

It is, of course, crucial to bear in mind that alongside the many dissatisfactions engendered by our bodies, it is through the physical self that we experience great and very various forms of comfort, pleasure and delight. These are not experiences we readily associate with older people and people with dementia, but we are beginning to wake up to the possibilities, and there is much scope for development of these ideas.

The self in relationship

We have already made the point that personhood can be seen as deriving from being in relationship with other persons. In this sense it is really not possible to separate all of the dimensions of personhood described here into those which are inherent in the self and those which depend on human relatedness. We have devoted a whole chapter in Part 3 (on themes) to relationships, but it is a subject which permeates all of the text.

The moral status of persons

Inherent in the idea of personhood is that persons are moral beings. Most people are concerned with issues of right and wrong, and are engaged in a struggle to do what is right, as they perceive it, in their own lives, in those of people they care about, and in the wider world. The notion of the internal moral voice – the conscience – is integral to our experience and understanding of personhood. Some people argue for the existence of absolute laws of right and wrong, whether these derive from systems of religious, cultural or pragmatic thought. Others argue that what is right and wrong is more fluid and complex, and has to be judged in relation to the characteristics of individuals and situations. Ideas change and develop, and come back full circle. The ancient discipline of moral philosophy has been chewing over the central question – How should we live? – for many hundreds of years. The debating continues. The big questions may baffle us, but on a more manageable level, we can acknowledge that as persons we have a sense of responsibility to others, and having this sense of responsibility is a basic part of being a person, whether and however this is expressed in behaviour.

What about people with dementia in this regard? Some may argue that such people lose their right to moral consideration, and justify this position by arguing that dementia undermines a person's ability to make full moral choices which are based on an understanding of a situation, and to take responsibility for their own behaviour. We can make a distinction here between the person's own capacity for living in a moral way, and the status in which we hold ourselves in relation to them. Stephen Post makes a clear statement of his position:

> people with dementia have heterogeneous disabilities that confer on them a preferential moral significance based on the magnitude of their needs. They are the socially outcast, the unwanted, the marginalized, and the oppressed.[34]

Here he is making two related points. First, that we should accord people with dementia special moral status on account of their disabilities, and second, that they deserve this status because of the disadvantages suffered by them through the attitudes and behaviour of others. Whatever the merits and difficulties inherent in this position, those of us in the dementia world have not yet reached the stage where discussion of these questions has found its place.

For our part, we are very conscious that any work which engages with people at a deep level is inherently moral, and that this is especially so with people who are undergoing such a radical and mysterious process as dementia. Communication work in particular raises many moral questions, and we address these both at points throughout the text, and also at the end of the book.

The pursuit of meaning

Human beings have a great need to try to make sense of their world and their experience within it, to find satisfactory ways of explaining things. Our lives are dominated and driven by this search for pattern and meaning from start to finish. We cannot live within randomness and chaos. As we shall discuss at greater length in Chapter 6, we explain events and experiences with reference to a set of personal beliefs, and our minute-to-minute thinking processes are a kind of ongoing effort of interpretation, which in turn influences the way we feel emotionally and what we do.

In our work with people with dementia, we need to recognize that the search for meaning within experience does not stop when dementia develops. Indeed it is likely that the changes and confusions that dementia brings intensify the need for meaning. This is forcefully expressed in the quotation that heads this chapter. Also, in order for us to do the best job of understanding the needs and experiences of people with dementia, it is necessary for us to attempt to try to 'get inside' their way of seeing the world, their subjective reality, and empathize with what follows from this. Our own efforts to make sense of their words and actions depend to a large extent on the sorts of assumptions and values we hold, and in-depth communication work should prompt us to question, modify and perhaps even throw a few out altogether.

Emotion

What makes life worth living? Could we be content with anything – people, ideas, things – if they did not appeal to that indefinable, multifaceted dimension of our experience we call emotion? Emotion is what makes things matter. It stimulates, motivates, irritates and generally drives us. When we feel emotion we know that we are alive. Those whose experience is characterized by an absence of emotion often feel that they are 'dead' inside. The psychotherapist Piero Ferrucci stresses the importance of feelings thus:

> feelings are necessary ingredients in everyone's life: they are an inexhaustible source of enjoyment, they facilitate communication, they add power and colour to whatever we do, they vitalize ideas and reflect intuitions.[35]

Sometimes emotions are powerful, clamouring experiences. We may feel filled with anxiety or apprehension, or flooded by relief or joy. Sadness or despair may seem to drain away our energy or commitment to people or activities. Anger can spike us into action. An excess of strong emotion can seem unbearable, and people go to drastic lengths to avoid it. At other times emotion is more like a background rhythm or texture, less noticeable but still present. This aspect of our subjectivity is tied up with what we call mood, that internal climate of emotional disposition which can act as such a powerful mediator of experience. Sometimes we seek experiences which are designed to stimulate heightened emotion – a sad film, a hair-raising fairground ride or a place of sanctity and peace. Our tireless pursuit of happiness, however that is conceptualized, is surely one of the dominant themes of our lives.

Emotion can be a solitary experience, but feelings are also often shared – we feel and project our own, and take part in those of people we are close to or identify with. People vary in the extent to which they see emotion as being something which they can control and take responsibility for, or whether they feel that emotions have a life of their own, as when we say '*I can't help the way I feel*'. Another dimension along which people vary is the degree to which they see others as being responsible for what they feel, and this will have a bearing on their behaviour, particularly in relationships.

Whatever our specific views about the nature and role of emotion, it is undeniable that emotion is a potent force, and life without this sphere of experience would be unimaginably different. Relationships would have a flat, formal quality, and activities be mechanical. Despite the crucial role of emotion, however, in our hypercognitive world it takes second place to the kingpin of reason. We dismiss an argument which is 'emotional', and often distrust as biased or suspect the information with which our emotional antennae provides us.

Where people with dementia are concerned we observe that emotion often seems to play a heightened role in their lives. The fact that they are undergoing such a profound process is bound to stimulate strong emotion, and a shifting pattern of abilities (that is, away from those relying on remembering and reasoning) may bring the emotional dimension of experiences more to the fore. In the past this would have been labelled automatically as a symptom of the condition. Such a point of view reflects the dominant medical frame, and again our hypercognitive values. In order to encounter the personhood of the individual with dementia, understand their world of feelings and respond with compassion we have to enter into a deeper level of emotional experience and expression ourselves. As Frena Gray Davidson, who has written about the experiences of relatives providing care, says:

> In many ways, the deepest revelation of the Alzheimer journey is that it is a kind of passage from the mind into the heart.[36]

Faith Gibson writes:

> Dementia strips people down to the essence of their being and frees them to be in more direct touch with their emotions. They communicate with greater authenticity than our customary conventional reliance on controlled emotional expression.[37]

Agency and autonomy

A corollary of the idea of a self is that of having the capacity to take action – agency, and having control over what one does – autonomy. This is related to the basic human capacity to form and hold intentions, and to make plans towards goals, whether in the short or long term. This includes the opportunity to take risks. Although we can never be fully in control of the events in our lives, in order to maintain physical and mental health we need to have at least a reasonable degree of control, and certainly a *feeling* of having control. We all know the sense of violation when someone disregards our preferences or takes away our ability to make choices. It is often felt as an assault on our sense of personhood, and accompanied by a particular feeling of outrage.

The idea of empowerment, finding ways to help people with dementia to take a greater role in decisions which affect them, is a recent development in the field of dementia care. Any attempt to achieve this must rely heavily on attention to communication.

Choices and preferences

Closely related to the matter of autonomy is that of opportunities to express preferences and make choices. We all have likes and dislikes, pertaining to every aspect of life, ranging from mundane decisions such as what to eat and drink, what to read or watch on television, through to the big issues such as our choices as regards work, relationships, political affiliations and spiritual or religious practice. These dispositions may remain stable throughout life, or they may change. Indeed the right to change our mind about what we favour or reject is another aspect of exercising choice. These facets of life are very much part of what makes us unique and recognizable as individuals. It is through the very exercising of choice, and the opportunity to make decisions that we experience ourselves as persons in a deep sense. In his book about soli-tude, the psychiatrist Anthony Storr is describing the vital role of decision-making for prisoners kept in solitary confinement:

> Even the prisoner who agrees to be totally at the mercy of his captors can retain some degree of autonomy: by for example deciding whether to eat the bread that he is given, or to save it for future consumption. On such apparently trivial decisions may depend whether or not the prisoner retains any sense of being an independent entity.[38]

As regards people with dementia, historically the assumption has been that through the erosion caused by the condition the capacity and even need to make choices has been lost, and indeed that the very experience of being faced with a choice will be stressful and potentially damaging. We tend to think of people with dementia as being basically vulnerable, and this causes us to reduce opportunities for decision-making for fear that this will lead to what has been termed a 'catastrophic reaction'. We can easily produce such a ration-ale for the limitation of choice on these grounds, especially if the person has, in the past, become distressed when faced with a decision point. It may be argued that the fact that distress has arisen on one occasion, however, does not justify something so basic to personhood being routinely withdrawn or cur-tailed. It is also important to recognize the risk of limiting opportunities for choice ostensibly to protect the individual when it is actually for our own ben-efit. Jenny Croft, whose husband has dementia, makes this point:

> Often I don't feel that I qualify for the title [carer] because 'I don't care' is a phrase I have been guilty of using when Ted's personhood forces me to accept things happening which I feel will make things difficult for both of us.[39]

With the realization of continued personhood, we have to address both the practicalities of how we can learn about and honour the individual's prefer-ences and support them in making decisions.[40] At a more general level there is a need to reflect on the ethical dimension of choice in terms of how we approach this issue, for example how we weigh up conflicting preferences – between ourselves and people with dementia, and also between people with dementia and their relatives, and between people with dementia themselves.

Occupation and creativity

The human body and mind are fundamentally designed to be active; they become the way they are through being used, and often we feel at our peak when we are engaged in a challenging and meaningful activity.[41] The impulse towards occupation manifests itself over a whole range of actions, from staving off boredom by performing domestic chores at one end of the spec-trum, to initiating and completing complex projects, whether in a work or pri-vate role, at the other. Activity provides structure and meaning for our lives as a whole, and puts into perspective those periods of rest, reflection and solitude which are also necessary components of living. And the kinds of things we like doing and are good at constitute an important facet of our identity. Speaking of his feelings when he was hospitalized after a leg injury, the neurologist Oliver Sacks observed:

> I had to relinquish all the powers I normally command. I had to relinquish, above all, the sense and affect of *activity*. I had to allow – and this seemed horrible – the sense and feeling of *passivity*. I found this humiliating, at first, a mortification of my self.[42]

But Sacks knew that for him this state which he called 'Limbo' was a temporary one. That essential aspect of one's outlook we call confidence comes about through doing. Once people with dementia begin to be denied opportunities to remain active they are unlikely to be able to recover the skills which have been lost. It becomes another assault on their very selfhood.

Creativity can be regarded as one form of activity, where the qualities of inventiveness and novelty are uppermost, and the special human capacity we call imagination is engaged. They are the very core characteristics of the inner life, but will remain largely dormant where opportunities for occupation are artificially blocked. We shall see in Chapter 4 how creativity in language is a notable characteristic of some people with dementia, and there is a growing body of evidence which suggests that intuitive and artistic talents are not always damaged by the condition. Indeed, it may be that the experience of dementia is actually a time when heightened creativity is possible. Such capacities can only be developed, however, if we learn to recognize and cherish them, providing the right kind of encouragement. This requires a sea-change in attitudes so that we begin to see people with dementia as ongoing, rather than defunct, persons with a unique and precious contribution to make to society.

Dignity and privacy

It is hard to define exactly what constitutes dignity, but we always feel hurt and undermined at a deep level when it has been infringed. Respecting someone and upholding their dignity involves honouring all of the above – the individual's uniqueness and complexity, their preferences and choices, their need for control over aspects of their lives, and also accepting their need and right to privacy. Dignity is also closely related to independence, something on which our culture places a great premium. Being able to do things for oneself, especially intimate physical tasks, plays an important part in maintaining dignity, which is in turn linked to self-esteem. Being seen and treated as an adult is another important facet of dignity. Privacy is a similarly complex issue. Having control over what we reveal about ourselves is terribly basic, and again the sense of violation when this is infringed hurts deeply.

People with dementia are often casualties in respect of both dignity and privacy. So much of their lives becomes the concern of other people. Their life histories, their feelings and moods, their cognitive and practical abilities, and the quality of their relationships become the subjects of discussions and reports. Increasingly their bodies become the business of others. The experience of having someone act upon one's body, if this is not accompanied by a regard for the person, must be highly threatening and alienating.

The effort to establish genuine communication itself confers dignity, and is the principal way in which we can learn about what a particular individual needs in order to maintain these vital aspects of personhood.

The role of memory

Some would argue that our sense of self and identity is based on being able to construct and maintain a self which is continuous and consistent, at least in some respects, over time. The perception that an individual loses their status as a person as their memory for events and information apparently declines is implicit in the way we think about dementia. The erosion of memory is often used as a metaphor for the very unravelling of the self, the descent into fragmentation and randomness.

Along with others we challenge the view that an intact memory, at least in the sense of being able to remember facts and hold a conventional framework of time, is basic to the idea of personhood. In the chapter we devote to this subject we explore complex possibilities around what is actually happening in the memory of the individual, and how this seems to affect their sense of self and the external reality of people and things. We also raise issues which prompt us to rethink our hypercognitive view of memory – that memory for information is the most important function of this facet of the individual – and think about the importance of memory for sensation, action, emotion and aspects of relationships.

Humour

Humour is a quality we all prize enormously. Those who have a special talent for bringing laughter and fun into our lives have always been sought after and rewarded. Existence can seem so grim so much of the time, and we have a deep need of the capacity of humour for lightening and cheering, pointing up our hypocrisies and absurdities, and offering new perspectives on situations and challenges. Although it is possible to laugh alone, humour is fundamentally a social and interpersonal phenomenon, and is a great catalyst and cement in the sphere of relationships. It can also be a source of controversy. Patch Adams, a doctor who has dedicated his life to treating ill-health with humour, says:

> People crave laughter as if it were an essential amino acid. When the woes of existence beset us, we urgently seek comic relief. The more emotions we invest in a subject, the greater its potential for guffaws. Sex, marriage, prejudice and politics provide a bottomless well of ideas; yet humour is

often denied in the adult world . . . The stress is on seriousness, with the implication that humour is inappropriate.[43]

Dementia is not a subject which readily brings smiles to people's faces. Some might even think it is wrong to laugh about an issue which occasions such enormous pain and suffering. While not at all wishing to deny this reality, however, we suggest that there is great potential for humour in many different aspects of living with dementia. Anyone who has spent a lot of time in the company of people with the condition, and is willing to recognize and uphold their personhood, must have shared many experiences of a comical nature, perhaps laughing together over a misunderstanding, false start or unintended pun, or a practical mishap. In our experience many people with dementia are highly sensitive to the humorous aspects of a situation, and are more ready to enjoy this than the rest of us, who may be too busy or preoccupied to notice a stimulus to laughter.

Humour can also serve as an important form of coping. This is from a woman who is in the early stages of Alzheimer's Disease:

> When I can't find something that I have put in the wrong place, I blame it on Al. When I say the same thing or ask the same question twice in a short time, I blame it on Al. When I start to say a word and it won't come to my head, I blame Al. Al took it! When I tried to make change for a purchase and couldn't, it was Al's fault. The line 'Al did it' has become a joke at my house.
>
> My son, Ricky, gave me a sweatshirt for Christmas. On the front it said 'I remembered'. On the back it said 'I forgot. Al took it.' Who is Al? Al is Mrs Zheimer's son, Al Zheimer. I know it's corny, but it beats dwelling on the sad side of the story.[44]

With more careful attention to communication, both verbal and nonverbal, we believe that there is enormous potential for humour and fun to become a much larger part of our relationships with people with dementia, with all the benefits to well-being that offers to all parties. We return to the subject many times throughout the book.

Sexuality

We are all sexual beings, and the ways in which we experience and express our sexuality are intimately interwoven with our sense of self and our individuality, and our relationships with others. A person's sexuality is, of course, a much larger and more mysterious and complex entity than the ways in which it finds physical expression in sexual behaviour. Sexuality motivates communication, and provides a kickstart to relationships, whether or not they go on to have an overtly sexual element. With many of our nonsexual relationships, it nevertheless plays a largely unconscious element in interpersonal dealings, ways of sizing up others and forming impressions of them.

Most people would agree that our society is obsessed with the subject of sex (sex more than sexuality) and that we are bombarded with messages, images and ideas which are sexually loaded. It is also undeniable that the preoccupation with sex carries a powerful subtext, which is that sexual feelings and experiences are for young, attractive and healthy people. Issues pertaining to sex and illness or disability are much less openly addressed, and where older people (over 50!) are concerned there is a huge stigma attached to the idea of sexuality which is expressed in disgust or mocking humour.

Where do people with dementia figure in this? Research is beginning to address the subject of sexuality.[45] Some of this work is orientated towards valuing this aspect of the person, but much is problem focused. It does raise deep and difficult issues, and certainly puts our shallow systems of values to the test. If we are to recognize and respond fully to people with dementia we must learn to acknowledge, and even celebrate, this aspect of continuing personhood.

Spirituality

Humankind has always looked beyond itself, and what is known and understood in conventional terms, for answers to the 'big questions' of life: Why are we here? How should we live? Is death the end? Historically, answers to these questions were provided by the dominant religions, and although the number of people who are regularly involved in organized religious activity is declining, most of us remain interested in and moved by such issues. Spirituality is a difficult term to define, but we can say that it is concerned with questions about what are the core aspects of human beings, perhaps called the 'soul', what we share at a fundamental level, and whether and how we relate to something larger, unseen and inherently mysterious. This should not be considered as being synonymous with the 'religious', however.

There is, of course, great variability between individuals in terms of their attitudes towards and experience of this aspect of life. But most of the people who currently have dementia are from a generation when religious belief and observance was common. For those from a Christian background, familiarity with scriptures, going to church, saying a Grace before eating and prayers at night, and specific rituals around major festivals would all have been an integral part of life. Other religions have similarly distinctive ritual observances. As well as the outward expression of faith, there is the deeply personal sense of meaning and connection it engenders. The implications of this aspect of the person's identity is something we need to think more about in the way we interact, and how care for people with dementia is organized and provided.

Historically, beliefs about dementia destroying personhood encompassed the assumption that whatever the nature and expression of religious or spiritual beliefs, the need for this aspect of the person to be recognized and affirmed was over, and certainly the capacity to take a full part in observance was lost. Although arguments about the persistence of personhood have only lately influenced the world of dementia care, the recognition of the importance of the spiritual dimension is even more recent.[46] The potential of the spiritual to transcend the apparently fractured nature of cognition, emotion and action is demonstrated in an account from the neurologist Oliver Sacks. He has a patient with Korsakov's Syndrome (damage to short-term memory caused by alcohol abuse) and the symptoms appear severe and all-pervasive. His care is being provided by nuns:

> 'Do you think he *has* a soul?', I once asked the Sisters. They were outraged by my question, but could see why I asked it. 'Watch Jimmie in the chapel,' they said, 'and judge for yourself.'
>
> I did, and I was moved . . . because I saw here an intensity and steadiness of attention and concentration that I had never seen before in him or conceived him capable of. I watched him kneel and take the Sacrament on his tongue, and could not doubt the fullness and totality of Communion, the perfect alignment of his spirit with the spirit of the Mass . . . There was no forgetting, no Korsakov's then, . . . for he was no longer at the mercy of a faulty and fallible mechanism . . . but was absorbed in an act, an act of his whole being, which carried feeling and meaning in an organic continuity and unity, a continuity and unity so seamless it could not permit any break.[47]

Sharing and enlarging personhood

We have already discussed the idea that if we accept that personhood is an inherently interpersonal construct, it then follows that to deny or ignore the personhood of any individual is to put our own at risk. When John encountered people with dementia for the first time, part of his distress was awareness of the threat to his own sense of being a person which arose out of his inability to see them truly as persons. This means that acknowledging and responding to the personhood of people with dementia has the potential to expand and deepen our own sense of worth as persons. Debbie Everett, a hospital chaplain in Canada, says:

> [People with dementia] are magic mirrors where I have seen my human condition, and have repudiated the commonly held societal values of power and prestige that are unreal and shallow . . . Because people with dementia have their egos stripped from them, their unconscious comes very close to the surface. They, in turn, show us the masks behind which we hide our authentic personhood from the world.[48]

If we are to recognize and celebrate the fact that contact and communication with people with dementia has such great potential benefits in terms of our own personhood, it is only realistic to accept that there may be dangers too. The risks which are inherent in work of this sort are explored in more depth in Chapter 15 on ethical implications.

Ethical implications

Power

At the heart of all the ethical issues we have to consider in relation to thinking about work with people with dementia is that of power, specifically the fact that people with dementia are so much less powerful than we are. Of course imbalances in power are a feature of many relationships, but when dementia is a factor the inequity is likely to be much more pervasive and stable. Our dealings with those with the condition have traditionally been constructed exclusively within the frame of their dependency on us and our responsibility for them.

People with dementia are lacking in power in all the following respects:

- *Status* – in the eyes of society and in those close to them, and, probably as a consequence of this, in their own eyes too. They are not taken seriously. Their label of dementia means that their actions are interpreted within expectations of incompetence, their words are assumed to be confused, and their preferences and choices likely to be disregarded or treated as irrational or unreliable.
- *Capacity* – whether through core features of the condition, or as a result of the way they are treated by others, people with dementia are limited in what they can do. These constraints operate at the cognitive, practical and physical levels.
- *Access to resources* – the access that people with dementia have to resources such as information, money, material goods and the kind of interpersonal contact we all rely on so much is often severely restricted. They suffer not only from the immediate consequences of these limitations, but also the indignity and injustice of the knowledge of them.

Across all of these dimensions, we need to recognize that feelings of powerlessness and the recognition of dependency are deeply frightening and threatening to one's identity. This cannot be overemphasized, and for all we know, the effects of these realities may be a much more dominant influence on the well-being of the person and the course of the condition than we have hitherto appreciated.

The manifestations of this power differential permeate the business of communication as they do with everything else. The chance of an interaction taking place at all is often beyond the control of the person with dementia, as is the length of the encounter, the subject matter of any conversation, and the manner of its closing. The question of how the individual's words or actions are interpreted, and whether anything else happens as a result are also in the hands of others.

It is vital that we recognize this, and become more aware of the many and subtle ways it finds expression and has effects. This is an interesting area because although we can recognize in theory the existence of the power differential, and the fact that it works in our favour, the minute-to-minute and hour-to-hour experience of staff and carers is often anything but that of being powerful. Indeed they may feel at times it is the person with dementia who is wielding much of the power, and that they are frequently being stymied or manipulated. The sheer difficulty of the caring role and the sense of exhaustion it often engenders also serve to minimize the feeling of power, and promote that of being trapped or even being in an impossible position. What is experienced by the person with dementia as a radical loss of power, may be felt by those around them as an oppressive form of responsibility. So this means that although there is a marked power differential, often no one feels powerful and therefore its workings are allowed to unfold without being checked by conscious awareness.

Having recognized imbalances in power, the next step is to try to redress them. But this is no simple matter. Since efforts to do so must begin from a position of power, any attempt to give back power must be a further expression of being powerful. Close attention to the word 'empower' reveals it to be a reinforcement of the reality of the imbalance. However while recognizing the complexities of the situation, we must still work towards restoring power to the person with dementia, and the particular ways in which this is attempted will depend on the person themselves, their relationships with others and many facets of their character. Attempting to establish opportunities for genuine communication functions both as a way of empowering the person in its own right, and also as a means for finding other ways in which this can be most effectively done.

While there is a danger of becoming hopelessly tied in knots with questions like these, we do feel that it is essential that we develop our awareness of them and become more accustomed to reviewing our attitudes and behaviour with reference to them.

What do we expect of persons?

Part of what constitutes an imbalance of power in a relationship relates to who is able to give, and who is positioned as being the person who receives. Where people with dementia are concerned, our views are quite categorical: we see them fundamentally as having nothing to give us. There is an assumption that relationships cannot be reciprocal, that we must provide everything ourselves. Dependency is a word which is used a lot in relation to people with dementia, and it is one which carries very negative connotations in our society. As well as very likely being experienced as degrading by the person with the condition, this quality of onesidedness is often highly burdensome for those who are called upon to provide and support. The question is, must it be this way?

Thinking about reciprocality in relationships takes us to the heart of questions about personhood. For if we are saying that personhood is constructed and maintained through relationships, and that relationships are inherently reciprocal, then this means that we must ask what we can expect from the person with dementia. Should we, at the very least, expect our own personhood to be recognized and respected by them? Should people with dementia be expected to take responsibility for their own actions? How do we understand the relationship between their difficulties and their capacity for taking an active part in relationships, for giving to others? We have no answers to these questions, but there is fuller discussion of them and many related issues later in the book.

Our motives

The woman whose words form part of the title of Chapter 15 ('What I want to know is, what is this doing for you?') was pinpointing a fundamental issue for those of us who work with people with dementia. It is important that we take time to think about why we are doing it, and what we get out of it.[49]

We appreciate that there is a range of routes into working with people with dementia, some of them involving conscious choice and some influenced more by pressure of necessity or circumstances beyond one's control. Total choice regarding the work one does is rare. But by the time anyone has found themselves in the position of doing this kind of work, and is interested enough in it to be reading a book like this, then there is definitely scope for useful reflection.

From an outsider's point of view, working with people who are ill or have disabilities may seem to indicate one of two things. Either that the individual who does so is some kind of saint or else that they are unable to find alternative employment. There is an immediate assumption that the work is inherently unpleasant. We are only too used to others' reactions when they find out about what we do, and it normally involves statements and questions like 'I don't know how you can do that!' or 'Don't you find it depressing?' or even 'Dementia? Now there's a case for euthanasia!' Such situations may prompt us to reflect on what it is that motivates us.

Despite perceptions (or feelings) of saintliness, it is important to acknowledge here that alongside what we would consider to be the 'best' motives for doing such work – helping others, alleviating suffering – everything we do has a self-serving element, however deeply buried or convoluted it may be. This is not a matter of choice, it is simply a given. Indeed perhaps it is true that it is in the sphere of effort which is, on the face of it, expended in the service of others that the workings of our selfish motives are most complex.

As we discussed earlier in the chapter, we all have a need to see ourselves as decent and deserving, to feel that we are making a contribution. The particular ways in which we do this will depend on a range of factors including personality, interests and experience. But for some the most obvious way to have a positive role is to work in a caring capacity. Deep-seated needs are also met by doing things that we do not enjoy or even find difficult. Part of our cultural and religious inheritance is the notion that overcoming one's resistance to something is 'character-building' or laudibly self-sacrificing. This complicates the matter of what motivates us to do the things we do enormously.

Although we use terms like 'help' and 'care for' in a routine way, they are far from simple, and there are many ways to interpret them. Within our culture the idea of helping has strong suggestions of the notion of protection and doing things for people. It carries connotations of the helper being more powerful than the one being helped, and perhaps also an expectation of gratitude. Alternative, but less prevalent, interpretations of the term include the notion of supporting the person in continuing to do whatever they can and exploring new possibilities and experiences. We need to be aware that there is a fine line between helping someone and adding to their disability by removing from them opportunities for making choices and decisions, pursuing activities and taking risks, which are, as we have seen, the sorts of things that reinforce our sense of personhood.

Some of these issues are touched on in the following passage by care assistant Laurel Rust.[50] She is describing her relationship with one of the residents in the nursing home where she works, Amy. On one particular day, Amy, during an extended general tirade, remarked:

> 'and I'm tired of people who come by just to be nice and say hello, goodbye!'

Later Laurel asks Amy:

> 'Do you think I come here just to be nice?'

Amy replies by saying:

> 'Well I think maybe you do, because I've seen you doing things you don't really want to do.'

But she concludes this statement by remarking:

> 'But you don't know what this means to me.'

Later Laurel reflects:

> But I drove home wondering if Amy trusted me, if I was another intrusion, some kind of macabre voyeur. She was right: I often do what I do not want to do. She'd blown the whistle on my little story. But not this, not seeing her, not coming to know her. I began to see the ways in which I needed her.[51]

The sorts of questions it might be useful to ask oneself in this regard include the following:

- To what extent does our basic sense of worth as persons depend on being able to 'do good' for others?
- What do we feel are the essential elements of 'caring' or 'helping' in this context?
- What do we look for in terms of responses from those for whom we care? What effects does it have when we do get them and how does it feel when we do not? How do we feel towards those people who do not give us the responses we look for?

- How might imbalances in power express themselves in our caring relationship(s)?

These are questions that everyone must answer for themselves. Like most ethical issues they are somewhat painful to engage with (we discuss this further in Chapter 15). Nevertheless communication work of the kind we advocate inevitably brings us up against them. We are confronting a condition which remains fundamentally poorly understood, and we are therefore opening ourselves to uncertainty and complexity. But as we shall discuss further in the ethical implications section of Chapter 6 on interpretation, it is vital to recognize that the reasons we do what we do are inextricably tied up with the values we bring to bear on the work.

3 Nonverbal communication: 'I just want to hold and hold you one minute'

The poet, David Wright, who has been totally deaf since the age of 7, speaks of his experience as follows:

> as somebody waiting impatiently for a friend to finish a telephone conversation knows when it is about to end by the words said and the intonation of the voice, so does a deaf man . . . judge the moment when the goodbyes are being said or the intention formed to replace the receiver. He notices a shift of the hand cradling the instrument, a change of stance, the head drawing a fraction of a millimetre from the earphone, a slight shuffling of the feet, and that alteration of expression which signals a decision taken. Cut off from auditory clues he learns to read the faintest visual evidence.[1]

Sometimes it seems as if we are all living according to the slogan 'Words come first!', so heavily is our culture dominated by verbal communication. It is true that language has played a crucial part in human evolution, and underpins our dealings with the complex world of people, things and ideas. As our sophistication in terms of electronic means of communication develops, we seem to become more and more wedded to the power of words. Yet there is in all of us a deep reservoir of self-expression and communication which does not rely on language at all, and this also goes to the heart of what it means to be human. Giving separate chapters to both nonverbal communication and language could foster the false impression of a clear distinction between the two. Although there are forms of nonverbal communication which do not involve words at all, in the majority of instances the two dimensions are intimately intertwined. Facial expression, qualities of voice, and gestures help the listener to decode and interpret words, and to refine and accentuate the messages they themselves give out. We have placed this chapter before that of language, however, to counteract the assumption that words are necessarily the highest form of communication, and in recognition of the fact that words often fail to do justice to the subtlety of our experiences, particularly when something as complex as dementia enters the frame. We echo the view of the ethicist Stephen Post in this context:

> Words are terribly limited; they can neither capture the ineffable depth of solicitude that shapes the caregiver experience nor convey the shaken existential foundations of the individual who confronts the journey into forgetfulness.[2]

We shall briefly review the specifics of nonverbal communication, and then discuss some of the ways in which we use these channels in everyday life. Then we go on to consider aspects of special significance in work with people with dementia. It is not possible to deal with these matters without straying a little into the realms of interpretation, but a fuller discussion of this subject is reserved for Chapter 6.

The nature of nonverbal communication

Nonverbal communication is, by its very nature, hard to talk about. Of this two experts from the field of communication with people with learning difficulties, Melanie Nind and Dave Hewett, say:

> Our knowledge of human experience has not yet reached a stage where we can precisely and scientifically choreograph people's use of body language. We all have a great deal of use and understanding of body language – much more than any of us can express in words. Such knowledge is sometimes referred to as 'tacit' – unspoken or silent, inferred or unconscious.[3]

The following is a list of the various aspects of nonverbal communication. The order of items does not denote their importance but you may be surprised by its length and complexity:[4]

- the eyes, including eye contact, eye movements, direction of gaze, degree of pupil dilation

- facial expression and facial movements
- touch and other physical contact
- gesture, and other bodily movement
- body posture and orientation
- voice, including tone, pitch, volume, intonation, rate of speaking and non-verbal vocalizations
- physical appearance, including dress and adornment, and smell
- use of the environment, including how the self is positioned in space and in relation to objects, barriers and so on, in the choice of environment where communication takes place, and how one chooses to arrange and decorate one's own environment.

Although for the purposes of discussion we can single out particular channels of nonverbal communication and talk about them in isolation, in reality they convey meaning by interacting with each other in complex ways. It should be noted that when certain features of nonverbal communication are absent, for example there being no eye contact between two people having a conversation, this also carries meaning.

The heightened use of nonverbal communication

We all communicate nonverbally all the time whether we are aware of it or not. Even when alone, our faces and hands and movements convey information about how we feel and the kind of relationship we have with our surroundings. Sometimes, however, we enter into a heightened use of nonverbal channels of communication, when it seems to take on a particular importance.

Difficulties with language would be an example of a time when we make more explicit recourse to nonverbal communication. Gesture or use of objects in the environment may increase when words do not spring to mind or are temporarily inaccessible, or when we find ourselves trying to express an idea and realize that we do not know a specific form of words for it.

• In times of intense emotion we may find it impossible to speak, either because of the difficulty in regulating our breathing and controlling articulatory muscles during deep crying, or because words are inadequate to convey the strength of our feelings. Our vocabulary for emotions is not well developed, but in any case there is something about powerful feelings which seems to impede access to words. Certain emotions are best conveyed nonverbally, where a gesture or facial expression can do the work of many words, and in a much shorter time. Putting a hand to the face in a covering motion when embarrassed would be an example of this.

• Tiredness may be a factor in the heightened use of nonverbal communication. Finding and using words can be quite demanding of energy, whereas a gesture such as a shrug or pointing can carry a message in a more efficient way.

At times we find ourselves in environments which hamper the use of verbal communication and force us to rely more heavily on nonverbal channels.

Very noisy places or situations where there is a barrier to sound (such as when one person is on a train and the other on the platform) would be examples of this. Where vision is reduced, there may be a greater use of physical forms of communication, and greater attention to qualities of voice.

In situations where humour is a part of an interaction, nonverbal communication can be a crucial part of the comic exchange. There are many times when attempting to express an idea or feeling in words would deaden the joke. This links into the more general idea of rapport. When two people in interaction seem particularly in tune with one another, and when the effort required to exchange meaning is minimal, we may say that they are enjoying a high degree of rapport. Sensitivity to the use of nonverbal communication plays an integral part in this quality of relatedness.

Intimate interpersonal scenarios are examples of times when the use of verbal communication can be inefficient, even distancing and undermining the mood. Touch, eye contact and, if words are used at all, tone of voice would be the dominant features.

Other situations where there is a strong element of physical contact, not necessarily in an intimate manner however, include dancing and some sports. The predominance of physical forms of expression may dispose us to use other nonverbal channels of communication in a heightened way as well. The presence of music or other sound may also have a role in reducing the use of language.

Finally, there are the times when we can enter into a special quality of companionship which has no need of words, as described here by the writer Anne Morrow Lindbergh:

> At home when I meet my friends in those cubby-holed hours, time is so precious we feel we must cram every available instant with conversation. We cannot afford the luxury of silence. Here on the island I find I can sit with a friend without talking, sharing the day's last sliver of pale green light on the horizon, or the whorls in a small white shell, or the dark scar left in a dazzling night sky by a shooting star. Then communication becomes communion and one is nourished as one never is by words.[5]

Dimensions of nonverbal communication

It is important to draw attention to certain dimensions of nonverbal communication which operate at a more general level. One of these is the distinction between communication which is deliberate and that which is not. An example of the former would be a facial expression which is clearly intended to answer a question or convey a feeling, and one which occurs in a more automatic way. Some nonverbal signals are predominantly physiological in nature, for example sweating or blushing, and as such are not intended as forms of communication. Since we all continually 'leak' nonverbal signals in this way, this leads to the 'marketing' of nonverbal communication as a reliable way of learning about a person's real thoughts, feelings and reactions.[6]

A related distinction is that between nonverbal communication which is conscious and that which is not. It is thought that a significant element of nonverbal communication which occurs between two parties is unconsciously transmitted and received. These dimensions overlap, but are not identical. It depends on the degree of awareness we have about our behaviour as we interact. In any case, it is in the nature of nonverbal communication that there is a great deal going on of which we do not maintain conscious awareness, and that this is probably closely related to its potency. This is also the reason why much of what is happening evades verbal description.

We should draw attention to the complex relationship between all the subtle ways in which nonverbal communication is used and a person's unique individual style, that which makes him or her a distinctive and recognizable person who elicits particular emotional reactions in others. The way a person presents continually projects information about his or her attitudes and values, and on encountering another person we in turn are engaged in a process of trying to discern meaning and patterns in what we find.

As well as the subtlety of the ways in which individual people use nonverbal channels of communication, many of its features form part of a cultural identity, and as such carry values about ways to behave and interact that are seen as right or wrong, or at least more or less desirable. For example in some Muslim cultures, certain patterns of rules exist in order to guide the ways in which men and women who are not related should interact. Infringing such rules would be seen as a cause for disapproval or offence. Where people from different cultures communicate without knowing these norms, there is potential for misunderstanding and breakdown. This is an area in which we have much to learn.

Clearly, then, nonverbal communication is a complex but fascinating subject. We turn now to thinking about its place in work with people with dementia.

Nonverbal communication and dementia

Nonverbal communication in dementia has received little attention so far[7] but if nonverbal aspects form such an important part of one's unique identity and way of relating to others, what happens to these channels in the context of dementia? Some believe that they may acquire even greater significance. Tom Kitwood expresses this in the following way:

- Dementia sufferers sometimes seem to have a heightened awareness of body language, and often their main meanings may be conveyed nonverbally. In the case of those who are very severely impaired it seems probable that the words and sentences are at times more of an accompaniment or adornment than the vehicle for carrying the significant message.[8]

If this is true, why should it be so? One reason is that for many people, the use of language becomes progressively more difficult as the condition develops.

When access to words and skills in putting them together deteriorate, the person may find it easier to express their meaning in nonverbal terms.

There is also the fact that as the facility for understanding the language of others declines, energy may become increasingly devoted towards interpreting meaning through nonverbal channels. The neurologist Oliver Sacks describes this shift in a woman with a specific difficulty in making sense of speech following a stroke:

> Since voices now lacked expression, she had to look at people's faces, their postures and movements when they talked, and found herself doing so with a care, an intensity, she had never shown before.[9]

For some people with dementia there seems to develop a greater awareness and sensitivity to the emotional dimension in life generally and relationships in particular. It could be that nonverbal channels of communication provide the richest and most immediate way of experiencing and exploring this. So often our words strive to mask and reshape our emotional lives, but if it is true that we express our emotional selves much more authentically through non-verbal means, then this becomes the obvious focus for communication. Oliver Sacks, again writing about the altered language and communication abilities of survivors of strokes (whom in this context he refers to as aphasiacs), writes:

> One cannot lie to an aphasiac. He cannot grasp your words and so cannot be deceived by them; but what he grasps he grasps with infallible precision, namely the *expression* that goes with the words, that total spontaneous, involuntary expressiveness which can never be simulated or faked, as words alone can, all too easily.[10]

A further reason for the enhancement of nonverbal communication in the context of dementia is the need for the individual to find better ways of sizing up the intentions and dispositions of others. People who are relatively powerless must develop skills in reading subtle signals, judging moods, and sensing when is a good time to approach the more powerful other, when to ask for help or favour. Sadly many people with dementia, by the very fact of their condition, occupy the markedly less powerful role, and may need to develop such strategies in order to strive to meet basic needs. One man said to John:

> *I'm watching your face – I can tell what you're thinking – it's going on all the time in your head. It's one of those things: 'Was he right? Was he right?'*
> *That's what you're thinking.*

Anthea McKinlay provides the following example of this kind of thing from her book about her mother. The conversation took place the day after she arrived in a psychogeriatric assessment ward:

> *mum, it's me, how are you?*
> I know what they're thinking,
> it's written all over their faces

do you mean the nurses?
whatever they call themselves
what are they thinking?
they think I'm skadoodley, but I'm not.[11]

If for all these reasons people with dementia become super-experts in nonverbal communication, seeing through us and our pretensions, cutting through our projected selves and encountering what lies beneath, then we have, in our interactions and relationships, rare opportunities to encounter *ourselves*. What might this mean? We explore the issue of personal exposure and authenticity further in the ethical implications section at the end of this chapter.

Examples of nonverbal communication

In this section we provide some examples of the role of nonverbal channels in communication and relationship with people with dementia. It is obviously a challenge to describe their richness and complexity in mere words, but we hope they paint a picture you can elaborate for yourself.

Meeting with Cath Waters

John had enjoyed many interactions with Cath, and on one of those occasions a number of photographs were taken of the two of them. He is describing one of these here:

> In the photograph we are standing in the unit, my left hand clasping Cath's. I being the much taller am leaning forward; our heads are almost touching. We are laughing. Cath's eyes are closed, with, I guess, the intensity of the feeling. It is a shared joke – one of many – but since she uses little language it may be something we have noticed and looked at. Or it may be that one of us has thought of something and merriment has spilled over onto the other. As always there is a complicity that goes beyond words.
>
> Bodies play a big part in our relationship: we hold hands and hug side by side. We are always on the move: walking or dancing – exploring our environment. She never seems to tire of new places and faces; or rather the old places and faces seem to her ever new.
>
> Photographs are amongst her favourite things. Her face mirrors the feelings they evoke in her, and she keeps up a constant commentary, though I cannot follow. I can tell much by the tone of her sounds, however. Her discourse is full of exclamations accompanied by gestures.
>
> When I come on the unit and she sees me in the distance we play one of our games. Cath walks towards me slowly pointing all the while, and I do the same. When we meet our hands touch. Then she says to me 'Oh you!' over and over again, in the most intimate and joyful manner, and I join in. Our relationship is full of such rituals, based upon affection and jokiness.
>
> I know hardly anything about Cath's past life, but a great deal about

how she feels and acts in the present. It gives us more than enough to go on in maintaining and developing our relationship. I have never felt a closeness with anyone where words mattered less.

Maria Tobin talking

As we shall discuss later, there are times when the person's use of language ceases altogether, but more often language and nonverbal communication coexist, and in our efforts to achieve a rapport with individuals, we shall be faced with the challenge of trying to interpret and respond to a complex combination. Words can easily trump nonverbal signals, so it can take a special degree of attention to prevent this.

Black Daisies for the Bride is a film by Tony Harrison shown on TV in the early 1990s. It was made in a long-stay ward of an English hospital, and features real people with dementia. One of the women who is shown, Maria, has a monologue to camera. It begins with the words:

> *We're all happy, we're all knotting.*
> *I went in the other day and pushed the . . .*
> *. . . my knitwell for the two . . .*
> *two men and the bends at the back,*
> *that were dying, crying, almost crying . . .*[12]

The full text is five times this length and has similar characteristics throughout. The use of unusual words like 'knotting' and 'knitwell', the trailing away of sentences, and the seemingly abrupt change of mood in the last line make interpretation on the page difficult. It is a challenge, too, to find meaning when you hear the words spoken, but the absolute conviction with which they are delivered, and the clarity of their enunciation hold you even though you are watching a screen. The emotional intensity with which Maria invests the last line of the utterance quoted confirms one in the view of its significance. Later on Maria imitates someone she calls Queen Mary, and here again her performance is convincing. She tells a story which obviously has a punchline, and her own amusement comes across with great naturalness. Soon afterwards she touches her hair as if preparing herself for some important occasion. One is conscious of being in the presence of someone whose verbal and nonverbal expressions are fully integrated, and also very normal in character. And if the sound were turned off and the nonverbal aspects of her presentation viewed alone one would hardly be aware of any trace of dementia. Clearly here is an instance of the nonverbal communication carrying the main message and convincing the viewer of the authenticity of the words.

Beyond words

Some people reach a point in their condition when words are no longer used at all. Too often in the past such individuals were simply considered no longer able to communicate, and other aspects of expression were ignored or discounted as meaningless. Our cultural inheritance is a disregard and suspicion of those who do not speak. Deeply ingrained in our idea of a person is the ability to use a voice, and when we encounter those who do not do so we have to struggle with powerful feelings of stigma and differentness.[13]

When a person stops using language we need to ask ourselves whether this derives directly from their dementia, or whether there are other influences which could be operating. Depression may be a factor for some. Loss of confidence or the repeated effects of being ignored or dismissed may cause someone to give up speaking simply because their efforts go unrewarded. It has been known for some people to respond to experiences of trauma by becoming mute. But people whose wordlessness does not seem to be due to mood or social factors, and who remain interested in being in interaction with others, present us with special challenges and opportunities. They invite us in the most full sense to develop our own powers of nonverbal communication.

A common assumption is that the loss of words marks a transition of the person into an unreachable and incomprehensible realm, somewhere we can no longer accompany them or try to understand their experience. On the contrary there are times in all of our lives when words can actually prove to be a barrier: we use them to distance ourselves from others; they keep our communication at a more superficial level than it could or maybe should go. Of this Michael Ignatieff, author of the novel *Scar Tissue*,[14] has said:

> I learned as much from my mother when she couldn't speak to me, when she couldn't communicate, when she simply stared and received our kisses on the cheek, as I learned when she was joking and laughing.[15]

It is undeniably difficult to enter into this realm of wordless communication. Our recourse to language is so strong, it takes effort to resist. For some people it may be that dementia brings with it experiences which those of us without the condition do not have, and for which there are no words anyway. In her novel *Cereus Blooms at Night*, Shani Mootoo talks of the state when Mala, a woman with dementia, has stopped using words:

> Eventually Mala all but rid herself of words. The wings of a gull flapping through the air titillated her soul and awakened her toes and knobbly knees, the palms of her withered hands, deep inside her womb, her vagina, lungs and stomach and heart. Every muscle of her body swelled, tingled, cringed or went numb in response to her surroundings – every fibre was sensitised in a way that words were unable to match or enhance. Mala responded to those receptors, flowing with them effortlessly, like water making its way along a path.[16]

This idea that words can get in the way of a more basic, direct and resonant form of responsiveness to our surroundings, and perhaps communication with each other, is fascinating. It seems that Mootoo is describing the kind of sensitivity to the environment that animals rely on for their very survival. Our biological inheritance surely means that we are equipped with such potential, however vestigial it may seem in our hypercognitive world. Is it possible that people with dementia, either as a result of cognitive change or through height-ened anxiety responses which unfortunately occur for some,[17] find themselves able to appreciate and respond to subtleties which are lost on the rest of us?

The need to become more aware of our own nonverbal communication

Of course in discussing the place of nonverbal communication with people with dementia we cannot simply focus outwards. In order to understand and enhance opportunities for establishing and developing relationships, we must focus on our own style of nonverbal communication. As was mentioned earlier, aside from the actual words we utter, part of what makes each of us unique and recognizable are the ways in which we use our faces, bodies, voices and the environment around us to express ourselves. We are therefore talking about something which is very personal. To become more aware of how one comes across to others in this myriad of subtle and interacting ways is a very difficult thing. Most of the time we are unaware of our own personal style of presenting and interacting, we just get on and do it. Bringing it into more con-scious awareness can induce an uncomfortable sense of self-consciousness or even embarrassment. And then of course if you are aware and thinking about what you are doing when you approach and interact with someone, this very awareness will interfere with the attention and absorption required to engage and communicate fully.

It is a challenging area, but we have both found that a little awareness and reflection on this matter can actually go a long way, and the process of both heightening awareness and losing oneself in naturalness can be practised and developed in all sorts of ways. We explore this further in Chapter 6 on interpretation, and in all of the practical chapters.

Some people have a special knack of communicating effectively with certain people with dementia. Others may try very hard, but simply not be able to achieve the same level of ease and rapport. These differences have at least part of their basis in different styles of nonverbal communication. Of this Melanie Nind and Dave Hewett say:

> It is frustrating that some people are obviously so much more naturally good at body language than others. Even when you know it and observe them, it can still be difficult to put into words what it is that they are doing which is so different and magical and effective.[18]

Despite this, we can probably all learn to improve our sensitivity to the other person's preferred style, and enter into a communicative space which is empowering and enhancing for both parties.

Mirroring

When developing relationships with certain people who do not speak, John has found that in general the most effective way of establishing and developing contact is to confine himself to using only those channels of communication the person with dementia uses. The practice that we have called mirroring has developed in a natural way in the course of John's work, as a response to individual people and situations, and has become part of his overall approach. Others have developed similar approaches in related fields, such as work with people with learning difficulties.[19] It can include words, but it is most powerful and moving when it occurs in a purely nonverbal manner.

Put simply, it involves being engaged in a one-to-one interaction, focusing closely on the person's movements, and reflecting back what they do, and in the style they are doing it, essentially following the leads that they give. So if the person looks at something and points, you would do the same. If they rock their body and stroke the arm of the chair you would do so also. As well as doing what the other person is doing, mirroring demands that you do it in a similar way so that attention must be given to the speed at which the person moves, the degree of muscle tension or relaxation involved, and the way one movement or gesture merges into another. It requires a great deal of concentration and attention, and being highly sensitized to the whole range of nonverbal channels of communication.

The lead-in to this style of interacting is of great importance. If it is begun in an insensitive way, then it may come across as being crudely imitative, even mocking. If the person you are interacting with is not used to close contact with another person, they may find it intrusive or even threatening. It may be an approach which is not suitable for some people at all.

A crucial aspect of this style of working is that the other person should be the one who is leading and largely controlling the interaction. We have already said that people with dementia are radically disempowered, and one of the major ways they are disadvantaged in relationships is through losing control over how interactions and communication arise and unfold. The practice of mirroring is one important way in which we can begin to give back to them something of the power they have lost. Even doing this for a short time on a regular basis may be a significant way of keeping the channels of communication and relationship open. In doing so we are demonstrating our recognition of their unique personal status, and joining them in their experience of the world. It involves an unspoken deference to the other person, conferring upon them a dignity and authority which the condition, or the way we respond to it, so often appears to deny.

Another facet of this is that the practice of mirroring demands that we limit ourselves to the range of communicative channels the person with dementia is using. This means not speaking at all if they do not speak, something which can be quite hard. Giving up, even for a very short time, our dominant and preferred mode of communication, however, is an immediate way of getting some idea of how it might feel to be the person with dementia. There is a quality of 'at onceness' which is unlike other more formal modes of communication.

The following is an example of mirroring taken from a journal entry of John's. It happened also to be filmed by a camera crew:[20]

> I had never seen her before and knew nothing about her. I met her in a corridor where she was sitting with a vacant seat in front of her. I asked if I might sit there. There was no negative reaction, but she showed no enthusiasm either. I asked her if she would like to talk to me. There was no answer to any of my enquiries. She consistently looked past me. There was no discernible expression on her face, and her body language was inscrutable. After two or three minutes I excused myself and left for the dining room.
>
> About ten minutes later she came in through the door. She was moving purposefully, and showed immediate recognition when I turned towards her. I asked if I might take her hand. She said 'Yes' and pointed to a chair. I walked her to the chair and helped her to sit down. I asked if I might sit next to her. She again said 'Yes'. We immediately engaged in eye contact which was startlingly intense. This was maintained for long periods of the interaction, which lasted for about four minutes. At first I talked, drawing her attention to some flowers on the table. At that point, she put her finger to her lips to enjoin silence, and I did the same to show that I would observe the rule. At all other stages of the 'conversation' she led and I followed. She pointed to the vase of flowers. She stroked my hand. She shook my hand in a long-drawn-out gesture of playfulness. She sat back, nodded and said 'Yes'. These actions were repeated more than once, and at all times I instinctively followed. A sense of deep intimacy quickly built up between us, but the effort of concentration rapidly tired us both. To close the interaction the lady let both my hands drop, lent back in her chair, nodded profoundly, and pronounced the word 'wonderful'.
>
> When I reflected on the encounter, I can only describe it as powerfully spiritual. It combined silence and mirroring in a potent manner, and I would like to believe that after experiencing it the lady came away feeling a little less alone in facing her condition. I certainly felt privileged to have been permitted to come so close to another human being.

It can be extremely moving to participate in a practice such as this. You may find it an emotional experience, and need to seek out support afterwards. It certainly demands a great deal of energy, so expect to feel tired. When mirroring works well, however, the sense of connection and meaning engendered by this can be extremely uplifting. At its best as John indicated it has a spiritual quality, and as such it can leave you feeling changed.

We now turn to further aspects of nonverbal communication, and the possibilities available to people with dementia.

Communication through the arts

The arts provide human beings with many expressive outlets which do not involve words – painting, sculpture, music, dance – and there is increasing reason to believe that those who are proficient in a specific art form before the onset of dementia may be able to continue to practise it.[21] Some who have no previous aptitude can learn artistic techniques and find satisfaction from exploring their creative potential after dementia has become a part of their lives.[22]

Selly Jenny and Marilyn Oropeza in California set up a project for people with Alzheimer's to provide opportunities in the visual arts, particularly water-colour painting. In the book they published about the project they comment:

> As we stand before their paintings they call out to us in a way we cannot ignore. They tell us their stories in a language we all understand, transmitting feelings and emotions trapped inside. Slipping beyond the language of words, their paintings show us glimpses of who they were and who they still are.[23]

It has been noted by many commentators and researchers, and is a matter of common observation by care staff, that music occupies a special place in the lives of many people with dementia.[24] It seems to speak widely to individuals irrespective of the severity of the condition and impairment of other channels of communication. This would be equally true of the capacity to create music in an improvisatory manner. By way of example of how this art form can be used as a powerful alternative to language, here is an account from Helen Finch, whose mother had dementia:

> My mother's speech was affected quite severely from very early on in her dementia; in fact that was how it first manifested itself. About six years after the onset of Eve's condition, she was admitted to hospital for assessment and within a few days collapsed with what the doctors thought was probably an ischaemic attack. My father and I rushed to the hospital and discussed with the doctors what should be done; at that point it looked as if she might not survive.
>
> The next day we went to visit her. She was in bed and awake but rather drowsy. She started to mouth something and didn't seem able to verbalise normally, but something told me that she was trying to sing. My father and I were in total disbelief when we realised that she was singing 'The Funeral March'. It was very dramatic, and I had to go out to recover my composure. I think we felt that this was her way of telling us that she was going to die. In retrospect we concluded that what she was probably communicating was her fear of the possibility of dying.
>
> My mother had always enjoyed family sing-songs and loved opera, so we then encouraged her to sing when she couldn't find the words. A few days later when she had recovered a little she tapped on my hand what she was later able to confirm was 'The Skye Boat Song'. It seemed as if she was telling us that she wanted to be somewhere else.

She didn't seem able to provide the words of the songs, only the tune or the rhythm, but I came to realize that the words were significant even though she couldn't sing them. Looking back through my diaries I see that there were well over twenty songs sung over that period of a year. She sang 'The Funeral March' again after suffering another collapse after entering a nursing home. One day she started singing it a third time, but suddenly stopped as if she realised that it wasn't appropriate. I think this was very significant: the insight was there into what the music might be communicating.[25]

Humour

We referred earlier to the role of nonverbal communication in humour. In our hypercognitive culture we tend to think of laughter as something verbally provoked, but then we recall examples of famous mimes and clowns, and all those silent filmstars with their exaggerated gestures, pulling of faces and slapstick. Physical humour can also be extremely subtle and sophisticated too, of course.

In our experience many people with dementia laugh a great deal, and often the cause of this is something seen, an amusing incident, the expression on a face, sometimes perhaps an imagined episode which cannot be shared. As with Cath, who was described earlier in the chapter, much of what occasions smiling, and even outright laughter, appears to come out of relationship. A shared intimacy will often find expression in characteristic gestures, little rituals, and movements which appear to trigger remembrances of past humorous encounters. One has only to observe some people with dementia together to perceive exchanges of a comical nature. From these we can learn to encourage our own moments of sharing the sheer fun of existence, often without a word being spoken.

Bernard Heywood, in his account of caring for Maria, a longstanding family friend, says:

> I've also devised a new aid to good relations and her well-being by making her laugh. This is achieved by indulging in antics – acting, gesticulating and walking in odd ways as one would with a child, or indeed like a real comic doing a routine. So far it's been very helpful.

Reflecting on this at a later time, he wrote:

> These antics remained helpful on and off for a considerable time, and my repertoire increased. It included wearing one or two comic or comically arranged, hats, and odd ways of dressing. Just as she could sometimes cry excessively, Maria could also laugh excessively. It was nice, though, when this happened.[26]

Related to the role that humour can play in communication, there are the possibilities of the 'game'. What we mean by the idea of a game is some kind of activity or interaction that takes place within a set of rules (however loosely defined), and which constitutes a kind of frame which is distinct from normal activity and interaction in life. Such activities need not be restricted to nonverbal communication, of course, but we have heard some interesting accounts from staff and relative carers of nonverbal interaction which seem to take this form.

Sensory stimulation

One area of development in dementia care which may have considerable potential in enhancing well-being and communication is that of providing stimuli to the senses, either through specialized environments or less structured approaches using familiar objects, scents and so on. We do not have much experience of sensory work, but believe it has real potential for providing what could be pleasant and evocative triggers to memory and starting points for communication, much of which could be nonverbal in nature. It could be used as a way to promote communication work, supplying structure and lessening self-consciousness for staff. Of this, psychologists Julie Ellis and Tania Thorn say:

> Perhaps multisensory stimulation rooms provide a safe environment for us, as staff, to unlearn our dependence on verbal communication, to work through our discomfort at communicating non-verbally, and provide the opportunity to communicate with our patients in a setting free of failure and the humiliation of getting no response.[27]

Touch in particular seems to have very positive potential to enhance well-being and possibilities for communication. Here is Beth Shirley Brough, writing about her relationship with a friend who has developed Alzheimer's disease, on this subject:

> I am delighted by the intimacy of touch that has developed between us since Reg's rationality has become fluid. These things are the real substance of our communication, confirmed and endorsed by the ephemeral word that sometimes broadens into wonderfully coherent sentences.[28]

The woman quoted in the title of this chapter was also attesting to the powerful reassurance which physical contact can bring.

Crying

Many people would shy away from considering crying as a form of communication, yet it is a clear nonverbal indication of distress or the upwelling of emotion. It can take many different forms: deep sobbing, wailing or a calm, silent shedding of tears. These variations may correspond to different emotional states. For many of us the sight of another person crying can be a powerful emotional experience, perhaps even bringing tears to our own eyes. Sometimes it will be obvious why a person is crying, at others the causes may remain obscure.

The ways in which we respond to someone who is tearful will depend on many things. Often our instinct is to try to stop them, as if by suppressing its expression, the underlying cause will be dissipated. In some instances, offering comfort in the form of taking the person's hand or perhaps giving them a hug will help. Where the reason for the tears is unclear, such an approach can also provide clues. Some crying, though, can be a private, internalized matter – a person giving way to grief over losses which will remain buried – and they may prefer to be left alone. In any case the tendency to encourage a person to stop crying is to be resisted: outward manifestations of inward hurts can provide welcome relief of tension. Where language is not attempted or words do not come easily the therapeutic value of crying may be even greater. We are reminded of one woman who pointed to John's notebook and said, rather mysteriously:

These are lines from my crying book.

Challenging behaviour

By challenging behaviour we mean the sorts of things that people do which others find unwelcome or even offensive. There is a set of such behaviours which are sometimes seen in people with dementia. Common examples include shouting, screaming, swearing, physical or verbal aggression, certain forms of sexual behaviour, undressing in public and so on.[29] These often have a strong nonverbal component.

It used to be thought that behaviours such as these were a direct consequence of damage to the brain, and therefore inherently meaningless. Responses to them included use of sedating medication or outright removal of the person, and their occurrence greatly added to the sense of hopelessness and burden engendered by the experience of caring. Of course the term 'challenging behaviour' (which has replaced even more negative expressions like 'problem behaviour' or 'disruptive behaviour') is itself highly loaded. The word 'challenging' is an attempt to redress the negative bias of words like 'problem' or 'disruptive', but we must still be cautious in its use. It should prompt us to consider to whom is the behaviour in question challenging? Whose problem is it? Should it always be approached with the objective of stopping or reducing it? And whose needs are being met by such efforts?

In recent years as part of the development of psychosocial models of dementia, new ways of understanding so-called challenging behaviour have become common. The person's actions are now more often considered to be a response to features of the social and physical environment and fluctuations in well-being, and as such can be very usefully conceptualized as a form of communication. Once we make efforts to enter into the subjective reality of the individual, instead of seeing the way the person is acting as being bizarre, disruptive or dysfunctional, we may suddenly be able to see patterns, and reclassify the behaviour as a perfectly rational response to an adverse situation. It may be an expression of pain or discomfort, or related to a strong emotion.

For some people, engaging in behaviour which others consider challenging is extremely positive – an expression of individuality and an assertion of the desire to be involved in their surroundings. But the most important thing is to try to find meaning. Dementia care trainer Frena Gray Davidson writes:

> When language and function betray the sick, leaving them without the ability to say what they mean, the only thing left is action. Acting out becomes a symbolic portrayal of their truth . . .
>
> In years of dealing with Alzheimer's sufferers in home care residences and skilled nursing facilities I have never come across a problem behaviour that did not arise from unmet needs or poor handling by carers.[30]

Alice, whom we met in Chapter 1, often went around the unit shouting 'Hee-haw-hee-haw!' and upsetting residents and staff. One day after engaging in this activity for a while, she turned to John and said:

> *When I do that I'm meaning 'Mind your own business'. But why don't you stop me doing it? It's much more interesting when you stop.*

Limitations on nonverbal communication in dementia

As well as recognizing the possibility of heightened capacities in this sphere, we need also to appreciate that there are various features of dementia, and other conditions which may accompany it, which interfere with nonverbal expression and interpretation.

Physical disability

Physical disability need not have any direct connection with dementia *per se* (except for those in the very late stages when physical capacity is extremely diminished), but it is nevertheless a serious problem for many older people. In many ways the whole body is involved in a significant proportion of nonverbal communication, and when physical capacities have been affected, say by a stroke or through difficulties in muscular control, then this will obviously affect how a person is able to convey meaning, particularly through posture, orientation and gesture. It may be that some of the frustrated expressive energy will be channelled in other directions, and partners in communication will need to adapt to such modifications.

Delays in responding

For many people a generalized effect of dementia is to slow down responses and actions. This can apply as much to nonverbal communication as to the use of language, perhaps even more obviously if the initiation and control of movement is impaired. It may therefore be that some people will take much longer to express themselves and respond nonverbally. One of the main ways in which people with dementia are disempowered in communication is that of being continually outpaced, having others speak, move and act move quickly than they are able to understand and match.

A woman who Kate has known springs particularly to mind in this context. On seeing her and offering a greeting, May would make eye contact, but this was relatively inexpressive. She would stare with unchanging facial expression for perhaps 10 or 15 seconds. However, if aspects of the greeting (particularly body orientation, eye contact and smiling) were maintained, eventually her face would break into a warm smile and she would respond verbally as well, albeit in a very limited way. The delay often felt very long, and there was a self-consciousness in holding the nonverbal features or repeating the verbal ones. The reward of it being reciprocated and obviously enjoyed by May, however, was well worth the extra effort.

Experiences such as these prompt us to reflect on the many occasions when people with dementia are greeted in the conventional way, but a delay is taken for lack of responsiveness. In the busy world of services, most staff would be long out of the room or down the corridor before such an individual had had a chance to respond. This sort of thing happening on a repeated basis must have an emotional and eventually a behavioural impact on the person. If, after many similar instances of unsuccessful communication, the person does actually give up trying to respond, then this may be as much the result of learning as of the progress of dementia itself.

Facial inexpressiveness

The faces of some people with dementia are consistently inexpressive and unresponsive even when the person experiences and wishes to express emotion and is given time to respond. Certain types of dementia may be more likely to give rise to this feature, particularly Parkinson's Disease, which is associated with muscular rigidity. These may affect the mobility, and therefore the communicative function, of the entire body, not just the face.

There is a great danger that this sort of absence of expression and response will be mistaken for lack of interest, concern or awareness in the person with dementia. It may be that there are fluctuations in the severity of this problem, and therefore times when greater expressivity is possible. Vigilance for such intervals is vital. In the context of an ongoing problem of masking of nonverbal communication it may be that some individuals, in their profound need to communicate *somehow*, find extremely subtle ways of projecting their thoughts, feelings and needs through much reduced or narrowed 'windows' of expression. Again the need to be alert to and respond to any such communication is crucial.

The impact of sensory impairment

The prevalence of sensory disability in people with dementia, and its impact on communication is much overlooked.[31] We mention the subject here specifically because hearing and visual loss have the potential to affect the use of nonverbal communication in important ways. Clearly if someone's vision is markedly impaired then their opportunities to utilize all the visual channels of communication will be much reduced. They will need to give greater attention to qualities of voice and touch, if available. Similarly hearing loss will force a heightened reliance on visual cues. These are realities which should influence the way we use nonverbal communication in relation to them. We understand even less about how hearing and visual loss affect the person's own use of nonverbal communication.

We end this section with the words of family carer Murna Downs (in response to a question about envisioning a world without dementia) which sums up our position:

> I am not so sure that I would hope for a world without dementia, for in a world without dementia we would be without the ones we love who have taught us that remembering and planning and naming and knowing are not the key activities of human life, but rather that feeling and being and touching and singing have enormous riches and depths that we are often too busy to relish in our race to rationality.[32]

Implications for care

If we are to meet the challenges and participate in the delights which nonverbal communication offers, then we must be prepared to rethink our whole attitude to this form of relating, take a good look at ourselves, and create environments in which it is nurtured and celebrated. This means reflecting on existing beliefs and attitudes, raising our awareness of our habitual behaviour, and entertaining a whole range of possibilities in terms of new activities and alternative ways of doing ordinary things.

Humour and fun may be very powerful starting points for developing the use of nonverbal channels of communication. There is a whole range of games and activities used by teachers of dance and movement, drama, education, and by leaders in various sorts of personal and spiritual development.[33] Many of these could be used or adapted to engage people in exploring ways of expressing ideas, emotions and needs without words. Different sorts of activities will suit different personalities, or accord with different moods or styles of relating.

Those of us who are involved with people with dementia need to learn more about how we ourselves use nonverbal channels of communication, and how these are affected by factors such as tiredness, mood, stress and illness. It is unrealistic to deny that these very normal aspects of life at times impinge upon work, and certainly not respectful of the personhood of staff. Learning ways of enhancing and deepening our own expressiveness requires a particular quality of openness and trust of others. Good teamwork is also essential for this goal.

The potential of touch in enhancing well-being and promoting communication with people with dementia has yet to be explored properly. Most of us feel comforted and affirmed by touch which is employed in a respectful way, and for those with the condition it could make all the difference between being able to remain in meaningful contact with others, and losing a sense of connectedness. For those with severe sensory disability it may be the only way real contact can be made with another human being. For those whose relationship with their physical self has become severely fractured, it may have a crucial role in affirming identity and personhood.

As a consequence of our natural attachment to the use of language, we tend to rely on this as the dominant mode of communication until it eventually begins to present serious problems. Rather than waiting until the stage at which words frequently let the person down before thinking seriously about nonverbal communication, perhaps we could make specific efforts to develop parallel systems of communication, exploring possibilities for combining mime and gestures with words and phrases. As far as we know no such strategy has so far been tried with people with dementia.

The effects and potential of the physical environment must also be considered in the effort to heighten the use of nonverbal communication. Observing how people use their physical surroundings and how their ways of expressing themselves vary in response to factors like noise and the presence of others is important. Creating environments which people can use in order to express different aspects of their personality or mood is another possibility. The imaginative use of colour, and the availability of pictures and objects as stimuli to the expression of ideas could be a valuable way in to communication. Taking trouble to find out about the person's preferences in terms of colour and style of clothes, hairstyle and other aspects of personal grooming, and remembering about these aspects of their identity, is a fundamental way of affirming their personhood, including specifically self-esteem, dignity and sexuality. These factors could make a real difference to the person's willingness to enter into communication. Developing such habits could provide scope for helping the individual to use resources such as colours and clothes to communicate their feelings and moods from day to day. We consider the subject of how staff present themselves nonverbally, including style of dress, colour and so on in the implications for care section of Chapter 5 on memory.

Ethical implications

Authenticity and self-disclosure

If it is true that people with dementia develop an especially sensitive facility for reading information which comes through nonverbal channels then we must expect our feeling states, moods and intentions to be more transparent to them. What might this mean for our day-to-day interactions? Does it suggest that we need to be more open about what we are experiencing? If, for example, a member of staff is having problems in their personal life and they are aware that this is having a bearing on their behaviour at work (meaning that individuals with dementia are able to pick up on this), would it then be incumbent upon them to provide some kind of explanation for the situation? It would certainly be unfortunate if the other person were to become aware that something was amiss and be concerned that they had somehow caused it. At the same time, we do not normally expect to have to disclose information about a state of mind which relates to something from our personal lives at work, and staff could suffer from a feeling of being personally quite exposed, something we would all find difficult.

The drama therapist Paula Crimmens addressed this issue, using the term 'congruence' which she defines as the 'the image I am presenting matches what is going on inside'.[34] Discussing situations in which staff members are struggling with difficult feelings about personal issues, she describes how some colleagues have actually told the person with dementia how they are feeling. She comments as follows:

> There is a big difference between burdening someone and letting them know what is going on. Staff who have adopted this approach have been amazed at the responses they have received from residents, even people in the very frail later stages – entirely appropriate human responses to another human being who is in distress.[35]

Neither Crimmens nor we ourselves are advocating that we reveal all of our complexities, problems and emotional fluctuations to people with dementia. This would not be appropriate or helpful, but surely being a person alongside others means, at least at times, that we share our vulnerabilities, and allow the other to offer comfort and understanding. To deny people with dementia this would be to deny an aspect of our shared personhood.

This issue relates to more general questions about the extent to which our relationships with people with dementia can be reciprocal, and this is discussed further in the ethical implications section at the end of Chapter 12. It also bears on questions about how far we should expect people to go in terms of giving themselves to this kind of work, and we explore this at greater length in Chapter 15.

Also on the subject of transparency of feelings, we need to consider how this squares with the need for the person with dementia to have privacy regarding their own inner experiences. Becoming practised in reading nonverbal communication can be a great asset, but if used insensitively it could lead to behaviour which is intrusive.

4 | Language: 'Words can make or break you'

The following excerpt is from the novel *Moon Tiger* by Penelope Lively. The first speaker is an older woman in a hospital bed:

'What's that?' she whispers, pointing.

'What's what, Miss Hampton?' says the nurse. 'There's nothing – just the window.'

'There!' – she stabs the air – 'Thing moving . . . What's it called? Name!'

'Nothing that I can see', says the nurse briskly. 'Don't fuss, dear. You're a bit muzzy today, that's all. Have a sleep. I'll draw the curtains.'

The face, suddenly, relaxes. 'Curtain', she murmurs. 'Curtain.'

'Yes, dear,' says the nurse. 'I'll draw the curtains.'

Today language abandoned me. I could not find the word for a simple object – a commonplace familiar furnishing. For an instant, I stared into a void. Language tethers us to the world; without it we spin like atoms. Later I made an inventory of the room – a naming of parts: bed, chair, table, picture, vase, cupboard, window, curtain. Curtain. And I breathed again.[1]

Language has a central role in human life. It sets us apart from all other animals, and has played a pivotal role in our evolution. As we noted at the beginning of Chapter 3, we are surrounded by words. They are before our eyes, in our ears and they swim through our minds in an unstoppable, messy and sometimes seemingly inconsequential stream. At other times they shine clearly, illuminating our thoughts and pointing the ways forward. Talking is what we think first of doing when something important happens to us. It is the way to share joy and grief, to clarify and solve problems, it is the saving grace, the compensation when nothing else can be retrieved.

Our understanding of words and the ways in which we use them are inextricably tied up with the way we function in the world. Our relationship to language is not just intellectual; it is visceral and emotional. It does not simply occupy another 'department' of the mind, in the way that we think of functions such as seeing, hearing or smelling. Rather the ability to use language is a basic organizing principle of the brain. If we were not adapted to learn and use it we would be unimaginably different, another sort of being altogether.

Closely related to our language-driven nature is another example of human uniqueness – the voice. Although the use of the voice is not restricted to speaking, it deserves special consideration here since full participation in conventional language (as distinct from, say, sign language) relies on its use. It is important to recognize that far from being a mere utility, however, the voice carries enormous personal, cultural and even spiritual significance. The voice therapist, Paul Newham, describing a variety of situations in which people are encouraged to explore and expand their use of voice says:

> these people are using the voice as a channel through which to express or 'push out' something from the inside; and the voice is indeed a major bridge between the inner world of mood, emotion, image, thought and experience and the outer world of relationship, discourse and interaction.[2]

In a similar vein, the philosopher Jonathon Rée writes:

> Metaphysicians and mystics have always liked to associate the voice with an immortal soul or divine spirit; and although we may be impatient with such unmodern notions, we will still have to admit that individual voices have a rather special significance in human life. We respond to them as we do to faces: as immediate embodiments of personal character and sensitive indicators of fluctuating mood. At the same time, they are marked by an enigmatic inner divide: the elusive fault-line between the voice that simply makes sounds, and the voice that speaks and utters the words of a language.
>
> When a little baby whimpers or cries or yells, its voice gives uncontrived expression to its emotions; but when a child begins to speak, it is using its voice to participate in social communication in accordance with artificial linguistic conventions. Voices thus encode an intriguing human tension, even a contradiction: they are both expression and communication, both feeling and intellect, both body and mind, both nature and culture. The whole of us, it would seem, is included in the compass of the human voice.[3]

In political and social terms the notion of having a voice is bound up intimately with that of having power, being included and being known. Conversely our responses to those who do not speak are characterized by suspicion, even fear, and at times outright rejection.

About language

In a superficial sense we all know what language is – speech, words and sentences. But in another it is mysterious. The psychologist Stephen Pinker says:

> The workings of language are as far from our awareness as the rationale for egg-laying is from the fly's.[4]

We learn most intensively about language and how to use it in the first few years of our lives. As children we soak it up – our brains are primed to attend to and make sense of it from the minute we are born. But because our first experiences with language occur so early in our lives, it is impossible to remember them, and therefore by the time we are able to think about it, it has long been taken for granted. In order to appreciate more deeply its role in our lives, it is necessary to spend some time thinking about its characteristics. We limit our discussion here to spoken language.

The sounds of language – phonology

Speech is made up of sounds, and the human vocal tract (which includes the larynx, tongue, lips and teeth) is highly specialized for the purpose of speaking. We use these organs to harness the flow of air as we breathe out, which in turn enables us to generate a range of precise and subtly distinctive sounds. This process is normally smooth and effortless, and allows us to speak without being aware of the staggering intricacy of the coordination between brain and muscles required. Those who have witnessed the strugglings of a stroke survivor who has sustained damage to the language centres of the brain controlling speech production will appreciate that making the sounds of a language is no simple matter.

Firsthand evidence of this comes from a book written by a highly intelligent and literary man, Jean-Dominique Bauby, following a devastating stroke:

> Speech therapy is an art that deserves to be more widely known. You cannot imagine the acrobatics your tongue mechanically performs in order to produce all the sounds of a language.
>
> On my birthday Sandrine managed to get me to pronounce the whole alphabet more or less intelligibly. I could not have had a better present. It was as if those twenty-six letters had been wrenched from the void; my own hoarse voice seemed to emanate from a far-off country. The exhausting exercise left me feeling like a caveman discovering language for the first time.[5]

In order to speak, we need not only to be able to produce the sounds which are the ingredients of words, but also to speak at a speed and with a rhythm that is comprehensible to others. This includes putting emphasis on the correct part of the word, for example we say 'de<u>men</u>tia' rather than '<u>de</u>mentia'. All of these aspects put together make up the 'musicality' of speech, and each of us has our own distinctive style, which varies to reflect our moods and attitudes, and the capacity to interpret and remember the styles of others.

Sounds into words – semantics

Until you think about them, words do not seem very remarkable things. Again Penelope Lively draws our attention to the wonder of them:

> We open our mouths and out flow words whose ancestries we do not even know. We are walking lexicons. In a single sentence of idle chatter we preserve Latin, Anglo-Saxon, Norse; we carry a museum inside our heads, each day we commemorate peoples of whom we have never heard. More than that, we speak volumes – our language is the language of everything we have not read. Shakespeare and the Authorised Version surface in supermarkets, on buses, chatter on radio and television. I find this miraculous. I never cease to wonder at it. That words are more durable than anything, that they blow with the wind, hibernate and reawaken, shelter parasitic on the most unlikely hosts, survive and survive and survive.[6]

But what exactly *is* a word? A word is a symbol – the word 'chair' denotes an item of furniture which is designed to be sat upon. Speaking a language means that we share an agreement that this particular sequence of sounds will 'stand for' the object. However, the relationship may seem entirely arbitrary. While many words in our language advertise or connote what they stand for, as with noises (for example, bang, hiss, crunch), most lack such reminders of meaning. There is nothing in the word or sound 'chair' which bears any resemblance to the object. Words, then, can be regarded as symbolic, and the meaning we exchange by using them is symbolic.

In order to use words successfully, we not only need to know them, we also need a highly organized system for storing and finding them. Although we are all familiar with the experience of not being able to find a word when we need it (the 'tip of the tongue' phenomenon), this happens very infrequently compared to the number of tries when all goes well. Research indicates that words in the mental lexicon are linked to one another through both sound and meaning, so that on trying to recall the word 'calendar' one may come up with 'camera' which has a similar structure, internal rhythm and links in meaning.[7] It seems that when trying to find a word from our store, the mind works by activating a few which are potentially relevant. Usually just one of the words will be selected, but sometimes two are taken up and a 'blend' occurs such as instead of saying 'She's really frightened' or 'She's really scared' the two are mixed and the result is 'She's really frared'.

Words into sentences – syntax

We do not use words in a random fashion. There are rules which make certain combinations of words meaningful, while disallowing others. We need to know about and follow these rules when using language. So what are the rules and how do we learn them? The first part of the question is difficult to answer. The enterprise of trying to work out and write down the rules underpinning the English language is something which many have attempted to do, but failed. The reality is that this system of rules is so vast and complex it has proved too difficult to record in a complete way.

Yet in another sense we all know these rules without even trying. On hearing a non-native learner trying to speak English we often hear mistakes which violate syntactic rules. We know at once that an error has been made, and are usually easily able to correct the utterance. However, if the learner then goes on to ask why the first attempt was not correct, we are likely to find ourselves at a loss. Syntactic rules are not readily available for conscious examination and explanation.

Again, learning the rules of language is something which begins to happen in early childhood. Children adopt a systematic approach to learning syntax, and this develops rapidly and without apparent effort. As Steven Pinker points out:

> A preschooler's tacit knowledge of grammar is more sophisticated than the thickest style manual or the most state-of-the-art computer language system.[8]

The social rules of language use – pragmatics

Even as experts (albeit implicitly) on phonology, semantics and syntax, we can still go terribly wrong in using language. The reason is that there is yet another set of rules and guidelines we must learn in order to function effectively in using language in a social context. Some of these rules relate to ways of helping language to do its job of conveying ideas effectively, but since a great deal of talk is concerned with establishing and maintaining relationships, many of them are concerned with politeness and the consideration of other people's needs and feelings. Like so many other social situations, there is a kind of etiquette with language, which allows some things, puts others in a questionable zone, and absolutely disallows and condemns certain behaviour. If we wish to get on with people and to further our own ends, we have to know these rules.

Here the neurologist Oliver Sacks is describing his first meeting with Temple, a woman with marked autism:

> I was feeling somewhat exhausted, hungry, and thirsty – I had been travelling all day and had missed lunch – and I kept hoping that Temple would notice and offer me some coffee. She did not; so, after an hour . . . I finally asked for some coffee. There was no 'I'm sorry, I should have

offered you some before,' no intermediacy, no social junction. Instead, she immediately took me to a coffeepot that was kept brewing in the secretaries' office upstairs. She introduced me to the secretaries in a somewhat brusque manner, giving me the feeling, once again, of someone who had learned, roughly, 'how to behave' in such situations without having much personal perception of how other people felt – the nuances, the social subtleties, involved.[9]

Examples of social situations involving such rules include initiating a conversation, or, once already involved in one, changing the subject. We know that in order to begin an exchange with someone who is already talking to a third party, it would be impolite simply to walk up and begin speaking as if the other person was not present. If it is necessary to interrupt, there are ways of doing this which soften the impact of the behaviour, for example acknowledging the potentially unfavourable impression that could be created: 'Sorry to butt in like this, but your car is on a double yellow line, and is about to be towed away.' We know that certain ways of asking questions can be considered rude, for example 'What time is it?' as opposed to 'Could you tell me what time it is, please?' Taking turns to speak is one of the most basic rules of conversation. We soon notice if our conversational partner is speaking in such a way that it is impossible to respond with ideas of our own, and we would also feel very uncomfortable with someone who makes no effort to wait until we have finished an utterance before coming in with something else.

Another rule is that of relevance. We expect our conversational partners to say things which bear on the subject at hand. It sometimes happens, however, that while talking we think of something we want to say which is not directly related, and there are ways of dealing with this. We might say 'I know this is getting off the point a bit, but . . .'. This alerts the other to a change of subject and also tells them that the speaker is aware that one of the rules of conversation is about to be broken. If we have embarked on a story the point of which is not obvious or is going to take time to become evident, we might reassure the other by saying 'You'll see why I'm telling you this in a minute'.

In most conversations there is an expectation that both parties will contribute roughly equally to the exchange. If this is not occurring there is usually a specific reason, perhaps that something special has happened, and often there will be a reference to the fact that the balance is not equal. In specialized situations, for example in a counselling relationship, it is part of the implicit agreement that the client will talk much more than the counsellor.

Again, the business of knowing and following social rules is a very complex and subtle matter. We learn much of the basics in childhood, but are continually reviewing and revising our behaviour as we get older, as our social circles change and certainly if we move to another culture where the rules may be markedly different. Successful communication demands a constant alertness and flexibility, but, as with so many other aspects of language, most of us achieve this without awareness of the skill and effort required. This again underlines how deeply we are verbal beings.

The role of language in our everyday lives

Language permeates our lives so fundamentally that it is very hard to imagine being without it. The following account from Oliver Sacks may help us a little in appreciating our reliance on it. He is describing an individual who has been deaf since birth and has never learned language, although he is of average intelligence.

> Two years ago . . . I met Joseph . . . an eleven year old who had no language whatsoever . . . Joseph longed to communicate, but could not. Neither speaking nor writing nor signing was available to him, only gesture and pantomime, and a marked ability to draw . . . He looked alive and animated, but profoundly baffled: his eyes were attracted to our speaking mouths and signing hands, inquisitively, uncomprehendingly, and it seemed to me, yearningly. He perceived that something was 'going on' between us, but he could not comprehend what it was – he had, as yet, almost no idea of symbolic communication, of what it was to have a symbolic currency, to exchange meaning.
>
> Previously denied of any opportunity . . . Joseph was now just beginning . . . to have some communication with others. This, manifestly, gave him great joy; he wanted to stay at school all day, all night, all weekend, all the time. His distress at leaving school was painful to see, for going home meant, for him, return to the silence, return to a hopeless communicational vacuum, where he could have no converse, no commerce with his parents, neighbours, friends; it meant being overlooked, becoming a nonperson, again.[10]

Here Sacks is suggesting that the ability and opportunity to use language of some kind is fundamental to personhood, which leads in to our next point.

The role of language in personal identity

Language is at the centre of the way we maintain and develop our sense of self, and the self as continuous through the past, present and future. As we shall discuss at greater length in later chapters on memory and narrative, the propensity to tell stories to ourselves and others is basic to how we develop and maintain a sense of identity – how we know who we are and how we fit in to our social and physical world. The use of language is essential to this. An illustration of the difficulties that arise in someone who has never learned language is again provided by Oliver Sacks in describing Joseph:

> Joseph was unable, for example, to communicate how he had spent the weekend -- one could not really ask him . . . he could not even grasp the *idea* of a question, much less formulate an answer. It was not only language that was missing: there was not, it was evident, a clear sense of the past, of 'a day ago' as distinct from 'a year ago'. There was a strange lack of historical sense, the feeling of a life that lacked autobiographical and

historical dimension, the feeling of a life that existed only in the moment, in the present.[11]

The role of language in understanding the world

In order to function in the world, we need to be able to organize our perceptions of it into categories of objects or sensations and to give names to the constituents of our environment and experiences. The fact that all normal children go through a phase of demanding to be told the names of objects attests to this need. Knowing the names of things allows us to take control of the world in a way which would be quite impossible otherwise. Without it one is cast out, forced to occupy a much reduced and limited realm. Here Oliver Sacks is describing another deaf boy of average intelligence, Ildefonso, who is for the first time entering into a truly linguistic sphere of sign language:

> The repetition of movements and sounds, as Schaller [a teacher] tried to teach Sign to Ildefonso, continued without any sense that they had an 'inside', had meaning . . . And then quite suddenly and unexpectedly, one day he did . . . Suddenly it was not just a movement to be copied, but a sign pregnant with meaning, that could be used to symbolize a concept . . .

He continues, quoting Schaller:

> 'His face stretches and opens with excitement . . . slowly at first, then hungrily, he sucks in everything, as though he had never seen it before: the door, the bulletin board, chairs, tables, students, the clock, the green blackboard and me . . . He has entered the universe of humanity, he has discovered the communion of minds.'[12]

The role of language in acting in the world

Life continually presents us with challenges and problems. The ability to think, reflect and formulate solutions to problems, and then take action is a basic need. Philosophers and psychologists have long wrestled with the relationship between language and thought, but it is certainly true that our species has developed an extraordinary capacity for problem-solving, and that this has been made possible by language, which allows the conceptualization of relationships between things and ideas, and then has the potential to make things happen. The following passage from psychologist Charles Antaki vividly illustrates the active nature of talk:

> when people talk, they aren't out to tell you what's in their mind. They're out to actually do something. When you talk, you talk in an interaction, and you talk to move the interaction forward. You don't talk to reel off the contents of your memory. You don't express an attitude like you display the contents of your china cabinet. An utterance is more like a bomb than a printout.[13]

We use language to exert control over our environment, and many of our actions are perpetrated through others by the use of language. By having names for things and ways of describing relationships between them it becomes possible to ask another human being to influence the environment in a way that would not be possible, or only in a very crude sense, without language.

The role of language in maintaining relationships

As social animals, it is essential that we form and maintain relationships with other human beings. The capacity to get along with others depends to a large extent on our ability to communicate our inner state (beliefs, thoughts, feelings and desires) and to learn about those of others. Although nonverbal communication is important, the precision of language is necessary to handle the great complexity of human relationships. Even then, the scope for misunderstanding and breakdown is all too great. Without language we could relate to others only in the here and now, and any kind of reflection upon experiences and exchange of meaning would be impossible. This passage from the philosopher Daniel C. Dennett underlines this point.

> Conversation unites us. We can all know a great deal about what it's like to be a Norwegian fisherman or a Nigerian taxi driver, an eighty-year-old nun or a five-year-old boy blind from birth, a chess master or a prostitute or a fighter pilot. We can know much more about these topics than we can know about what it's like (if anything) to be a dolphin, a bat or even a chimpanzee. No matter how different from one another we people are, scattered around the globe, we can explore our differences and communicate about them. No matter how similar to one another wildebeests are, standing shoulder to shoulder in a herd, they cannot know much of anything about their similarities, let alone their differences. They cannot compare notes. They can have similar experiences, side by side, but they cannot really share experiences the way we do.[14]

Creative use of language

Human beings are inherently creative. All the time we are looking for and responding to novelty, and finding new ways of making sense of experiences. Where language is concerned, our culture of prose and poetry explores the huge variety of ways of playing with words, enjoying their sensuous qualities and seemingly endless possibilities for conveying ideas and meaning.

There is a particular sense of delight in finding or inventing an expression which captures the exact quality of an experience or perception. In so doing we transform our experience, making possible the appreciation of greater and greater levels of subtlety. All this would be impossible without language.

Of the possibilities for creativity through conversation, the philosopher Theodore Zeldin writes:

Conversation is a meeting of minds with different memories and habits. When minds meet, they don't just exchange facts: they transform them, reshape them, draw different implications from them, engage in new trains of thought. Conversation doesn't just reshuffle the cards, it creates new cards. That's the part that interests me. That's where I find the excitement. It's like a spark that two minds create. And what I really care about is what new conversational banquets one can create from those sparks.[15]

Language and dementia

Armed with a greater appreciation of the nature of language and its place in our lives, we now turn to thinking about what happens to language in the context of dementia. Language is often identified as a focus of change in dementia, but what do we actually observe? The common difficulties include:

- producing the right sound or combination of sounds
- getting stuck on one sound, and repeating it
- producing sounds which are 'speech-like' but do not conform to conventional patterns and therefore are not obviously meaningful
- finding the right word
- using words in the wrong way
- using pronouns (such as he, she, him, her) in confusing or ambiguous ways
- making statements which are incomplete or vague in content
- making repetitive statements or asking questions repeatedly
- speech which has meaningful elements, but does not adhere to normal structure or connections in meaning
- the progressive reduction in speech, so much that it may finally stop altogether.

Research investigating the nature of language changes in dementia has been undertaken in a variety of fields.[16] However, as with much of the investigation on intellectual functioning, often the approach adopted is that of studying one ability in isolation from others, and without taking the effect of interpersonal factors into account. This is an especially important deficiency in the case of language which has communication as its central purpose. Again, in common with so many other descriptions of dementia, there has been an emphasis on the nature and rate of negative change, and of the deterioration of general functioning and particular skills.

The observation of these difficulties has been too readily regarded as evidence of generalized incompetence with language. When problems are encountered in identifying meaning in what the person is saying, this has led to an early abandonment of effort to decode and interpret, and to help the person to maintain their currency in the exchange of symbolic meaning. From one study there is a quote about conversation with people with dementia as: 'being led across a bridge that suddenly drops into an abyss'.[17]

Another characterization is the following: 'fluent, irrelevant speech, with well-preserved syntax and words, yet for practical purposes the meaning is lost'.[18]

An alternative approach was adopted by the sociolinguist, Heidi Hamilton.[19] She undertook a four-and-a-half year study of the language of Elsie, in conversation with herself. She describes it in the following terms:

> This 'personal and particular' (Becker 1988)[20] study of conversations with one Alzheimer's patient is offered as a humanistic approach to language loss, one in which communicative breakdowns are analyzed not apart from details about the patient, her conversational partners, and the setting, nor from relevant social facts which may influence the interactions – one in which language is seen as an integral part of human life.[21]

Like Heidi Hamilton, our interest is in looking at language change in a more positive light. Despite the difficulties which dementia brings, very striking changes in the way people use language can be observed, and we are impressed by how resourceful people with dementia are in continuing to use whatever language resources are available to express things that are important to them. Although special efforts of attention and interpretation are required of us, as verbal beings people with dementia continue to use their linguistic powers to do all the things with language described above, and we have a responsibility to support them.

In his novel *Scar Tissue* Michael Ignatieff wrote:

> When you strip us right down, when illness pares us to our core, we remain creatures of the word. Nothing can save us but the word, the messages we send from deep in the shaft of sickness.[22]

He goes further, saying:

> [People with Alzheimer's] are on a voyage into deep space, sending back messages that it is our job to decipher.[23]

Examples of the language of people with dementia

In this section we offer a series of examples of texts and excerpts of dialogues which explore certain characteristics of the language of people with dementia. As with all other aspects of functioning, there is great variability both between and within individuals, but common features do emerge. Later we discuss some of the issues arising from these and other examples at greater length.

Lena Saunders

This is the first of several conversations John had with Lena. Her style was intense, and she held John's hand tightly throughout:

 1 *Are you the text-man?*
 2 *I need to wind the clocks. Take me to wind the clocks.*
 3 *I'm frightened. I'm frightened of being caught in a current.*

   4 *It's a breast-up. You're in need of a breast and I'm up.*
   5 *I'm a very unnecessary, different person. But you never lay the law down at all.*
   6 *I can't get comfortable, in my mind I can't get comfortable.*
   7 *How come you stop talking when you're talking? You shouldn't do that.*
   8 *My hair, I washed it, and now it's sulking.*
   9 *You're a barrican. You don't know what that is? I'll tell you. It's something that you*
  10 *don't expect to be good but that turns out better than expected. That's you.*
  11 *And now I'm going to ask you a question: would you like to live like this?*

Lena's talk is characterized by a series of short statements and questions. It has a brisk, staccato quality, and gives a sense of a rapid flow of disparate thoughts and impressions. The connections between subjects are not obvious, and she moves on without signalling changes. Once she has dealt with a particular topic, she appears not to refer back to it.

The majority of her words are conventional, but some words and phrases are unusual, such as 'text-man' in line 1, and 'breast-up' in line 4. The characterization of John as the 'text-man' is actually extraordinarily perceptive, and is a wonderful illustration of how sometimes people with dementia go to the heart of the matter. Her use and development of the statement 'It's a breast-up' exemplifies humour and perhaps an element of flirtation.

Alongside the lighter-hearted material, she makes what appear to be some more serious statements. In line 2 her clear remark about needing to 'wind the clocks' may be a direct articulation of her sense of having to do something practical. She follows it up with a simple request for help in this. Perhaps this is straightforward, but it could be viewed as an expression of a need to do something familiar and regular – the stuff of normal life with its predictable rhythms and markers.

The statements about being 'caught in a current' and 'being frightened' (line 3) seem to reflect more distressing aspects of her experience. They may be an explicit description of her emotional state, and the image is a vivid one. Perhaps this is how she conceptualizes the flow of changes which can characterize dementia, and her response is fear – including maybe the fear of being overwhelmed by it.

It is less clear what she means by her remarks about stopping talking in line 7. Perhaps on this occasion, John started to say something and then stopped and she is expressing her view of this. She may be giving a view about the conversational practice of interruption.

The term 'barrican' in line 9 is curious. This may be a local or idiosyncratic term as she acknowledges that John may not be familiar with it, then going on to explain what she means. In John's experience it is rare for people with dementia to explain their use of unusual language in such an explicit way. Her initial impressions of John, along with her sense of an unexpected pleasure, are conveyed pithily. Her honesty about her initial low expectations may be a reflection of her personality and style or may be an example of how dementia sometimes lowers inhibitions and allows people to give expression to their thoughts and feelings more easily.

In lines 5–6 Lena makes a series of comments about herself, and describes her state of mind in unusually physical terms. Nevertheless the words call up an image with which we can all identify. These unemotional, but perhaps personally very significant statements, are embedded in talk of other subjects, and she does not linger with these themes. The statement about her hair in line 8 is a vivid example of metaphorical talk. She describes her hair almost as if it were a young child who dislikes being washed and who gets its own back by sulking afterwards.

Her final statement is a direct challenge (and it is also unusual to have a change of tack signalled so clearly). The question implies an awareness that her present state is not a desirable one. It is not clear whether she expects an answer, or is content to have made her point with the question.

Bob Darley

Bob was a small man who 'button-holed' John. He spoke with speed and vigour, as if he had a lot to say in a short time:

 1 I'm fighting to win. There's so much stuff rassling about. I'm well on
 2 and off. There's not many bad days. But the Jimmies knocked me out.
 3 I'm from Glasgow, all over England, all over everywhere. My
 4 brother's Italy. We can't fall out, but he knows everything. Every time
 5 he has double he's single.
 6 When that accident happened that was the end of it for me. Crossing a
 7 bus. It happened in that town.
 8 She's absolutely weak, that lady. She's a very bad person. Nobody
 9 wants her, not a soul. And her partification is horrible, she shouldn't
10 be getting anything.
11 This place is good, but not too good, not five-star. I've roomed for
12 myself. There's some good ones and some bad ones here. There's
13 places where you can be good, and where you can't be good. And this
14 is somewhere where you <u>can</u> be good.
15 I've done so many of what you're doing this month that I'm out of
16 hand. I'm so mixed up I don't know where I'm going. But was that
17 good for you?

Bob tells us quite a lot about himself in this piece. Among the pieces of factual information are that he may be a Glaswegian, has a brother, and had an accident (lines 3–7). He also expresses his views: he does not like one of the other residents (lines 8–10), but he does seem to approve of the nursing home (lines 11–14). He seems to realize that he has difficulties with confusion (line 16).

There are some unusual uses of individual words ('rassling', 'the Jimmies' and 'partification'). Some of his sentences, while being structurally clear, are ambiguous in meaning. For example, 'Every time he has double he's single' (lines 4–5), 'Crossing a bus' (lines 6–7) and 'But was that good for you?' (lines 16–17). This last one, since it comes at the end, may well be a comment on the process, an enquiry of John as to whether he has fulfilled the expectations John had of him at the outset.

Lines 11–14 are particularly interesting. What Bob seems to be saying is that, while what the home provides is good it is not so luxurious that it makes him feel out of place. So he feels comfortable, 'at home', living there. It is somewhere with aspirations, but they are not so impossibly high that he would have difficulty in living up to them. This is quite a sophisticated concept and he articulates it well. 'I've roomed for myself' could mean that he is speaking from experience, or that he has single accommodation. Or perhaps he is referring to a previous lifestyle which involved living in hotels or boarding houses.

Despite his references to his accident (lines 6–7) and his perceived lack of coherence (line 16), Bob comes across as a person with strong opinions. He seems to despise what he regards as feebleness (line 8) and admires positivity (line 1). He attempts to provide an honest account of his position, and does so with conviction.

The two foregoing texts are examples of speech which is reasonably fluent. Our next example in this section is of someone for whom verbal communication has become more fragmented.

Emily West

This was the third conversation John had had with Emily. She was a quiet, courteous and gentle person, who clearly had a great need to express herself.

> 1 I can't tell people . . . things. With me the problem is . . . something
> 2 that's just ordinary . . . that's the problem.
> 3 The past . . . I think a lot about it . . . I'm thinking when . . . I'm not
> 4 saying anything . . . You . . . it's silverly, perfectly silverly.
> 5 Beryl, she's . . . lovely, she's gorgeous. Not raining or anything like
> 6 that . . . She's really good. And will be.
> 7 My room here . . . yes, lovely. You leave it and come back, and it's
> 8 perfectly . . . perfect. You go everywhere and . . . yes, welcome.
> 9 It's all right here, it's . . . nothing really. I don't know how many
> 10 people need . . . you know . . . and there <u>are</u> a lot of people.
> 11 Anyway . . . it was a real life, I think. Here now . . . life takes its
> 12 . . . you know. I don't think there's anything else.

Here much of the story is told by the pauses between sentences and the pauses within sentences. Emily is having great difficulty in gathering her thoughts. Her whole effort is going into the activity and apart from creating hiatuses in the text, this means that the creativity of language so marked in the speech of Lena and Bob is absent. She is struggling to make plain statements and only sometimes succeeding.

The statement about the past in lines 3 and 4 seems important. So often the silences of people with dementia are presumed to be signs of mental inactivity; here we have confirmation of the opposite.

Also in line 4, the repeated word 'silverly' is probably a reference to John's hair, at which Emily was looking at the time. Beryl, to whom she pays such warm tribute (lines 5–6), is Emily's daughter. The strange sentence 'Not raining or anything like that' may be an indirect way of referring to Beryl's sunny disposition. The very positive 'And will be' could be an expression of confidence that Beryl will go on behaving towards her in a caring manner.

The reference to other people shows an awareness of the accommodation being shared (line 10), and the sentence that tails away on the word 'need' may indicate that she realizes that her fellow-residents share a common condition.

Lines 11 and 12 are extraordinary. 'It was a real life, I think.' while suggesting a positive sense of authenticity it also carries a burden of sadness. Speaking of one's own existence in the past tense is a very rare phenomenon. The final sentence is typical of the ambiguities of this text: it could be a statement that there is nothing more to say at this juncture, or given that she has been talking about life in general, and depending on the thoughts behind the previous sentence which tailed away, she may have been referring to her feeling that there is nothing more to come after this life.

Beryl is also very positive, particularly about her room: how it is a relief to come back to it and find it the same as she left it (lines 7–8), and what a comforting place it is, as evidenced by the repetition of the idea of perfection.

Jean Copeland

Jean greeted John with enthusiasm, and was very positive about the idea of making a recording of a conversation. She immediately began to tell him her story. This is only a small part of it, and, as you will see, it was a major challenge to transcribe:

John: Would you like to tell me about yourself?

Jean: Well about the pentheless I was perten a bulder. The perten a bides narra ma mide. Ma bebs a blarry packen a bulder, and frackta muld nerm. Your packen a giesher. Will you becken a minda a caulda. Is that all right? Is it? I don't want you having to totter a buld!

John: And can you tell me about your mother?

Jean: My mother's very cheeribothers to the trip, five foot minnow, she must have been about five or six pie round the breast nun. How she'd be dub nupty but how olwra bulder.

Jean's language is packed full of remarkable and arresting features. One of its most dominant aspects is the sheer number of strange and apparently invented words she uses. These appear to be creations of Jean. Despite their apparent novelty, however, the sounds she makes are very word-like, almost as if they were from another language. It is also striking that the unconventional sounds are integrated with standard words and phrases, and adhere to normal sentence structures. Although the full text is not presented here, it is in fact very consistent in its mixture of familiar and strange.

Her response to all questions and comments is immediate and enthusiastic. She speaks with musicality, animation and colour, and proceeds at an unusually rapid pace. She laughs frequently, and demonstrates other signs of involvement with and enjoyment of the conversation on both verbal and nonverbal levels. Despite its strangeness in some senses, all of her talk has a remarkably normal conversational character. It is as if one is simply not quite catching the words, but it seems clear that at times she is remembering and describing something from the distant past, or reflecting on something for the first time, or making a statement with a resignatory or summarizing message. At no time does she show any awareness that her use of language is not conventional, and that John may have difficulty understanding it. However, it is clear that Jean is responding to John's question by telling him about her mother.

In those circumstances it seems better to let the person talk and to make one's responses as appropriately as possible. One can usually tell by the tone, facial expression and body language of the speaker whether a positive or negative reply is suitable. The occasional question such as 'Is that so!' or 'And what happened next?' is unlikely to interrupt the flow but to demonstrate one's continuing interest in the narrative.

What people with dementia say about language

Perhaps the most profound statement made to John on this subject was the following:

> *I want to thank you for listening. You see, you are words. Words can make or break you. Sometimes people don't listen, they give you words back, and they're all broken, patched up. But will you permit me to say that you have the stillness of silence, that listens, and lasts.*

We think that when this person made the statement 'you are words' she was not just thinking of John and that particular exchange, but referring to people generally and making the point that to a very large extent we are the language that we utter. We would therefore be committing a huge sin of omission if we neglect to take those words seriously. Of course it would be easier for us to listen if what was said, and the way it was said, was easily comprehensible. In this chapter we have begun to address some of the difficulties, however we understand so little about exactly what dementia does to the linguistic capabilities of individuals, we must keep an open mind and be alert to a diversity of clues.

The following are some examples of statements about language from people with dementia:

> *I'm talking, talking, talking all the while. I didn't know if you would understand, with you living on the other side.*

> *I used to know some of the language, but I could never quite get a hold of it. Somehow or other I can't gather myself to be the same as I was.*

> *You and I, John, we speak the same language. Only you speak it straight and I speak it upside down!*

I used to be lovely. I would speak to anybody. Now I'm a cross patch: somebody's put a spoke in my wheel.

One day when John was working with a lady who was evidently enjoying the conversation greatly, she said:

I'm blethering, I don't usually do that, but it's all from beneath the surface.

'Blethering' is defined by the Oxford English Dictionary as 'loquacious nonsense' and 'from beneath the surface' carries the suggestion of a 'stream of consciousness', where the mind supposedly reveals meanings from a deep level untouched by the intellect. Maybe the talk of many people with dementia, often described as 'rambling' or dismissed as 'nonsense', is a tapping into thoughts and feelings which had hitherto been hidden and which now pour out in an unremitting and uncensored stream?

Of this Beth Shirley Brough, describing occasions with her friend, Reg, writes:

To my shame, I was often far too slow to tune into what was the real and most important issue of the day. Once I learned to treat what he said as the relating of a dream, once I listened for images and took them very seriously, we were able to explore very deep reserves within each other.[24]

Characteristics of language of people with dementia

Here we explore some of the features of people's use of language which are of particular interest. As usual we have to be selective in what we cover, but we return to some of these themes in the section later on implications for care.

Creativity: the inventive use of language

We have already introduced the idea of symbolic language in our commentaries on the above texts. Put simply it is talking about one thing in terms of another, often by the use of images. In a simile the comparison is made explicitly, for example, 'as fit as a fiddle', whereas in metaphor the link is left out – one thing appears to become another – 'the apple of his eye' . In order to derive meaning from such expressions we have to engage our imagination. A logical approach to interpretation will yield little. Shakespeare probably provides the most audacious and copious examples of symbolic language in English. His famous sonnet likening his lover to the weather begins with the line:

Shall I compare thee to a summer's day

Here are some examples of the figurative use of language from the speech of persons with dementia which come from John's work:

It's a lovely day – I feel like playing with all my flaps open.

The circle of life is shot away.

My eye doesn't half bother me – it comes out as if it's going to walk through that door!

I've been playing in the House of Ages.

My mother pulled it in – the string of humankindness.

From the work of a writer in residence, Trisha Kotai-Ewers, in Australia we have the following:

> The first words of Irene's that I recorded were 'I've worn the bottom off me!' She had been leaping around the lounge room batting a balloon back to the Occupational Therapist. She was tired! Language like this is no doubt what attracts a writer to this kind of work. Since then Irene has been a source of delight with her inventive replacements for words no longer readily available to her. A 'handkerchief' or 'tissue' is always a 'sniff-sniff'. No doubt what she means![25]

By any standards these are examples of the creative use of language. They do not rely upon cliché or conventional structures, but convey their meanings vividly and emotionally. It is unfortunately not possible to compare the speech-patterns of these individuals prior to their having dementia with their present characteristics. It seems unlikely, though, that they would have contained such poetic expressions in adult life. What about further back, though, in their childhoods? The linguist Jean Aitchison has observed:

> [The] spontaneous use of metaphor decreases with age, according to one study. It fades fastest amongst children who attend reputedly good schools, and more slowly among those who go to supposedly bad ones. This suggests that education channels children towards conventional usages and less colourful speech.[26]

If our education system rewards the logical uses of language and undervalues creativity it is hardly surprising that conventional adult discourse is plain and inexpressive. But what if dementia affects those pathways of the brain which process thought in logical ways, while leaving relatively intact those which respond more creatively to the world? Sound-patterns, association of words and ideas, and the symbolic uses of language through simile and metaphor could then come into their own. It is frequently observed that people with dementia retain their appreciation of music until quite a late stage of the condition, which would appear to complement this idea. If we add to the increased use of the emotional properties of language the sometimes disinhibiting nature of dementia, there are perhaps fewer social barriers to the individual producing unusual and original combinations of words and images.

Oliver Sacks lends support to the possibility of new creativity:

> While one may be horrified by the ravages of developmental disorder or disease, one may sometimes see them as creative too – for if they destroy particular paths, particular ways of doing things, they may force the nervous system into making other paths and ways, force on it an unexpected

growth and evolution. This other side of development or disease is something I see, potentially, in almost every patient[27]

Variability in language use

It is a common observation of those working closely with people with dementia that there can be marked variability in their use of language. Sometimes words seem to come easily, and talk is fluent, whether or not it is readily comprehensible. At other times the person may struggle to produce even a single word, with a great sense of effort and perhaps frustration. Such variations can occur within even relatively short periods. John has had many experiences of failing to strike up a conversation with a person in the morning (perhaps concluding that the individual has severe difficulties with language), only to have a very successful encounter in the afternoon. It has occurred that a fascinating exchange with a woman on one day was followed up by an agreement to talk again the next, only to find that by the next day, her speech was painfully halting and she was apparently exhausted by the effort to capture and articulate even a few words.

We have little understanding of what underlies these variations, although it is likely that mood, tiredness and other physical states such as pain may play a part. For some people it may be that a set of factors needs to coincide in order for them to achieve their potential for verbal expression. Traditionally we have assumed that the factors that underpin variability in language use (and other functions) are internal to the person, but as part of a psychosocial understanding of dementia we need to recognize that they may be much more interpersonal in nature. We think it likely that our own attitudes and behaviour play a much greater role in facilitating or undermining the individual's capacity for expression and communication. The implications of these ideas are explored further in the next section.

Altered pacing

People with dementia often take a much greater length of time to speak than most people. It seems to take longer for the person to decode the utterance of another, and to formulate and express a response. Whether this feature arises as a direct consequence of brain damage, or through psychological mechanisms, or both, unless this is understood by others and allowances made, the chances of successful communication are much reduced. If there is an assumption that the reason for the person's failure to demonstrate understanding and produce a reply within the usual length of time is that they are simply no longer able to do so, the withdrawal of effort is liable to follow. One woman demonstrated her awareness of this problem by saying:

People haven't time to talk to me now because it takes such a long time.

In order to maintain communication with people with dementia it is necessary radically to rethink the pace and rhythm of conversation. John has spent much time in silence with people, waiting, uncertain whether they are going to prove able to articulate thoughts and feelings, but at all times attempting to convey the message that what the person has to say is worth waiting for, and that being with the person is itself important, even if the words do not come.

Sometimes the reply to questions or statements may come so long after the original utterance, however, that the connection in the mind of the listener may be lost altogether. Caroline Keegan, a nurse studying her conversations with Jean, a resident in a long-stay hospital ward, found that on examining transcripts, utterances of Jean's, which had appeared nonsensical to Caroline at the time, were actually reasonable and sensible follow-ups to themes and questions which had arisen in the conversation minutes earlier.[28] All too often we ourselves will have moved on in our minds and the memories of what went before will not be readily accessible. If we learned to extend our range in terms of timing then much more of what people with dementia say to us might become easily comprehensible.

Confidence

We are increasingly inclined to wonder whether lack of confidence underlies a large part of the difficulty people with dementia have in using language. We have discussed the fact that as fundamentally verbal beings we experience significant distress if our ability to use language is compromised. It is such a vital link both with other people and in the internal processes of creating meaning, accessing memories and retaining a sense of mastery over the world, that powerful feelings of anxiety are bound to be generated.

As we have described, people with dementia demonstrate considerable resourcefulness and creativity in their attempts to convey meaning. But if the person repeatedly experiences distress, or finds that despite great effort others do not take the time to encourage the person to find means of expression or even dismiss utterances as meaningless, there is bound to be an eroding of confidence and a decrease in efforts to talk. This in turn will have a negative effect on self-esteem. One woman said to John:

> *I seem daft, awfully stupid . . . when you were young you just opened your mouth . . . and now . . .*

Difficulties finding words

As we have noted before, a common feature of the use of language by people with dementia is difficulty finding the right words to express their thoughts and feelings. The potential for frustration and anxiety in these circumstances is very real, and this scenario can give rise to discomfort on the part of others, both through feeling for the person who is having such a struggle and also due to uncertainty as to how to help. Offering words which seem likely candidates may be irritating or distracting to the person with dementia, or the message may be so unclear or partial as to render such a strategy infeasible.

Sometimes it is not that the person cannot find a word at all, but rather that the way they use certain words is unusual. The work of communication scientist Jane Crisp provides helpful pointers to the unravelling of meaning in these circumstances.[29] She explains that because words are stored in our minds according to links in both sound and meaning, it is often possible, with some imaginative awareness, to trace these links. Another general tendency is for people to choose words for a higher order category, for example 'dog' rather than 'Dalmatian', or to use one word, for example 'dress' to refer to all items of clothing.

Many of the ideas we have discussed here are illustrated in this example from Kim Zabbia's book about her mother:[30]

Mom blurted out, 'Yesterday! A food!'
'What, Mom?' I asked.
'An old food', she said. 'Hand, hold it.'
'A sandwich?' I offered.
'Yes! Old sandwich, used to.'
She was again searching for that exact word until 'Piano punna!' she yelled.
'Not another piano', I said.
'No, peanu punna!'
'Peanut butter?'
'Yes! That's it!' Mom was excited.
'Kate, write that down. That's perfect,' I said.
'That's it: peana putta, peana pinna, oh. . .'
Mom still couldn't say it.[31]

Awareness of linguistic change

People vary in the extent to which they seem aware of changes in their ability to use language. Sometimes a person is only too conscious that they are struggling to form sounds or to find and put words together. Sometimes, as with Jean Copeland, even though their speech is highly unconventional the person will talk with fluency and confidence, and there will be no indication that they realize anything is amiss. Why should this be so?

The person's longstanding habits and preferences regarding talk as an activity may have a bearing here. For someone who has always enjoyed verbal interaction, spending a lot of time talking to others, the sense of familiarity in the conversational context may carry them along, distancing them from the awareness that their language has changed. Again, perhaps Jean is such a person. Some people are naturally more concerned than others with precision and economy in their use of language, choosing words carefully and with attention to form and the finer points of meaning.

For such an individual, the changes which can accompany dementia may be much more keenly felt. In some cases this may lead to the person falling silent, in a similar way that someone who can no longer play a musical instrument with the same skill as previously refuses to go on trying. Sometimes there are fluctuations in an individual's apparent degree of awareness of difficulties. This might be related to the subject of the talk, the particular feelings surrounding it, or the sense of urgency they have in getting their message across. Physical health and wellbeing, mood, the actions of others or aspects of the physical environment may also have a part to play in this.

Humour

We find many examples of people using language in a humorous way. Here are some one-liners which arose in the course of John's work and, in our view, are perceptive, witty and can even involve plays on words:

> I had a bath this morning, and I felt like a ship-wrecked mariner.

> What good pasture there must be here – we're full of fat nurses!

> Up to three tons my licence. And now I can't even ride a bicycle!

> Spending my time? I never earn any!

> I've got financial cramp – it's a very well-known condition!

> Is it one o'clock yet? That's Shock, Horror and Murder Time! I mean The News!

Some examples are more extended. Here a man follows through a joke in a most convincing manner. He is addressing John:

> Now don't stand there laughing or they'll think you're a policeman, that's for sure. And I'll let you into a secret: I'm one too. When you go these locals'll yap, yap, they think you're a policeman all right. It's the notebook: they think you're taking statements. If anybody asks me I'll tell them you've been promoted Detective Inspector!

There is another aspect to humour, more complex and probably highly significant as an expressive outlet and evidence of personhood. That is where individuals appear to be using humour in an attempt to come to terms with their condition. This may take various forms, for example irony, scorn, caustic wit. Here is a man who has just entered a nursing home. He plainly does not want to be there, is angry and bemused, and takes his frustration out on the architecture:

> This isn't a building, no way is this a building! I'd describe it unkindly. Somebody came along and stuck three rooms together and called it 'a home'! Then 33 other people came along and tacked a piece on. In short, it was thrown together and the bits didn't meet, and'll never be got right!

Here is a woman talking to John and asserting herself in a situation where it is all too easy to feel patronized and humiliated:

I don't mind you writing it down – I can always alter it . . . Who are you – a gentleman? No, go and look for one . . . Between you and me, you know, it's a battle of wills. Why don't you just lose first!

Music and language

In Chapter 3 we made mention of the importance of music in people's lives generally and also in communication. In many ways language is inherently musical, for instance through features of rhythm and timing, and the urge to combine words and music in song finds expression in every culture. For some people with dementia this can become a deeply important means of communication. We know from neurological and psychological research that singing as a means of expression can remain available to those who have lost the power of speech, for example through stroke or head injury. It seems that for some people with dementia there is a similar effect.

One woman, Ella Jackson, whom John met was particularly memorable in this regard. She could hardly communicate at all through speech but she used to work as a singer, and was happy to be taped. She was happier still to hear herself singing. Her voice quality was still beautiful, but the words were impoverished and there were few which were recognizable. A straight transcript reads rather like an Irish or Scottish folksinger when they are improvising Gaelic in 'mouth-music': for example Ella sang:

Ay to the boy to the way to the way
At the way to the way at doder doder may
At the doder little ohti doder day
At the old wey hey the idle didle day
At the older deedle day!

When she heard herself on the tape she was able to sing along, and the syllables she pronounced were an exact match for those she came up with the first time round. It was an extremely positive experience for her, and a clear demonstration of how language can be used creatively to convey mood and meaning.

The potential of rhythm and music both to comfort and to serve as a kind of 'warm-up' for speech is described by Beth Shirley Brough:

My heart was rent by the gobbledegook, the rhythmic running together of sounds, but the mumbo-jumbo served a purpose. I wondered if it provided a comforting chant-like state from which other words and phrases could arise. Was it a minimalist massage on the tender interface of the conscious and the unconscious?[32]

Dialect and language

Part of the richness of language is the way that it varies in accordance with locality, culture and time. The words, expressions and rhythms of speech used in one part of the UK vary widely from those from other areas, and these features of language also vary according to social groups, age groups and over time. The particular dialects of language people use form part of their identity, both personally and in a deep social sense. This is something we need to understand when communicating with people with dementia, both in relation to the words and expressions we use ourselves, and also in thinking about their language. If you are unfamiliar with the area of the UK the person with dementia is from, it is easy to mistake local words or expressions for the effects of dementia upon language.[33]

Britain's increasingly multicultural society also means that more and more we are meeting people with dementia who come from other cultures, and whose first language is not English. We have had very little experience of this ourselves, but it is something we all must become more sensitive to generally.

A small piece of research by Naina Patel and colleagues has looked at barriers to communication among ethnic minorities.[34] They found that providing interpreters was not necessarily the answer to the problem. Although it could assist first generation minority ethnic older people there was a tendency for them to lapse into a mixture of English and mother tongue, making it difficult for them to be understood by careworkers, relatives and interpreters. It was even suggested by some professionals interviewed that this language confusion might be a deliberate ploy to hide their dementia from others. Turning dementia into a language problem may be a form of denial practised by those for whom English is a second language. It is important that more studies be undertaken to explore these possibilities further.

Language and identity

Above we touched on the relationship of language use and one's sense of identity. What is the nature of this link in dementia? Sometimes people with dementia can be observed talking, perhaps for brief or sustained periods, in a way which appears not to be intended for others to hear. It is as if they are talking to themselves. What could be the function of this? One possibility is that the individual's thought processes – the kind of internal monologue which is going on in all of our heads all of the time – has become externalized. Instead of thinking inwardly, they speak their thoughts out loud. If this is true, then it means that not all talk is intended to be part of an interpersonal encounter, and we must find ways of affirming it without attempting to make it part of an interaction.

We end with the following quote from care assistant Laurel Rust describing Amy, which seems to make this point:

> Talking is Amy's way of knowing she is still alive. It is her intense, continuous engagement. It is one of the very [few] means of creative expression allowed her. It is a way of creatively adapting to a monotonous and

inhuman environment where no one really talks with her. If she stops talking, she'll 'just stop.'[35]

Implications for care

We have seen that despite the challenges that dementia poses to language, there are great possibilities for helping people to continue to use and enjoy it. As with nonverbal communication, a large part of this involves creating an atmosphere where the use of language and appreciation of its qualities are fostered and celebrated.

John has had experience of various ways of doing this. One was in a nursing home where staff had established the practice of displaying in a prominent place a different quote from one of the residents every day. The quote (which was obviously chosen with respect for privacy) was put up on a board, together with the name of the person who said it, where it attracted the attention of staff and residents. Discussions about the words, phrasing and meaning were stimulated, with the resultant boost in self-esteem for the speaker, and the general message that people's words and ideas were valued and felt to be interesting and important.

We have seen that many people with dementia express themselves using figurative or imaginative language. Having a place where words of an evocative or stimulating nature are displayed (perhaps on a large distinctive board) is another possibility for reinforcing a message about their value and interest. These could be grouped in themes which reflect current events or concerns. Well-chosen quotes from poems or novels could be displayed, again with the purpose of triggering imagination or discussion, and communicating a general respect for the power of language. Dialect words and expressions provide another rich source of interesting language, and inviting people to talk about their local ways of speaking can have the additional benefit of reinforcing identity and encouraging storytelling.

Part of making the most of linguistic communication means reflecting carefully on the way we ourselves use language. We all have our verbal mannerisms, some of which are expressive, others of which hamper the conveyance of meaning. There can be no hard and fast rules here, but things to watch out for include the use of words and expressions which are clearly unfamiliar to the person with dementia, and trying to tune into the ones which have particular meaning for them. For example, we have heard about one woman who used to say that she was going to church when she meant she was visiting the toilet. Adopting her convention for referring to the toilet in this way would obviously be helpful.

Many people with dementia seem to lose confidence in using their voice, which is an obvious hindrance to communication. Musical activities often seem to provide a way to ease the person back into using their voice, either through simple humming or actual singing. Encouraging people to talk in the time immediately after activities like this can prove very successful and enjoyable.

Ethical implications

Humour

The subject of language use does not appear to present many ethical issues, but the role of humour definitely does and we have chosen to include it at this point. We have placed this section in the language chapter, but it could also have been in the chapter on nonverbal communication since humour can take either form.

Like anything which has the potential to do good, there are dangers inherent in the use of humour. In our everyday lives we use it for a wide variety of purposes – to break the ice, to make a point, to dispel embarrassment or to put another in their place, to pinpoint just a few. The situation where people with dementia is concerned is similarly complex. We need to ask ourselves questions about what constitutes respectful and constructive forms of humour, and in what ways it might be used to demean people and undermine personhood. We make a distinction between laughing with someone and laughing at them, but at times this may be difficult to discern, especially if we are uncertain as to the understanding the other person has of a given situation.

Our values (see discussion in Chapter 6) very much guide what we find funny, and what we think is acceptable for other people to laugh at. In our dealings with people with dementia it may well be that we will encounter some who enjoy a form of humour which is very different from our own, and may even be offensive to us. Such tensions can also arise between different people with dementia. These scenarios raise interesting ethical issues.

Some forms of humour touch on issues about dignity, and this in turn can have implications for the extremely complicated dynamics of dependency and responsibility in relationships. The following excerpt is from Margaret Forster's novel *Have the Men Had Enough?*[36] The story is told from the point of view of the granddaughter, Hannah. Bridget is Grandma's daughter, and her main carer:

> Grandma is laughing too, she knows she is a good turn. She has taken the tea cosy off the teapot . . . and she has put it on her head because she says she can feel a bloomin' draught. She has one ear poking out of the hole for the spout and the other out of the hole for the handle. The vivid reds, blues, greens and yellows of the tea cosy stripes straddle her large head. Adrian is crying with laughter and I am almost as bad. Then Bridget arrives. She snatches the tea cosy off Grandma's head. Grandma yelps and tells her to get lost. Bridget's face is red and angry. She *hates* Grandma to be a laughing stock even though Grandma loves to be the cause of mirth.[37]

This scenario prompts us to reflect on issues around whether we have a duty to intervene when a person with dementia is presenting themselves in a way which seems to compromise their dignity, whether this is through humour, the exposing of a lack of competence or through emotional expression. Of course where we would draw the line and say that something had gone too far is a matter of judgement and values, and it is necessary to balance the risk inherent in the possible embarrassment caused by allowing the situation to develop unchecked, against the assault on the person's sense of dignity caused by the intervention, by taking it out of their hands. If we say that it is necessary to intervene, then this must mean that we are assuming the person with dementia to be unable to take responsibility for themselves, at least in respect of self-presentation, and perhaps other respects as well.

Part of the notion of taking responsibility for someone is the sense that their welfare and perhaps even behaviour is a reflection on oneself. Was it that in the above scenario, Bridget was angry because she felt that, in albeit an indirect way, she was being laughed at as well? That as someone who, by becoming her main carer, had in a sense 'appropriated' Grandma's personhood, and therefore Grandma's welfare and behaviour had somehow become an extension of her own? These reflections draw us quickly into deep water about the nature of human relationships.

To come back to the example, she was certainly angry with Hannah and Adrian for allowing Grandma to behave in this way and for laughing with, even at, her. The fact that they all found the situation funny was a reflection of how their values differed from Bridget's.

However, looking at the scenario more dispassionately, might we not wonder whether Grandma's behaviour had some element of powerlessness underlying it? That playing the fool was one way in which to be noticed and given attention by others? It is often observed that those who feel themselves to be less powerful than others, seek the acceptance of others through the use of humour. Could this apply at times to people with dementia? In which case, what should our response be? We often enjoy the role such individuals have, but does this amount to a collusion in a form of social injustice?

The following passage is also from Margaret Forster's novel. It is again told from Hannah's point of view, and here her brother, Adrian, is attempting to justify why he has such a minor role in Grandma's care:

> He says he does his bit in providing that background Male Presence she finds so comforting and asking her if his tea is ready. And he laughs at her jokes and antics. I hate the way he does that. Grandma shows off when Adrian is there, getting sillier and sillier, and his laughter is patronising. He treats her like a Good Turn and is only seconds away from presenting her to his friends as My Batty Grandma from the Funny Farm.[38]

'If I wasn't laughing, I'd be crying' is a statement we make and hear from time to time. It is a recognition that laughter can be an outlet, a way of coping with something and not necessarily a pure response to humour.

Groups of people who share similar experiences, and face similar difficulties, often engage in a form of humour – sometimes called 'gallows humour' – which plays a specific set of functions. These include creating a sense of cohesion, acknowledging common difficulties, cutting those who are more powerful down to size and dispelling emotional and physical tension. This kind of humour may very well be used by people with dementia themselves, but if we think about it in relation to staff we can focus on some interesting behaviour. We can probably all think of times when our response to a tense situation has been to laugh, perhaps to laugh in quite an intense way, even when, on the face of it, this has seemed inappropriate, even cruel. This can happen to otherwise perfectly sincere and serious people.

It is as well to admit that contact with people with dementia in all their complexity, pain and ordinariness will, at times, push us to our limits, and a certain kind of laughing can be a way of coping with this. While we can readily admit that it is not right to laugh at someone, or their situation or their difficulties, since we are all only human, this situation is bound to arise from time to time. Perhaps the best way to respond is first and foremost to accept that, although it may seem dreadfully out of place, such laughter is a genuine reaction, and it is important to think about what might have contributed to it. Has there been particular strain or anxiety around? Have support measures not been in place? Do certain people stimulate complex or poorly understood reactions in others?

Humour itself has a way of going to the heart of things in life, and this certainly appears to hold true where our relationships with people with dementia are concerned.

Finally, in-depth analysis always kills a joke. Sometimes it is better just to laugh, enjoy it and move on to the next thing.

5 | **Memory:** 'Playing in the House of Ages'

The neurobiologist Steven Rose writes:

> Memories are our most enduring characteristic. In old age we can remember our childhood eighty or more years ago; a chance remark can conjure up a face, a name, a vision of sea or mountains once seen and apparently long forgotten. Memory defines who we are and shapes the way we act more closely than any other single aspect of our personhood. All of life is a trajectory from experienced past to unknown future, illuminated only during the always receding instant we call the present, the moment of our actual conscious experience. Yet our present appears continuous with our past, grows out of it, is shaped by it, because of our capacity for memory. It is this which prevents the past from being lost, as unknowable as the future. It is memory which thus provides time with its arrow.[1]

Most of us, at least from time to time, think about our memories and how they work. We are most likely to wonder about memory when it lets us down – when we fail to retrieve someone's name or realize too late that we should have been somewhere or done something. From time to time we experience the very distinctive sensation of knowing that we know something but not being able to put our finger on it. There is also the curious experience of forgetting what you were going to say a second or two before actually saying it – as if there is a crack in the pavement and every so often the thought we are about to express falls down it. But memory can also surprise us with its efficiency. Sometimes, as described in the quote from Steven Rose, it presents us with information we did not know we knew, and with very little effort. Unexpected triggers like smells or music can reawaken memories for events that have long lain untouched, at least by our conscious mind.

The subject of memory has fascinated humanity for thousands of years. We can trace writings and reflections about its nature and place in the intellectual, emotional and spiritual life of humankind from the writings of the ancient Greeks, right through to a range of current academic journals, modern philosophical writings and a huge variety of different sorts of literature from poetry to fiction to autobiography. All sorts of theories of memory have been advanced over the ages. The Greeks thought of memory traces as writing on a tablet, and that over time all traces would disappear completely. The harder one pressed the longer the trace would last, but it would still go eventually. Freud advanced the 'total memory hypothesis', which maintains that our memories retain all information we encounter in our lives, but that we are unable, for a variety of reasons, to retrieve it. The idea that hypnosis can help to enhance recall is based on this view of memory. Modern ideas about memory rely much more on computer analogies and notions of information-processing. Instead of seeing memory as a kind of container into which information is collected, the memory is seen much more as a system that processes the information, discarding some of it, but allowing some of it into 'long-term' memory, which is continually being updated and re-organized.

The academic study of memory is now the province of psychology and various forms of neuroscience, and academics who investigate memory are often also interested in how we think, reason and make decisions. As well as trying to find out how memory works, they study the way we organize and store information in our brains, and what factors influence its successful or unsuccessful retrieval. There is a lot of interest in how memory works in real life situations, such as the role of memory in eye-witness testimony, how we remember commercial information such as that presented in advertisements and so on.[2]

Important distinctions

The subject of memory is obviously highly relevant in work with people with dementia. This chapter is concerned with exploring the relationship of memory functioning to communication, and discussion of how we can use this understanding to enhance relationships. We shall therefore begin with a section which discusses distinctions in different types of memory and some of the factors which influence the way it works.[3] Although not specifically about dementia, the relevance of this to work with people with the condition will become clear.

Different stages of memory

The memory is best thought of as a kind of system – active rather than passive – and interacting in important ways with other aspects of psychological functioning such as thinking, reasoning and decision-making. The system has three distinct stages: encoding, storage and retrieval.

Encoding

In order to be able to remember something, it is obviously necessary to get it into one's memory in the first place. This involves a certain level of attention and concentration – new information has to be 'worked on' which involves some effort to assimilate it. There are various ways of working on information and these are likely to influence how well it will be remembered. Memory theorists encourage the 'elaborating' of information, perhaps by linking it with something we already know or by converting it into a visual image.

Storage

Clearly if information is to be retrieved later it has to remain in the circuits, to be stored somehow, and located within a reasonable amount of time. If you think of just how much knowledge you have accumulated over your lifetime, and yet how quickly you can answer a question like 'What is the capital of Spain?', this shows that the information we hold in our memories is highly organized.

Retrieval

There are two main modes of retrieval: recognition, where the target is chosen from a set of possibilities – for example trying to find the name of a place by looking at a map, and recall, which involves producing information without any help. By and large it is easier to recognize than to recall.

The act of remembering something successfully involves the efficient operation of all three stages. Sometimes when memory fails we are aware that we have never properly absorbed the information in the first place. At other times we have the conviction that we do know the answer but cannot at that moment put our finger on it. Sometimes it comes back when we stop trying.

Long-term and short-term memory

A distinction is often made between 'long-term' and 'short-term' memory, but this is frequently done in a confused way. When psychologists speak about short-term memory, they are referring to the span which is occupied by consciously rehearsing material, such as the digits of a phone number, between looking at the telephone directory and dialling the number. If we repeat or rehearse this information sufficiently it can be transferred into long-term memory, but the amount of data that can be held in short-term memory is extremely small, and very fragile. Thus long-term memory holds information which was absorbed as much as a lifetime ago or as little as a few seconds ago. It is therefore not correct to talk about memories for events the previous day as being part of short-term memory. If the person remembers, they are retrieving information from long-term memory, albeit information which has been there only a short time.

Autobiographical and semantic memory

Another major distinction is that between information which relates to our own experiences, for example what you had for lunch or where you went for your last holiday, and that which has no personal connection. The first is more complex in that it has an emotional dimension, subjective meaning and is linked with other experiences. It is called autobiographical (or episodic) memory. Memory for information, for example the number of calories in an egg, is referred to as semantic memory.

Knowing that and knowing how

Finally, we should distinguish between memory for actions and memory for knowledge. The first is called 'procedural' memory, and includes skills such as walking downstairs, riding a bicycle or knitting. Information in procedural memory is implicit, almost impossible to articulate, and can be fairly resistant to decay. The other sort of memory here is referred to as 'declarative' memory. This is the type of knowledge which can be put into words.

When you think about these dimensions of memory in relation to people with dementia it is clear that not all sorts of memory are affected in the same ways. We shall explore this at greater length later.

Memory and context

Whenever information or skills are learned, they have a context – physical, temporal and personal – and this context can have important effects on subsequent recall of information. You may feel that you have forgotten much of what you were taught at school. Undoubtedly this is true. But if you were able to go back to the classroom where you were taught about, say, the river systems of Britain, and to have the familiar features of the room – its appearance, layout, smell and the particular social atmosphere reinstated – you might be surprised by what comes back to you.[4]

Memory and emotion

We mentioned above the influence of context on the working of memory. It is possible to think of emotion as an aspect of this context.[5] Think of the last time you felt especially sad or even depressed. What sorts of experiences came most easily into your thoughts when you were in this frame of mind? Most probably the things you remembered and thought about when sad were other experiences or subjects which induced similar feelings. Being in this mood state enhanced your access to other memories with a similar emotional tag. This applies to other emotions too. When we are angry about something, we are more likely to remember and think about other things about which we feel or have felt furious. This can lead to the 'and another thing . . .!' phenomenon during an argument. You start off quarrelling about one subject or incident, and in no time there are a host of other issues which feel just as important, and these are dragged into the exchange. This pattern can have a powerfully reinforcing effect on our emotional state. The linking of memory and emotion creates a kind of filter. We remember and think about other emotionally congruent material, and this reinforces our sense of the validity of the way that we think, feel and behave.

Another feature of the relationship between memory and emotion which deserves mention is the observation that people who are anxious or depressed, or otherwise experiencing emotional disturbance, perform more poorly in the area of memory functioning than they would under conditions of normal mood. It appears that these conditions negatively affect the ability of the person to learn new information, and sometimes to retrieve well-established material.

Memory and interpretation

We do not take in, store and retrieve new information in a vacuum. Our memories are intimately linked with other facets of our mental life, including our interests and preoccupations, beliefs and assumptions, hopes, desires, fears and expectations. Our minds process information in line with our fundamental need to make sense of our experiences, to find patterns and achieve a sense of meaning. The chances of assimilating new information into memory, and the way it is understood, are affected by all of the above factors. If you are busy and your mind is occupied, you are unlikely to pay attention to something which is of no interest to you. If, however, in the welter of information which surrounds us you see something which is relevant to a current concern, it is more likely to catch your eye and start you thinking, which heightens the chances of it being remembered. If the new information is in any way ambiguous or incomplete, the likelihood is that you will interpret it according to your 'take' on that particular subject, although you will probably not be aware of having done so. This kind of thing underpins the common experience of having picked something up differently from someone else, or being surprised to find that the original source of information is much fuller or more complex than it first seemed.

Just as we interpret and remember new information in the context of our concerns and interests, the act of recall is similarly affected. We have all had the experience of listening to someone describe an event of which we ourselves were part, and wondering if they are talking about the same experience. We may be amazed to hear them telling what seems like a completely different story from the one we would tell ourselves. Most of the time (storyteller's licence apart) there is no intended distortion of the facts. This phenomenon is another illustration of how much the way we remember is influenced by individual factors. Our memories are not like video recorders receiving, storing and replaying information in a neutral and standardized fashion. The psychologist Frederick Bartlett, a pioneer of the study of memory, wrote:

> Remembering is not the re-excitation of innumerable fixed, lifeless and fragmentary traces. It is an imaginative reconstruction, or construction, built out of the relation of our attitude towards a whole active mass of organized past reactions or experience, and to a little outstanding detail which commonly appears in image or language form. It is thus hardly ever really exact, even in the most rudimentary cases of rote recapitulation, and it is not at all important that it should be so.[6]

Memory and dementia

Of all aspects of change in dementia its effects on memory are the most obvious and strongly associated with the condition. Indeed when we wish to refer to it in euphemistic terms we often describe it as someone having 'memory problems'. The other changes which are observed may be considered as secondary to the progressive failure of memory (the person forgets words and their meanings; they forget how to get dressed; they forget the difference between night and day) or we may see change in these other areas as arising from direct damage to the parts of the brain that control these functions (the organic explanation) or the effects of the social and physical environment (the psychosocial explanation).

However, the role of memory loss in dementia is defined, it is clear that when we interact with the person we are usually encountering someone with significant, perhaps very severe, memory difficulties. This can be expressed in a variety of areas:

• finding words
• asking the same question more than once in a short time
• talking in a repetitive way
• not being able to remember the names of close relatives or friends
• difficulty remembering recent events
• not being able to recall why they attend a day centre or why they are not still living at home

- getting lost
- failing to remember that they have just seen someone.

These various forms of memory disturbance overlap and interact in complex ways, and may be affected in different measure by factors such as mood, motivation and environmental influences. The following excerpt from Linda Grant's book about her mother gives a vivid illustration of difficulties with repetition in a conversation:

> Apart from the physical wasting, the diminution of her body to the size of a large doll, she looked normal – she looked like a sweet little old lady – and people would start up conversations with her which would proceed as they expected until a question answered a moment before would be asked again – 'No, I must interrupt, you haven't told me yet where you live.'
> 'As I just said, Birmingham.'
>
> And then asked and asked and asked until you lost your patience because you thought you had been entering a dialogue which had its rules of exchange, and it turned out that what you were really talking to was an animate brick wall. Questions asked over and over again not because she couldn't remember the reply but because a very short tape playing in her head had reached its end and wound itself back to the beginning to start afresh. She knew the conventions of conversation – these had not deserted her – but she could not recall what she had said herself a few moments before. Sometimes the question was repeated before the person asking had finished getting through their response. There were little holes in her brain, real holes in the grey matter, where the memory of her life used to be, and of what she had done half an hour or even a few minutes ago.[7]

As we encounter these sorts of difficulties in the person, we find ways of explaining them which are based on certain beliefs about memory and how it works. It may be helpful at this point to make explicit the sorts of assumptions which often underpin thinking about memory in dementia:

- that memory is progressively destroyed by dementia
- that memory is a simple all or nothing matter – you can either remember something or you cannot
- that people with dementia are unable to remember recent events
- that events in the past are better recalled than recent events, at least until the later stages of the condition
- that in the final phase of the condition even long-established memories are destroyed
- that people with dementia are unable to learn new skills
- that, at least up until a certain point, people make up stories to conceal the extent of their problems with memory.

We shall be better able to subject these assumptions to scrutiny in the context of what follows, but first let us turn to thinking about the words of people with dementia on this subject. As with other topics, we are most interested in the person's own perspective, and on focusing on how we can best support people in using remaining abilities.

What do people with dementia have to say about memory?

John has found that this is a major theme in his conversations with individuals. The following are some examples:

> *Lack of memories is the worst of all my troubles. I had a lovely life until this happened. I can remember things from long ago. But recent things I can't recall.*

> *I've got to the stage where it's difficult to decide what is from now and what is from the period.*

> *It's the memory that's really defeating us, and I actually am not in this world at all.*

These are all very explicit statements about individuals' perceptions of their difficulties and how they feel about them. Alongside clear evidence of awareness, themes of loss, helplessness and exclusion emerge from these apparently simple statements. The following provide perhaps a more slanted commentary on memory and its difficulties:

> *The years go down quaint – I don't understand it.*

> *The old days are baffling me to get them right!*

> *It's like a gone past everything. I'm not able to take it on as I used to. I shall be very glad to have a picture of what is with us. I cannot remember as night falls.*

Finally, although the expression is enigmatic, the person whose words gave this chapter its title seemed to us to be talking of her pleasure in remembering the important experiences of her life.

We now turn to examining a longer text for its lessons about memory.

Joe Steer

John met Joe Steer for the first time in his room in the nursing home. He was extremely friendly but also with a wistful air about him which intensified his distress towards the end of the conversation when he began to experience confusion:

> *The last few months I've got very forgetful. It's not all recent things. I'm pretty good on memories of my schooldays. I used to be, but I'm not so good now, I think.*
>
> *. . .*
>
> *I was born in Madeley. I myself, and all the family too went to St Mark's Church in Church Road. And there's like a lych-gate getting towards the*

pavement. It was a shelter for anyone standing, you know. And I went to St Mark's School. It was about a quarter-of-a-mile lower down the road from the Church. Our Headmaster in those days was a bloke called Harry Jackson. And later on his brother came to help him. I called him Sir. He also lived pretty well on the job. The schoolhouse was built right there. When we were lads we lived down on the road by the crossings. They were poor days then. We either went into employment in the ironworks or into the local brickyards. In point of fact there were two collieries as well. My father got killed in one of them. They brought him home on an open cart, horsedrawn. It belonged to a little man who used to deliver our coal. It was on a Friday, I actually saw him. No covering, just lying in the dirt – there were no pitbaths. And, of course, they did work hard in sweaty weather. I would never go down the pit: the nearest I got to it was peering down the shaft, which isn't very exciting.

. . .

Are you married to that lady you came in with? Oh, she's the boss, is she? I shouldn't have asked you, I can see who she is anyhow. But, see, I'd forgotten who she was for the moment. Except I made as if I knew her. And, of course, I do know her. Only by saying 'Good morning' and things like that. I think I know her, but who is she? I'm very often like that. But I never used to be.

It's a pretty terrible awful thing this being forgetful. I never used to be. What was I going to say? We're in a mess already, just going from here to there!

Joe appears to have no problem in accessing memories from his early life. He is confident about the details of his childhood, naming people and places instantly, and telling the story of his father's death. His language is fluent throughout. It is when he is trying to cope with his present circumstances that he runs into difficulties. The woman who enters his room is actually the home manager, and though he must encounter her on a daily basis, he does not recognize her. His seeing her in relation to John can be considered an attempt to make sense of the relationship between individuals he comes across. Later in the conversation (not supplied here) he gets into a tangle with the identities of his brother and son. He expresses clearly the struggles to make connections in this area and puts his finger on the nature of the challenge he faces – one of 'just going from here to there!'.

Issues arising

In the following sections we discuss some of the important issues which arise from the role of memory in communication with individuals with dementia.

Variability in memory performance

It is a common observation of those working or spending time with people that memory functioning is not always constant. Sometimes people surprise us by being able to retrieve a piece of information from long term memory which normally eludes them, and on occasion we are struck by the fact that certain experiences or ideas from the recent past seem to have been assimilated into a person's memory, and are later recalled. The person may be able to remember part of a story or some details of a situation, even if they do mix this up with information about a different subject or scenario.

There is for all of us a normal degree of variation in mental and physical performance subject to a range of factors including physical influences such as general health, tiredness, hunger, pain or discomfort, and psychological ones including mood, stress or anxiety, our level of confidence and our perception of how important or relevant our effort is. The behaviour of other people and characteristics of the physical environment also exert influences on our performance. Where memory is concerned, however, our functioning is reasonably stable. It seems to be fairly resistant to the vicissitudes of our day-to-day ups and downs.

When dementia is present, however, the situation is more complex. As yet we understand relatively little about exactly how memory is affected by the condition, and we are only beginning to appreciate that other influences (such as those detailed above) can act to impair or enhance the performance of the individual.

The following account from John's experience is an example of how memories for certain sorts of events can, with the right kind of support and encouragement, emerge from what seems to be an empty mental landscape:

> I was working on a unit where one of the residents, George Watson, was a retired clergyman in his mid-eighties. His wife requested that she and I spend some time with George in an attempt to establish some conversation and stimulate his powers of recall. For nearly an hour she fed me questions which I then proceeded to ask George. Despite an immense struggle, which found expression in groans and stutters, he was unable to answer any of them. I seriously began to doubt whether I should be causing the man this degree of frustration.
>
> Then George's wife said 'Do you remember, darling, when at the age of eighty you went paragliding for the first time?' At this her husband, who had been slumped in a chair all the while, suddenly stood up to his full height of six foot three or four and addressed us as if we were a congregation. He boomed:
>
> > There were the three of us in the boat, and I was the first to do it. It was the flying, it was the feeling free. And when I flowed like that I was astonished. And then I flew again. One, two, three! When are we going again?
>
> And then he collapsed back in the chair as if all the wind had been taken out of his sails. He was unable to respond to any more of our queries and remarks.
>
> Afterwards his wife told me how deeply she had been moved by this episode. She regarded it as a miracle. I felt that it was as if the clouds of

confusion had parted for a minute or two, and a clear memory had shone through. George had re-assumed the bearing of his calling. His personal preaching style had been clearly evident, and he had temporarily regained verbal fluency. All, it would appear, in the service of some powerful surge of memory and emotion.

We have much to learn about how and why episodes such as these occur when it is often taken for granted that dementia causes irreversible damage to the brain. Simplistic observations and assumptions must be challenged. We need far more openness, more careful and sensitive observation, and efforts to make sense of the subtleties of the individual's functioning. We should also give greater consideration to how our own behaviour and environmental features may impact on the person. We discuss the potential for acting to support instead of undermining the person's remaining abilities later in this chapter.

We should recognize here, that (as with the issue of awareness which we explore in Chapter 13), it sometimes suits us very well to make certain assumptions about the memory functioning of the person with dementia. If we take it for granted that new experiences are immediately forgotten, then if something unpleasant happens to the individual we can tell ourselves that there is no need to attempt to address this. And that if we let the person down in some way, for example by not visiting them at an agreed time or not doing something they have asked, this is not important because they will have forgotten about it anyway. The reasons for our investment in certain beliefs is something about which we need to be constantly vigilant.

Reminiscence

Despite the many and radical difficulties with memory observed in people with dementia, there are still exciting and important possibilities in working in the area of remembering. Of the positive potential of people with dementia in this regard, the psychologist Marie Mills, talking about a research study she conducted, says:

> Autobiographical memories were found in some abundance, but these memories might be more appropriately described as memories of the self (Brewer, 1986), as opposed to memories of the world. It is argued that memories of the self remain strongly present throughout life, and even for long periods throughout a dementing old age. It is recognised that semantic memory, or memory of the world, declines in dementia (Parkin 1987, 1993). This study suggests that memory of the self has a greater durability.[8]

In recent years there has grown up a whole movement around the use of reminiscence. Prior to the 1990s, reminiscence as an activity was often frowned upon since the zeitgeist was Reality Orientation, and the importance of reinforcing information about the here and now.[9] This has now changed, and reminiscence (and related approaches such as Life Story Work)[10] have taken their place among the range of activities and therapeutic approaches used with people with dementia.[11] It has done a great deal of good – providing enjoyment, enhancing the self-esteem of people with dementia, and encouraging others to listen to and to value their experiences.

Despite its rehabilitation and widespread acceptance in the world of dementia care, however, reminiscence as a practice does still carry some negative associations, such that when an older person (any older person) starts to say 'When I was young' or 'In my day', eyes will roll and hearts will sink. Younger people may laugh at themselves for talking about times past, and label it as evidence of getting old. These attitudes are underpinned by values about the importance of being aware of new trends, keeping up with change and generally being 'in touch'. Our negative perceptions of the practice of talking about the past are dismissed as 'nostalgic', and are part of a wider culture of ageism and disparagement of older people and their experiences.

While acknowledging the value of reminiscence-based activities, however, we must beware of defining people predominantly in terms of events and activities from the past, with the consequence of undervaluing talk related to the present or future. It has been John's experience that, given the freedom to choose what to talk about, many people have as much to say about how they are feeling, and what is going on around them in the here and now, and also what is likely to happen in the future, as about where they lived, people they have known, and what they did in years gone by. This reminds us that people with dementia are ongoing human beings, actively engaged in constructing the present and projecting into the future.

That said, it is certainly true that talk about the past does figure in conversation with people with dementia, as indeed it does with all of us. Sometimes it is clear that reminiscence activity is going on, at other times historical themes are blended in such a way as to mean that very careful attention is required to distinguish meanings which relate to the past and those which pertain to ongoing circumstances.

When people reminisce about their experiences, it is easy to label the activity and see it as being just that. However, sometimes what people talk about and the way they talk about it should prompt us to ask deeper questions. For example, why is the person talking about this subject at this particular time? Are there themes which could pertain to current concerns? We return to these issues in Chapter 11 on narrative.

Also, although reminiscence activity can be highly enjoyable and affirming to the individual and those around them, it is not necessarily the case that people want to recall everything from their past, and in emotional terms it is an activity which carries some risk:

> Recall activity should not be taken lightly – the facilitator needs to be aware of sudden and completely unexpected consequences of a given direction within the conversation . . .
>
> Reminiscence needs to be taken seriously, as it has the potential for shared pleasure or individual distress.[12]

Confusion

As we shall examine in greater depth in Chapter 6, the need to understand what happens to us, and therefore of being able to exert a degree of control over events is fundamental to human beings. Our memories play a central role in helping us to maintain this sense of order, continuity and predictability in our lives. So what happens to people when memory function begins to fail, and a sense of confusion is an increasingly prominent feature? Again people with dementia have much to say on the subject of confusion. Some of the statements are relatively straightforward (and non-confused!):

It's the terrific confusion of things that worries me more than anything else.

In my mind I only came here yesterday. I have no clue whatsoever.

My thoughts – they go away and come back again.

Some statements are bursting with distress and urgency:

I can't place this place at all – isn't that terrible? What street is this, what town? I can't find that label with my address. Find me, please tell me where I am!

Another aspect of confusion is that of talk which is puzzling or disjointed. Often this is dismissed as 'rambling', and there is the assumption that it is the expression of random thoughts or fragments from memory which are essentially meaningless. The reader will not now be surprised to hear us urge that the speech of people with dementia should never be ignored or discarded as meaningless. It is true that there may be occasions on which it is difficult to discern structure or meaning in what is being said, but this is not justification for labelling the speech as nonsense and the person as unable to communicate.

At such times it is helpful to bear in mind that the person may be recalling incidents and information which are connected by emotional links, rather than logical or chronological ones. Again the psychologist Marie Mills says:

The characteristics of emotion and duration of memories, which are associated with autobiographical memory, imply a relationship between emotion and available long-term memories in older people with dementia. Moreover, a certain strength and durability is indicated in the emotional autobiographical memories of informants that was not apparent in other aspects of memory.[13]

Confabulation

This is the term given to the unconscious act of filling in gaps in memory by 'making up' new material, rather than recalling actual information. It is a practice which has been identified as characteristic of quite a wide range of different groups of people with neurological or psychiatric difficulties. Here Oliver Sacks is describing a man with severe memory problems caused by alcohol-related brain damage:

> Mr Thomson, only just out of hospital . . . was still in an almost frenzied confabulatory delirium . . . continually creating a world and self, to replace what was continually being forgotten and lost. Such a frenzy may call forth quite brilliant powers of invention and fancy – a veritable confabulatory genius – for such a patient *must literally make himself (and his world) up every moment.*[14]

Clearly this man was responding to an acute situation with very florid instances of confabulation. Most examples occur in a less intense way. Sometimes confabulatory material has a quality which differentiates it clearly from other talk. On other occasions it may be much more conventional in nature, only identifiable through the possession of in-depth knowledge of the person and their circumstances. But in general, the labelling of talk as confabulation suggests that the content of the story is fantasy, nonsense or otherwise essentially unreliable and best dismissed. This is an assumption we should avoid. Although the details of the talk may be factually incorrect, confabulation could be regarded as an example of a creative response which gives clues to the underlying concerns of the person, and is therefore an important resource for communication. There is also the danger that, in order to let ourselves off the hook in terms of trying to understand, we assign the label 'confabulation' to talk which is worrying or otherwise difficult to interpret. This allows us to ignore it, seeing it merely as a symptom of the condition, instead of giving it proper consideration and response. Sometimes so-called confabulation can be an important function of the way a person copes with or makes sense of their experiences. The psychologist Lauren Slater commenting on the process of writing her autobiographical account *Spasm* about her experience of epilepsy says:

> Spasm is a book of narrative truth, a book in which I am more interested in using invention to get to the heart of things than I am in documenting actual life. The text I've created uses, in some instances, metaphors, most significantly the metaphor of epilepsy, to express subtleties and horrors and gaps in my past for which I have never been able to find the words. Metaphor is the greatest gift of language, for through it we can propel silence into sound. And even if the sounds are not altogether accurate, they do resonate in some heartfelt place we cannot dismiss. That is why it is in this book, although not always factually correct, that I feel I have finally been able to tell a tale eluding me for years.[15]

Memory for people

A person constitutes a multisensory stimulus, encompassing the way the individual looks, how they sound, how they smell, and what they say and do, and the emotional associations they engender. This may mean that the chances of the person with dementia being able to hook onto and remember something, and thereby recognize the person, is heightened. It is a regular observation of staff that while from day to day it is often not clear whether a person knows and remembers them or not, if they are absent for a while and then return, there are clear signs of recognition, including sometimes the use of their name. Where people have achieved a deep bond through communication this can prove remarkably lasting. John provides the following example:

> I worked with Judy Phillips on four separate occasions about a week apart. When I met her for the first time she immediately expressed a pessimistic view of the possibilities of relationship in the words, 'Nobody cares about anybody really.' However, conversations that were memorable and mutually satisfying ensued, and on the fourth occasion of meeting she greeted me with the words 'I remembered you were coming. I ran in the house and told my mother', which I took to be a metaphor for joy. She ended the encounter with the words, 'When I'm with someone talking like this it fills me up.'
>
> A period of six years then elapsed before I was able to revisit that nursing home. I did not expect her still to be alive. But when I opened the door of the unit there she was, sitting in the same seat in the corridor where I had seen her and spoken with her before. As I approached her, her eyes lit up and she held out her hands to take mine. 'So you've come back to see me, and we're going to have another of those wonderful conversations,' she said. I found her much changed: physically more frail, her language more impoverished, and she had difficulty accessing her memories, but we experienced a closeness as palpable as before.

Nonverbal aspects of memory

We referred above to the fact that memory for actions and skills is separable from that for facts, information and stories. It is said that once we have learned to ride a bicycle, we will not forget the knack. There is evidence from research and experience which indicates that people with dementia often hold on to old skills, and are, given the right kind of support, able to learn and retain new ones. We have examples from John's work in the field of communication through the arts of people with dementia being able to acquire new skills, such as those required for watercolour painting, and through this activity finding real satisfaction and opportunities for communication.

Nonverbal memory encompasses the whole rich sphere of sensory experience too. Think of how evocative a smell can be. The merest whiff can trigger a powerful and complex recollection, some aspects of which may be verbalizable, while others will evade description. The smell-triggered memory may also have a powerful emotional component, on account of the very direct brain connections between the smell and emotional circuits. Since the senses of smell and taste are closely related it may be that tastes can have a similar effect.

Visual memory may be more vulnerable to loss in people with dementia, but the sense of hearing enables people to partake in one of the most consistently striking ways in which they demonstrate that some forms of nonverbal memory persist – music. We see over and over again people responding powerfully to music, demonstrating their recognition and recall of familiar tunes and often even lyrics, when musical cues are present. Touch is another sense through which profound experience can be relived. Of this the psychologist Marie de Hennezel, who works with people who are dying, says:

> It is a fact familiar to me from frequent observation that the simple reality of being touched with gentle respect can sometimes unleash the most powerful emotional reactions. For even the skin itself possesses a memory, and a simple touch, if it feels *good* and *reaffirming*, can trigger the re-experiencing of the most deep-rooted deprivation and distress.[16]

Trauma

We have all had experiences which are painful and upsetting, and remembering them triggers a reliving of similar feelings. Some of us have had experiences which were so severe (for example involvement in an accident or being assaulted) as to give rise to specific emotional problems, some aspects of which are manifested in the area of memory. Traumatic experiences can be associated with highly distinctive and powerful memory phenomena, and we need to bear in mind that the people with dementia in our care may have had such experiences (for example during wartime or in a domestic situation) and still be struggling with its effects in the here and now.

Some traumatic memories take the form of an ongoing form of background awareness and recall of distressing experiences, but for others a very acute form of remembering can occur. Such a memory (sometimes called flashbacks) may surface suddenly, and stand out in terms of force, vividness and time sequencing. There is a quality of re-immersion in the nature of the original experience, and although the actual duration of the re-experiencing may be very brief, a subjective slowing of perceptual processes may produce a slow-motion sequence which feels much longer. And of course afterwards there is the time it takes to reconnect with current reality and calm down emotionally. Such experiences can be overwhelmingly frightening and distressing to the person, and to those around them. Many people who experience flashbacks worry that they are going mad, and even when the nature of the difficulty is understood it can precipitate enormous distress. Imagine how much more unpleasant such an experience would be for a person with dementia. If the individual is unable to describe the experience, their response may take a behavioural form, perhaps even as aggression.

Related to the earlier discussion of the relationship between emotion and memory functioning, research has been carried out in Japan following the Kobe earthquake into its effects on people with dementia.[17] The main focus was on the extent to which people, who at the time of the disaster already had significant dementia, could recall events surrounding the earthquake. In line with other evidence about the effects of emotion on the registration, storage and retrieval of information, it was found that these people were able to give a much clearer and more accurate account of the events surrounding the earthquake compared with other, less emotionally charged experiences (for example medical examinations) which took place close to the earthquake in time. This is an extreme example, but it serves to remind us that the functioning of memory in dementia is far from straightforward, and that similarly heightened memory performance may well occur in other situations which are, for whatever reason, traumatic to the individual.

This is a specialized topic, and we cannot go into detail here about ways of working psychologically with people experiencing these sorts of difficulties,[18] but in the course of any kind of communication work and relationship development, the possibility of trauma and its likely effects should be borne in mind.

Emotional effects of memory failure

We all know the frustration of not being able to recall a piece of information when we need it, and the dismay of realizing that we have forgotten to do something we were meant to. There is not only the inconvenience or embarrassment which results from the lapse, but also the sense of vulnerability which derives from the realization that our memories are fallible, yet play such a pivotal role in our lives. This is generally a fairly fleeting feeling, however, and one which can have the positive effect of motivating us to find new ways of supporting our memory.

The situation for the person with dementia is far more serious. We need to consider what might be the emotional, even existential, impact on an individual who is undergoing repeated and radical memory loss. How does someone in such a situation cope? How do they feel? How are their emotions expressed? The extent to which the person is aware of their difficulties is another important issue, and one which is explored further in Chapter 13.

Memory and identity

We introduced ideas about personhood and identity in Chapter 2, and here we explore the connections between that sense of selfhood which permeates our being – and the capacity to recall the past. This is a profound topic, and we will raise more questions than we can answer.[19]

Part of the idea of identity is that it persists over time. We do not have one identity at one instant and another the next. In normal circumstances we perceive a quality of stability – indeed stability is an essential part of the notion of identity. Despite considerable flux in one's physical and psychological self, there is the feeling of being the same person throughout.

Memory must play a large part in this sense of consistency. We must be connecting the self as presently experienced with the self of five seconds, five minutes and five years ago, perceiving some essential quality of continuity. It may be helpful to see memory as a kind of glue that holds the self together. With its help we are enabled to find meaning in our lives. So what happens when memory begins to fail? Does the glue unstick and the sense of identity fall apart? What is the experience of people with dementia in this regard? Writing about the mother of the central character in his novel *Scar Tissue*, Michael Ignatieff wrestles with these questions:

> I began to think that there was something wrong with the idea that her memories were localised and that illness was obliterating them one by one. It was not that she was forgetting discrete events; she was unable to place herself in a meaningful sequence of those events. She knew who she once had been, but not who she had become. Her memories of childhood were intact, but her short-term recollection had collapsed, so that past and present were marooned far from each other.
>
> I suspected that the breakdown in her memory was a symptom of a larger disruption in her ability to create and sustain a coherent image of herself over time. It dawned on me that her condition offered me an unrepeatable opportunity to observe the relation between selfhood and memory. I began to think of my mother as a philosophical problem.
>
> My mistake had been to suppose that a memory image could subsist apart from an image of the self, that memories could persist apart from the act of speaking or thinking about them from a given standpoint. It was this junction between past and present that she was losing. She was wondering who the 'I' was in her own sentences. She was wondering whether these memories of a blue beer mug in a warm suburban garden were really her own. Because they no longer seemed to be her own, she began to throw them away.
>
> In spite of all this, her gestures, her smile, her voice remained unchanged. A blurred vision of her charm survived, together with hints of her sense of humour. She was suffering from a disturbance of her soul, not just a loss of memory, yet *she* was still intact. I was back where I started.[20]

Memory loss and its effects on the sense of self is one of the biggest challenges to the practice of communication we are advocating in this book. It would be foolish for us to claim that we have a formula which will enable a person to hang on to their sense of coherence. What we do believe, however, is that being with the person, encouraging them to share what memories remain, helping them to tell their stories to themselves and to us, and in so doing promoting meaningful relationships, must be the sorts of things that can make a difference. It may involve an act of faith on our part, but if we behave at all times as if the person's identity is still there uniquely manifesting itself, who knows what a stabilizing and empowering force this may be?

Experience of time

Perhaps one of the most profound things with which we have to come to terms in our work with people with dementia is that we seem sometimes to be operating according to different time-scales. It is a function of our memory that we have a sense of past, present and future, and maintain a sense of time passing in a predictable way. We are able to locate ourselves within this. If, however, dementia affects the ability to call up the past in a conventional linear way (at the same time as *knowing* it is the past), and to imagine the future, it may be that people with dementia live in an endless succession of present moments, which are nevertheless informed by material from memory.

A hospital chaplain, Debbie Everett, makes this point in the following passage:

> For those of us who are cognitively intact, time is like a stream of water in which we float with the current. For someone with Alzheimer's Disease time is frozen into individual snowflakes that touch the skin and melt.[21]

So perhaps the person with dementia experiences points in their past as if they were the present. We, on the other hand, cannot escape from our constant flitting between the past and the future – and often have a diminished sense of the present as a consequence – so it is difficult for us to imagine how they may see their world. Michael Ignatieff describes this in these terms:

> They are not vegetables, but primary selves. They are no longer like us, busy and full of purpose, bent on becoming something. Instead they are prisoners of the realm of pure being. In this realm there is only now, this instant.[22]

If Everett and Ignatieff are right then we must cease struggling to have people with dementia conform to our time-scales, and begin learning from them how to be content with existence in this most immediate manner.

Memory and communication

To come back to our main argument, it is our view that many people with dementia fall silent through the lack of an opportunity for talking. It is reasonable to suppose that this neglect has repercussions on their ability to recall events from their past lives. Regular interactions provide at the very least a stimulus for memory, and as we discussed at the beginning of this chapter, memory involves a process of continual revisiting and reconstruction of material. This impression is confirmed by people with dementia themselves. One woman, speaking of her talks with John, said:

> *I'm glad this has happened to me, because the memories are all here inside me waiting to come out.*

And a man said:

> *Your memories are more important that your limbs are, 'cos you can have conversations with all your faculties.*

But the most striking example of the way providing opportunities for talk can transform the communicative possibilities for an individual is provided by Alice. She reflected extensively on the effect of memory loss in the course of her conversations with John. Some of these thoughts are found in Chapter 1. Another not included there is the following:

> *It's really quite exciting having all these memories come back from you. But I'm getting to the point where I'm bound to admit that what I say is not necessarily gospel truth.*

Here she recognizes John's role in provoking recall, and also a degree of what may be considered confabulation. On another occasion she makes an honest appraisal of the current level of her faculties and pays tribute to his role in the process:

> *Hang it all, I cannot remember such a lot of things. I lose the thread so quickly, but it doesn't mean to say that I am dotty. And then you come and it helps quite a lot.*

Implications for care

The main point to make about memory is that we need to hold back with our assumptions about what is going on in the mind of the person with dementia. Despite the prevalence of the view that the mechanisms for moving information through short-term memory into the long-term store are damaged, we can never simply assume that what happens to the person in the here and now is invariably forgotten. It may be that as things happen from hour to hour and day to day, aspects of events are encoded (along with some understanding of their meaning), but that the ability to express that memory or understanding to others is lost or fluctuates.

Similarly we should never generalize from one particular incident – inability to remember something on one occasion – to the view that this information has simply been forgotten. As we have seen, there can be marked variability in the level at which the person operates, and for some it may be that the process of remembering does still work but takes so long that once the information is retrieved, it no longer seems to make any sense.

When talking to a person with dementia about events which have already taken place or people from the past, it is probably better not to begin a statement with a question such as 'Do you remember when . . .?' Starting in this way risks inducing anxiety or frustration in the person who knows that they are struggling in this respect. A more helpful strategy is to start the conversation by supplying information such as 'Last month, we all went out on a bus trip to the coast'. This sort of approach places no demands on the individual but rather provides them with information which may stimulate memories of their own. Careful observation of the person's response should give you clues as to their reaction, and whether there is evidence of recognition of the information.

We have discussed above the findings from the study of memory which indicate that restoring the context where information was first learned has a positive effect on recall. This has obvious significance for the person with dementia. If we are able to help people to have rich experiences, and if we can work to enhance the consistency of experiences and contexts, then we shall support the maximum functioning of the person's memory.

If you know that you are going to have a series of conversations with an individual, you could try to have the conversations in the same place, at the same time of day and as part of a regular routine. It can be difficult in the context of busy service settings, but you could try to work on enriching the context of the encounter by leading up to it in a consistent way – for example walking with the person to the room, noticing sights and textures, spending a minute or two listening to the same music before talking, burning the same scented candle, offering the same sort of food and drink. You may be very surprised at how much enriching the context of the encounter can help the person to access memories of similar previous occasions, even if they do not seem to be consciously aware of this.

Making things as memorable as possible for the person extends to the way we behave and present ourselves. We know how reassuring it can be for the person with dementia to have someone around who not only behaves in consistent ways, but also looks, smells and sounds distinctive. Many people with dementia seem to retain good sensory capacity and, say, by using colour and scent or other special features imaginatively, we can make this work for reinforcing memories in the service of relationship development.

Ethical implications

Hypercognitive values

The first issue here concerns our basic assumptions about the role of memory in personhood. As the quote from Steven Rose at the beginning of the chapter and that from Donald Spence (p. 216) suggest, our ideas about what it means to be a person are very closely tied up with the importance of an intact memory, and it is hard to get away from the perception that someone whose memory functioning is compromised is not somehow less than fully a person. These ways of thinking are woven deeply into our framework for understanding the world.

We need to appreciate that where thinking about memory is concerned, there is a very powerful tendency towards hypercognitive values. The whole concept is orientated towards seeing memory for information, which can be consciously recalled, verbalized and integrated with other knowledge, as being of primary status. The value our culture places on competence and independence under-lines this. We have a long way to go in fully exploring the value of other sorts of memory, for example memory for emotion, sensory and physical memory and memory which is expressed in action and habit. Recognizing our bias towards valuing intellectual aspects of memory, the ethicist Stephen Post says:

> Memory-based solicitude is troubling . . . because it seems to draw some line in time between the person who was present and the remnant that is now.[23]

This has important implications for our practice in terms of communication. If we were fully attentive to the focuses we create and sustain in conversation and interaction, we would probably be surprised at how much they revolve around themes of memory – asking people if they recall events from the past, encouraging people to try to remember items of information, somehow at times almost seeming to 'test' the individual, as if their performance in this respect were a kind of barometer of something deeper. This sort of thing can happen even when we do not mean it to, and is likely to be a function of our awareness that a good deal of the person's difficulties in the area of memory. It simply keeps springing to mind.

What might be the effect of these practices on the person? Earlier in the chapter we briefly discussed the emotional impact of difficulties with memory on the individual, and this is something which demands ongoing sensitivity and reflectiveness.

Of course sometimes it seems that people want to try to remember, and we have acknowledged that for all of us remembering information, events and experiences provides an important sense of mastery and power, reassurance, perhaps, that we are not stumbling around in chaos. Given the value we place on this it would seem wrong to deny people with dementia such oppor-tunities. However, it is also necessary to recognize that as a function of the power we, as people without dementia, wield in interactions it is easy to create a situation, a frame, where it could appear to the other person that the value we place on the interaction depends on their being able to remember specific information. The ways in which we set up these expectations are no doubt numerous, some extremely subtle, others more overt.

Reminiscence and life-story work

While these considerations apply to communication practice generally, they are of most acute relevance to reminiscence and life-story work, which have the activity of remembering in a central role. We know that people with dementia can obtain tremendous enjoyment and self-esteem from these activities, and relationships often blossom in the context of the deeper know-ledge and understanding of an individual's history and experiences which can develop. However, just as with any intervention which has real positive poten-tial, there are dangers too. The following are some questions to consider:

- To what extent should we should be placing a premium on remembering when this is one of the very greatest areas of difficulty?
- In carrying out reminiscence and life-story work are we at risk of communicating the message that the worth of a person lies in the domain of previous competence and achievement, rather than in their current state of being and doing? Is there again a hypercognitive subtext?
- To what extent are we aware and take account of individual differences in attitudes to reminiscence work? Research by Peter Coleman explored variability in the meaning and experience of reminiscence activity for older people generally, and this has direct implications for people with dementia.[24]

As with most things, it is not the activity itself which dictates the nature and meaning of the experience, but rather it is the way it is carried out. Those who are experienced in facilitating the best kind of reminiscence work bring to bear a sophisticated range of conscious and intuitive skills, and the results can be both magical and profound.

6 | **Interpretation:** 'After all, what is this lump of matter if you can't make sense of it?'

In his book of reflections on life, Robert Fulghum writes:

> a small town emergency squad was summoned to a house where smoke was pouring from an upstairs window. The crew broke in and found a man in a smouldering bed. After the man was rescued and the mattress doused, the obvious question was asked: 'How did this happen?'

> 'I don't know. It was on fire when I lay down on it.'

> As with most of what we see other people do, we don't know *why* they do it, either. If our own actions are mysteries, how much so others'? Why did he lie down on the burning bed? Was he drunk? Ill? Suicidal? Blind? Cold? Dumb? Did he just have a weird sense of humour? Or what? I don't know. It's hard to judge without a lot more information. Oh sure, we go ahead and judge anyhow. But maybe if judgement were suspended a bit more often, we would like us more.[1]

Our lives are driven by the question 'Why?' The most basic psychological characteristic of human beings is the need to try to make sense of the world and our experience within it. At the most grand end of the scale this has led to the great scientific feats of exploration and discovery, but it also finds expression in the most intimate mental processes of every one of us. As we go about our business from day to day, we are all engaged in the task of trying to explain things to ourselves and others, and to achieve a sense of understanding of what is going on both within and around us. It is as if, underpinning our conscious thinking processes, there is a stream of questions: what is happening? Is it normal? Have I encountered this before? What does it tell me about myself, other people, the world? In this way we keep a monitoring eye on events, classifying them and integrating them with previous experience, and checking them against our expectations. This is the activity we call interpretation.

The drive to understand what is going on is closely tied up with the need to have a sense of control over events, and this means that we have to identify patterns, to find out what goes together, what leads to what. In this way we can know what to avoid and what to seek out. Since in our highly social environment most of what happens involves other people, we need to develop skills in making sense of their behaviour. In order to do this we refer back to our own experiences. Of this, the psychologist Nicholas Humphrey writes:

> When we watch the behaviour of our fellow human beings, we seldom, if ever, see merely a mosaic of incidental acts: we see beneath it a deeper causal structure – the hidden presence of plans, intentions, emotions, memories etc – and it is on that basis we can claim to understand what they are doing.[2]

In normal circumstances most of what goes on around us is unremarkable, and these processes do their work below normal awareness. Encountering someone doing something unusual triggers a more overt process of sense-seeking. Our antennae are activated, and more conscious effort is brought to bear. We will go to considerable lengths to find some way of accounting for what is happening – to conclude that a person's actions are meaningless would be the least preferred option. The need to perceive meaning is so basic to our nature that to admit that there is none is to accept that the world is an unpredictable, and therefore dangerous, place. This is highly threatening.

As we shall explore further in Chapter 13 on awareness, individual people vary in terms of how deeply they need to understand their own behaviour and that of other people. Some are content with enough understanding to get by in a practical, day-to-day sense. Others have a need to look for pattern and meaning at a much greater depth and level of subtlety. Some people seem to have an ability to understand other people, while seeming relatively uninsightful about their own way of being and doing. Alice Jopling, who gave us the title of this chapter, was making a clear statement of her need for understanding.

Beliefs and assumptions

If making sense of our experience is so important, how do we go about doing it?[3] We do so with reference to what we already know, or, more accurately, believe. Early in childhood we start to develop a set of beliefs about ourselves, other people, and the world of objects and events. Some of these we learn immediately through experience – that hot things burn and ice cream tastes sweet. Some are passed directly on to us by others, perhaps in the form of advice or maxims, for example that if you work hard you will be rewarded. Others come to us through exposure to the myriad of ideas which abound in popular culture, literature and so on.

Although they may not always remember individual incidents, children are always learning from what they encounter. If, for example, a child is frequently in contact with people who behave violently when angry, he or she will learn to equate anger with violence. Or if as a child you received attention only when you did something special, you may come to believe that your worth depends on your achievements. We go on developing and refining our system of beliefs throughout life, but most are formed in childhood and tend to persist in guiding our subsequent interpretations and actions. Although our beliefs have a crucial influence on the way we interpret current experience, they occupy a quiet, largely unconscious role in our lives. We take it for granted that they are 'true', and tend to examine them only when it becomes clear that our ideas differ markedly from others or that a particular course of action will lead to difficulties or conflict. Relating to others who have different beliefs is a major way in which we learn about our own, and this forms part of how our personhood is constructed and maintained.

Interpretation and thinking

Just as our underlying beliefs rarely call attention to themselves, our thoughts and the process of thinking are not normally the subjects of deliberate reflection. However, the constant stream of images, words, impressions and ideas which make up the richness of our inner lives is so close to us that we tend to regard thoughts as a direct reflection of reality. Again, we assume that they are true. In fact the process of thinking is far more appropriately considered an ongoing form of interpretation, and as such should not be seen as reality or fact. Rather, an interpretation could be considered more or less consistent with the available evidence, more or less realistic. It is also vital to appreciate that the way that we think has a pivotal role in the way that we feel emotionally and in what we do. An example will illustrate this.

Say on arriving at work on Monday morning you meet a colleague and they seem offhand and reserved. If over the weekend you have been worrying about whether you are making a success of your job, whether people like you and hold you in high regard, you are likely to interpret your colleague's lack of warmth as a reflection of his or her feelings towards you personally. This way of making sense of the situation is likely to precipitate an emotional response. You may feel upset and anxious. These thoughts and feelings could then prompt you to act in a nervous, stilted way which in turn the other person may interpret as rejecting. All of this will exacerbate further your perception of there being a problem. If, on the other hand, you know that your colleague is having personal problems and often feels very depressed on Mondays, then you are likely to make a completely different interpretation of their behaviour, and one which is less liable to trigger anxiety and upset in you. As a result your behaviour is also likely to be different. You might even offer some comfort which could alleviate the other person's distress, and might lead to a completely different train of events.

There are three crucial points to draw out here: the first is that the way we make sense of events is influenced by our existing preoccupations. These act as a kind of filter guiding what we focus on. Things which do not seem relevant may not be noticed at all. The second is that the style in which we interpret the things which happen to us, has a direct effect on the way that we *feel* and how we *act*. This in turn affects the thoughts, feelings and behaviours of others. The third point is that given that a person's thinking processes are informed by their own unique set of reference points then it follows that different people will make *different* interpretations of the *same* set of circumstances. One person will make different interpretations of similar experiences at different times, according to mood, interests and as a function of competing demands on their attention. All of these points have a direct bearing on situations involving people with dementia.

Biases in interpretation

In examining the ways in which we make sense of our own behaviour and that of others, social psychologists have identified a set of biases to which we are all subject, in all sorts of situations.[3] There are three main types. The first concerns our tendency, when trying to make sense of someone else's behaviour, to assume that the main cause lies within themselves, for example personality factors or conscious intention. We tend to underestimate the extent to which the environment or the behaviour of others has influenced them. The second bias concerns the interpretation of our own behaviour, and here the bias acts in the opposite direction: we see environmental or other external factors as being more significant than ones relating to the self. The third type of bias also operates in relation to the self, and it concerns our basic need to see ourselves in a positive light. Such a bias will operate in relation, say, to seeing the reasons for our successes as being internal to ourselves, while we explain our failures in terms of external factors.

Making sense of dementia

How does all this relate to work with people with dementia? First, we need to recognize that as part of the belief that dementia destroys personhood, we have all assumed both that their pursuit of meaning has ceased (if there is no person, there is no need for meaning), and also that any attempts of our own to make sense of their words and actions are futile. A landscape of meaning-lessness has developed around dementia, and this urgently needs to be tackled.

We return to the subject of meaning or the lack of it in what people with dementia say and do later in this chapter, but for now let us think further about our own perceptions of meaninglessness in the lives of persons with the condition. We have a clue here as to why many people find those with dementia so disturbing. Indeed this feeling is described vividly by John in the account which opened Chapter 2. He felt frightened and alienated on being confronted with a group of people whose behaviour seemed to make no sense. This would be the reaction of many: people who do strange and incompre-hensible things are, by their very nature, disturbing. On an immediate level we fear they might do something to embarrass or harm us. On a more general level they are frightening because we cannot empathize with their motives, and therefore see them as fundamentally different from ourselves. They rep-resent a challenge to our need for pattern and order, and this in turn points to the unwelcome conclusion that the world is not ultimately a meaningful place. This is partly what engenders such a powerful stigmatization of people with dementia. One solution to the problem of people who do not make sense has been to say that they are no longer persons, not in the full sense, and then to lock them away and ignore them.

Another point which is of great importance is that just as we, without dementia, need to make sense of our experience, and do so with reference to pre-existing beliefs, people with the condition are engaged in the same pur-suit. Their search for meaning may be impeded by their problems with memory, reasoning and so on, but in all likelihood the basic need is the same, as are the ways in which they try to meet it. In order to understand an indi-vidual's thoughts, feelings and actions, therefore, we must make efforts to dis-cover more about the beliefs which underpin them. This sort of understanding comes about in a variety of channels – careful observation and genuine com-munication, and also the gathering of background information from relatives and previous carers.

Our beliefs about dementia

As with any other sphere of experience the sense we make of our dealings with people with dementia is constructed in the course of minute-to-minute think-ing processes, which are (as we have seen) guided by underlying beliefs. If we are to be successful in finding new ways of communicating and developing relationships with people, it is necessary to become more aware of what is hap-pening at both the thought and belief levels, but for now we focus on the level of beliefs. In the Introduction we listed some common beliefs about demen-tia. You may wish to look back at these just now, and spend some time think-ing about the extent to which they form part of your way of understanding dementia.

There is no point in denying that we all carry around a lot of unhelpful baggage where beliefs about ageing,[4] illness and death in general are concerned, and about dementia in particular. Our personal and family experiences will have sensitized us in this regard, our culture bombards us continually with negative messages, and our society is organized in such a way as to devalue, ignore and even ridicule those who are ill, disabled or old. We may wish to assert that all this does not affect how we behave in relation to specific individuals, that we can somehow rise above it, but the reality is that these assumptions are present and active, although they do operate below the level of normal awareness. Often it is necessary to observe our reactions to situations in order to discover what we think and believe about them. We explore this further below.

Learning new ways of communicating with people with dementia demands that first of all we acknowledge the existence of negative assumptions, and then work towards trying to pin down exactly what they are and to challenge them. This is not a simple task, but there are skills that can be learned which help. One way of doing this is using a technique called the 'downward arrow' method.[5] This strategy employs the metaphor which conceptualizes particular thoughts, which flash through our minds very rapidly and in relation to specific situations, as existing on the surface, while beliefs exist at a deeper level and are more enduring and stable. The beliefs are connected to the thoughts, and exert a predictable influence on them, even though there might not seem to be any direct link. Using the downward arrow technique is like catching and holding onto a thought on the surface and digging down to see what it is connected to underneath. An example set out in graphic form will make things clearer:

Situation
Mrs Black and some other ladies are sitting in a circle, and a care assistant, Gillian, is reading out quiz questions. As well as Gillian and the group members, there is a new member of staff, Emma, present. This is the first time she has been in the group and seen Gillian at work.

Normally Mrs Black has difficulty contributing any answers because she has problems articulating words, although she seems to quite enjoy watching what is happening. At one point, however, just after Gillian has read out a question, she sits forward in her chair, lifts her hand and starts to try to speak. Most of the other ladies notice this, and turn and look expectantly at her. Mrs Black is still looking as if she is trying to get some words out. At this point Gillian thinks she sees one of the others rolling her eyes impatiently, but she is not sure.

At last Mrs Black manages to say something, but it is not easy to make out her words. She goes on to say a few more but still in a very indistinct way.

At this point Gillian hesitates, glances at Emma and then says 'Okay, never mind that one. Here's another question,' and proceeds to read it out. Mrs Black slumps back in her chair looking upset, and Emma looks very concerned about her.

Afterwards Emma asks Gillian why she didn't give Mrs Black a proper chance to say what she wanted.

This was clearly a significant episode for Mrs Black and for Gillian. Emma also felt that she had seen something important happening. Gillian did not feel very happy with her performance in the group, but after Emma queried her response to Mrs Black she felt especially upset. She wondered how she could possibly have been so insensitive. Fortunately she decided to talk to a supportive colleague about the incident; he recognized its significance and encouraged her to give proper consideration to the experience. The first step was for Gillian to try to remember exactly what was going through her mind when she made the decision to move on with the next question. To do this she went back into the room where the group took place and tried to recreate the scene in her mind. After quite a lot of reflection, she managed to pin down the thoughts which were around at the time. One cluster which seemed particularly important was:

Oh no! This is embarrassing! What is she trying to say?
She won't be able to get it out. I'd better just move on quickly.

Having managed to identify the thoughts, the next step was to start digging down. In order to do this, her colleague suggested that she say to herself, 'Okay, let's say my thoughts in this situation are realistic, what would that mean?' This may seem like a strange thing to do, but it does enable you to access a deeper level of thinking. Sometimes a slightly different form of question such as 'And what would be so bad about that?' or 'And what does that mean I think about dementia?' works better. In doing this, Gillian came up with the following:

Original thought:
She won't be able to get it out. [meaning the words she wanted say]
(Say that was true, what would be so bad about it?)

That it was going to be embarrassing.
(Say that was true, what would be so bad about it?)

That she would be upset and it would be my fault.

That everyone, especially Emma, would think that I was rubbish at my job.

That if I can't do my job properly then I'm a waste of space.

Gillian found it quite hard to get going on this, but once she got the hang of it, it came a bit more easily. Then she started to wonder when she should stop. The guidance here is that once you have reached a point where the answer to the question is quite general, no longer relating specifically to the situation which gave rise to it, you are tapping into the level of beliefs. Another clue is that when you come up with an answer, you may experience a surge of emotion. This indicates that what you have struck on has personal significance.

It is important to note here that the value of this technique will be lost it in answer to the questions, Gillian simply came up with descriptions of emotions. For example, if in answer to the question 'And what would that mean?' she had said 'I would feel rotten', that response would short-circuit the process. The answers to the questions need to be thoughts, for example 'I thought that would mean I couldn't do my job properly.'

When Gillian went through this process, she was surprised at how quickly thinking about the incident in the group took her into a very personal domain. Generalized doubts about her own abilities and qualities sprang quickly to mind, and were accompanied by feelings of upset. She realized that she held the belief that unless she could do everything well, she was no use as a person.

The example given above explored just one aspect of what was a complex situation. After further reflection Gillian realized that alongside the need to protect herself, she had been very worried that Mrs Black would also suffer embarrassment. She examined this in the following way:

Original thought:
Oh dear, poor Mrs Black! She isn't going to be able to
get this one. It must be awful for her!
(Say that is true, what would that mean?)
↓

She is going to get embarrassed and frustrated.
(Say that is true, what would that mean?)
↓

That would be terrible for her.
↓

It would be better if I stepped in and stopped this happening.
↓

That it is more important to reduce the chances of Mrs
Black being embarrassed than to let her struggle to express
herself.
↓

That I think avoiding embarrassment is more important
than making space for attempts at communication.
↓

That I made that decision for someone else rather than
let them take the chance of making a mistake or getting
it right.
↓

That I believe that people with dementia basically need to be
protected from themselves.

Once Gillian got to this point, there was again a surge of emotion. She was rather shocked at what she had uncovered. She had heard about how important it is to recognize and respect the personhood of clients, and agreed with these ideas. She herself believed that she sought to empower people through the work that she did, and she was certainly convinced of the centrality of genuine communication.

Examining this particular incident, however, made her realize that deep down she did have strong views about people with dementia needing to be protected, particularly in situations involving the possibility of embarrassment in front of others. Further reflection on this enabled her to see that this was probably connected with the fact that she herself had a lot of anxiety about doing things in front of other people, which was probably related to several significant experiences in both her childhood and adult life.

Making these connections was a very important development experience for Gillian. Although she had been upset by the original incident, and found the process of working out what lay underneath it also rather painful, being able to set it in context like this had quite dramatic positive effects. It not only greatly expanded her understanding of that particular incident, but also raised her general awareness of how she functions in a professional context, and strengthened her self-esteem as a worker. Up until that point she had found times when she got upset in connection with an incident at work quite demoralizing and confusing. Although she normally loved the job, these occasions made her wonder if she should rethink her career choice. Being able to gain perspective in this way also gave her a stronger sense of connection with the clients, and to see their experiences and difficulties as being quite similar to her own.

By way of refocusing, the point of this whole exercise is to become more aware of the beliefs and assumptions which underpin our dealings with people with dementia. Sometimes it is very obvious that what you come up with using this strategy is part of a problem, but there are situations when it can be more ambiguous. In order to get a clearer sense it is often necessary to find ways of distancing yourself slightly from the belief, and there are various ways of doing this. One is to write it down (in fact it is advisable to try to write the whole process down). As we shall explore in Chapter 10, writing is a powerful way of getting perspective on thoughts and feelings. Seeing them on paper will probably enable you to evaluate them more objectively. Another good strategy is to imagine what you would think if you heard someone else expressing the idea. On doing this you might immediately be able to recognize that it is distorted or unrealistic. Once you are reflecting at this level, you may be able to identify similar or related beliefs and think of other situations in which they have been at work. The next step would be to watch out for further situations in which you think similar beliefs may be operating.

All this is quite a sophisticated strategy for examining thoughts and beliefs. You should not expect it to work smoothly at first, but with practice you will get the hang of it and it will start to work for you. The point about experiencing emotion as part of this process is especially important though. This approach has the potential for taking you quite deep into your own psychological make-up, and as well as brushing up against ideas, beliefs and memories that you already know about, there is the possibility of realizing new things too. As with so much of work with people with dementia, there is an element of risk and unpredictability. We advise, therefore, that you seek support while exploring yourself in this way, perhaps from a colleague or friend, certainly someone with whom you feel you could explore difficult feelings or conclusions.

Thinking about meaning

As we discussed in Chapter 2 and earlier in this chapter, until recently it was taken for granted that the words and actions of those with the condition were merely fragmented expressions of the breakdown in mental processes and ignored. People with dementia were seen as beings whose existence does not adhere to the normal patterns of meaning we all value. We know now that these perceptions need to be turned upside down. If we are to be able fully to explore the possibilities in terms of exchanges in ideas and feelings, we must commit ourselves to the assumption that what people with dementia say and do always has meaning, whether or not we are able on any given occasion to interpret and understand that meaning.

Work exploring these ideas, specifically the ways in which meaning is created between two people when one has very severe difficulties, has been carried out in Scandinavia by nursing researchers.[6] Drawing on ideas about communication between mothers and infants, it is suggested that what is happening is that:

> carers of people with severe dementia impute meaning to seemingly incomprehensible communicative cues, thus creating a feeling of contact with the carer in the person cared for.[7]

The comparison with interaction between infants and their mothers is made as follows:

> when the mother acts as if the infant's cues were comprehensible, it creates a feeling in the infant that what he or she communicates has a meaning. This constitutes the beginning of a two way communication.[8]

While we could question whether the comparison between people with dementia who have had a lifetime of expressing and receiving meaning with infants who are only just setting out is a helpful one, this discussion captures the idea of meaning being an essentially interpersonal construct, and this accords with more general ideas about the socially constructed nature of personhood. Questions about the origins of meaning in communication lie in the domain of philosophy – well outside our area of competence – but the main message here for us is that it is only by approaching the person with dementia with the assumption of meaningfulness that we will have any chance of engaging properly with them.

In addition to its practical dimensions, as we shall see in the final section of this chapter, this subject also raises ethical questions.

Not everything is caused by dementia

A primary point which applies to all of the following is that whenever we encounter a person in the midst of a condition such as dementia, and it is clear that many changes have been brought about in how the person manages, it is tempting to assume that *all* of their characteristics are a consequence of the dementia. Again as we discussed in Chapter 2 on personhood, each individual with dementia came to the condition as a unique person. Some of their characteristics will be altered by their dementia, others will remain the same or even intensify. We can never know what would have happened had the dementia never struck, and similarly we can never take it for granted that the condition is responsible for what we encounter now. Thus the person who says little, mumbles only very softly when they do speak, and who tends to curtail encounters by closing their eyes and bowing their head, may always have been a quiet and withdrawn person, uncomfortable with the close attention of others. A person whose speech is loud, pressured and insistent may always have been a strident conversationalist. The individual who gets stuck with certain words, and appears to give up in frustration, may have struggled with a stammer throughout their life. The relative of one person with dementia said:

> I've never noticed anything different about her language. To me it has always been difficult to understand. Sometimes now I can't understand her at all.

The person's subjective reality

We have already discussed the fact that people with dementia sometimes feel themselves to be younger than they actually are. Some seem to experience more general shifts and appear for a time to be inhabiting a different frame altogether. For example one woman appeared for part of the day to be in the role of a child. At other times she seemed to feel that she was a young adult out at work. It was clear from the way she spoke and acted that this altered frame was very real to her, and it had implications for how others behaved towards her. (This is something we discuss in the ethical implications section at the end of this chapter.)

Some people may maintain this altered perspective for long periods. For others it may fluctuate or cycle in predictable ways in accordance with events or other factors. Sometimes it is obvious that something is going on, at other times it may be more subtle with the person seeming to be experiencing an altered reality in a more inward way.

We do not understand much about why this kind of thing happens. No doubt it is highly personal and intimately tied up with what is significant to the individual and the way they see themselves and their life. Clearly, however, the effort of interpreting what the person says and does needs to take account of their subjective reality. Something which does not seem to make any sense in relation to the person's current self may be highly significant in the context of them being in the role of a young adult. Vigilance for occasions when a shift has taken place is necessary, and the more you can get to know about the way the person experiences changes in their subjective reality the better.

Understanding emotions

As part of the drive to achieve meaning, we not only have to try to make sense of what happens out there in the world of other people and things, we are also faced with the task of understanding our inner experiences. If, for instance, you notice that you are feeling especially tired, your mind will immediately start to search for an explanation: have I been working very hard? Did I have a late night? Am I ill? If you find an account which satisfies you, you will have explained your experience of tiredness. Similarly, if you were to experience a powerful surge of emotion, say anger or sadness, you would (after identifying the feeling) certainly want to be able to explain it to yourself. An inability to do so would be a source of concern.

   What about people with dementia in this regard? Is there, at least for some, alongside a continuation or even deepening in the capacity for emotional experience, a disturbance in the ability to label feelings and account for why they are occurring? If, for example, memory difficulties interfere with an individual's ability to recall that they had an acrimonious exchange earlier in the day, then it may be hard to account for feelings of anger and upset. We imagine that the experience of strong feelings without the ability to explain them is distressing. If we are right about the association between emotion and memory, then it could be that for such an individual the presence of anger may heighten access to other experiences of anger from memory, further confusing the situation. Perhaps the heightened emotionality we see in some people with dementia arises from the inability to make reliable sense of feelings. We need to bear these possibilities in mind when working with them, and it may be that at times we can make a direct contribution to helping people to understand their emotions.

The role of empathy

As individuals we are in many ways isolated in our own separate worlds. We can never truly know what it feels like to be another person. The extent to which you operate on the assumption that your world bears a resemblance to that of another, and that you can achieve a 'good enough' understanding of how it feels to be someone else and vice versa, forms part of your individual belief system and personality, and has a direct bearing on behaviour. When assumptions about similarity and differentness lie towards the extremes this may lead to serious problems. Someone who feels themselves to be so different from those around them that trying to explain what they think about things is pointless, will have relationships with others which are distant and superficial. If, on the other hand, a person assumes that others are very similar to them, then they may feel it is not necessary to consider others' feelings and preferences when making decisions that affect them. Such an attitude will also give rise to difficulties. Most of us lie somewhere in the middle. We know and feel ourselves to be different from others in some respects, but also share a sufficient sense of commonality to support satisfying relationships and straightforward effective interactions.

In order to make sense of the behaviour of others it is necessary to interpret what another person says or does within the context of their personality and general style of behaving, and to try to understand this with reference to their experience of the world of people, things and ideas. Skills of empathy help us to do this. Empathy is the ability consciously to enter into the world of another human being, and to try to see and feel things from their point of view. It involves effort, may be painful, and demands that we use our own experience in an imaginative way. Given that during this effort we remain ourselves, yet are striving to enter into the experience of another, it requires us to maintain a complex set of boundaries. The process of empathising involves the ability to soften those boundaries, at least temporarily, and to use our own experience to get closer to an imaginative understanding of another. At all times during this process we remain aware that we are not actually the other, and never will be. But we must believe that it is possible, and at times desirable, to find ways of expanding our understanding what it feels like to be another. Of this the psychologist Nicholas Humphrey says:

> Empathy means feeling simultaneously with others: not just imagining at one remove another person's state of mind but experiencing that very feeling in one's own person right now – seeing someone else in distress and having tears come to one's own eyes; hearing their laughter and finding oneself smiling with them.[9]

If effective interpretation in interpersonal dealings involves the ability to empathize with another person in their particular circumstances, how is this to be achieved where people with dementia are concerned? Some may think that without direct experience of the condition it is impossible properly to obtain a feeling of how it is to be in their place. In a strict sense, this must be so. However, we are firmly of the view that the minute-to-minute and day-to-day experience of the individual is probably much more influenced by the same sorts of physical, psychological, environmental and interpersonal processes which affect us all, dementia or no dementia. It should be possible, therefore, to use our experience and awareness of these processes in order to achieve a greater sense of their likely effects on the individual.

Tom Kitwood has the following to say on this subject:

As we discover the person who has dementia we also discover something of ourselves. For what we ultimately have to offer is not technical expertise but ordinary faculties raised to a higher level: our power to feel, to give, to stand in the shoes (or sit in the chair) of another, through the use of our imagination.[10]

Exercises in developing empathy

We now describe two major ways in which skills of empathy can be developed. No doubt there are others, and many possibilities for exploring variations on the basic approaches.

The first involves developing greater awareness of possible similarities between our own experiences of forgetfulness, confusion and incompetence, and those that characterize the experience of people with dementia. A simple example is that of not being able to find something. Perhaps you are standing at a till in a busy shop. You are convinced you have enough cash to pay for the item, but when you check your purse or wallet, there is not enough. Where else could it be? You start to rummage, aware that the shop assistant is rolling her eyes, and people behind you in the queue are fidgeting. At this point you could try noticing what you are experiencing. What thoughts are going through your mind? How would you label your emotions? Are there accompanying physical feelings? What do they make you want to do? Perhaps your thoughts and emotions are very similar to those experienced by people with dementia when a difficulty is encountered? Of course there are also dissimilarities. Presumably you are not encountering this sort of episode as frequently as someone with the condition, and you are aware that your inability to find your money is not part of a larger and more sinister pattern. But nevertheless there are parallel features which provide an opportunity for developing greater understanding. There is a whole range of experiences like this, from the trivial to the more serious (for example being acutely ill and unable to express your thoughts and feelings clearly) which can be creatively explored in the effort to empathize more fully with the experience of people with dementia.

An example of the second strategy would be to spend a period of time 'in role' as a person with dementia. This is most easily done within a service setting, but could also be tried within a family situation. It generally involves more planning, and will probably entail other people adopting certain roles towards you. A member of staff in a nursing home known to us tried being a resident for a day. For her this exercise was a powerful way of highlighting unanticipated but highly salient aspects of experience of being on the receiving end of care, such as the discomfort of spending long periods sitting, and the experience of being helped to eat.

The effect of prior knowledge about the individual

The possession of knowledge about the individual with dementia prior to the onset of their condition is generally upheld as a useful adjunct to care. Information of this sort may be obtained from the person themselves, or from relatives or other carers. While we agree that often background information can play a very useful role in understanding the person's words and actions, we all need to adopt a sensitivity and openness in using this knowledge to make sense of the person's current behaviour. Whatever information we have is likely to be incomplete, and perhaps to a degree distorted (if entirely unintentionally) by having been filtered through others, and their complex needs and motivations. There is also the fact that as people get older they can change, and what was previously a strong preference may no longer hold such attraction for an individual. Basically, the possession of background information can be an asset, but should be treated in a cautious way with an awareness of the dangers of fitting what we see too slavishly into old patterns and ways of behaving.

The distinction between observation and interpretation

Prior to any discussion of developing skills of actual interpretation, it is necessary to draw attention to a crucial distinction, and this applies both to verbal and nonverbal communication. The distinction is that between *observation* and *interpretation*. The skill of observation is that of attending to what can actually be seen, heard, felt and so on. The raw data of observation are that which would be available to anyone from your point of view, and stop short of actual interpretation, which (as we have discussed) involves going beyond that which is given and trying to make sense of it.

It is a common mistake to see someone behaving in a certain way and automatically to assume that you know what is going on in their mind, and proceed to behave accordingly. For example, if you were to observe someone pushing food around their plate but making no attempt to eat it, you might then think that they did not like the food or were unwilling to eat. This would be one interpretation, and if you did not question it further you might never find out that actually the person's dentures are a bad fit, and attempting to chew causes great discomfort. Leaping to the wrong conclusion and acting on it would serve only to muddle the situation further. It is important to develop the ability to observe carefully, and then to be more deliberate and cautious in the further act of interpretation. Again (as was explored above) it is necessary to make interpretations. We would all be overloaded with disconnected pieces of information, and paralysed in our actions if we did not, but it is possible to learn to interpret in a more flexible way, and to treat our interpretations as theories to be tested rather than as fact. We shall return to the distinction between observation and interpretation later in this chapter.

The role of intuition

Our advice so far has been to become more conscious of the processes of observation and interpretation, implying perhaps that we can reach the right answers through conscious reasoning. Actually, it seems unlikely that such a thing is possible. Much of successful communication work draws on a different kind of sense we call intuition.

We mean by intuition an implicit sense, which normally cannot be accounted for in conventional ways, for example by recourse to logic or by citing objective evidence. The *Concise Oxford Dictionary* defines intuition as 'immediate apprehension by the mind without reasoning'. Intuition as a way of learning about the world has tended to be disparaged in our modern, evidence-based ways of operating, and it has been seen as a feminine aptitude, and so all the more suspect for that. What role has it to play in communication work with people with dementia?

We are convinced that intuition plays a very significant role in this sphere. As we saw in Chapter 3 on nonverbal communication, much of what is happening is going on below the level of normal awareness. This may in part account for its usefulness in communication with people with dementia since it is less likely to be affected by the kind of loss of confidence many people experience. But it is also a faculty which is applicable to linguistic communication. Caroline Keegan, a psychiatric nurse with long experience of caring for people in advanced stages of dementia, says:

> I have noticed how my nursing colleagues seem to experience a strong sense of what is being *meant* when these people speak to them, even though the manifest content of what is said, and often the order in which the words were spoken initially, may seem bizarre and nonsensical.[11]

Work on the role of intuition as part of exemplary caring can offer some illumination. Studies carried out in Scandinavia report that although staff members who were considered to be outstanding in the area of interpersonal work with people with advanced dementia could not explain exactly how they understood those in their care, or why they behaved in certain ways towards them, they nevertheless had an extensive understanding about the conditions affecting them.[12] They described what were essentially efforts to maintain a sense of openness, humility about what they did not know and could not understand, and a loving regard for the people with dementia in their care. Of this specialist nurse Patricia Benner says:

> Intuitive grasp is never blind as a wild guess, but relies on prior experience. It should not be confused with mysticism since it is available only in situations where a deep background understanding of the situation exists, based on a broad base of knowledge and experience.[13]

We are only at the beginning of thinking about the role of intuition in communication and work with people with dementia, but it is a fascinating area and deserves greater attention. We return to thinking about the tension which exists between a more conscious approach to observation and interpretation and the less easily articulated intuitive approach later in this chapter.

Confusion

It is probably wise to accept that in the course of undertaking communication work the experience of being confused – this is you, not the person with dementia – will be quite common. But this is not necessarily a bad thing. In most situations in life we are quick to try to remove any feelings of confusion, and replace them with a sense of certainty, to make a decision and go with it. Being in a state of confusion or uncertainty is uncomfortable for a variety of reasons. It is cognitively demanding to have competing ideas in mind, or to try to clarify vague hunches or fleeting notions. At such times we are prone to fall back on old maxims which seem to offer more solidity, but are in fact too simplistic and do not take the complexities of an individual person or their situation into account. Other reasons for wishing to remove feelings of confusion relate to our need to see ourselves as rational, competent and decisive. We like to think that we know our own minds, and can analyse complexity and reach decisions, and our society praises and rewards those qualities. The experience of being confused, therefore, arouses a degree of emotional discomfort, and it seems preferable to make a decision and proceed with a course of action, even if it turns out to be the wrong one. There is also the fact that care processes as specified by organizations increasingly emphasize the need for conscious decision-making based on evidence, and this further marginalizes the role of intuitive approaches.

But what about the positive potential of the experience of confusion? Psychologists are beginning to recognize that a state of confusion may actually foster new learning and creativity in some circumstances, especially in situations involving complex phenomena which are not easily verbalized.[14] This is exactly the sort of scenario we are often faced with when involved with people with dementia. Being able to tolerate feelings of confusion long enough to allow transient impressions, apparently contradictory notions and hunches to develop is likely to be more helpful than recourse to explicit reasoning based on existing assumptions or 'knowledge'.

Another reason for remaining open to – even cultivating – experiences of confusion was mentioned above. Since this is the experience of so many people with dementia, our powers of empathy are likely to be heightened by such a practice.

Developing interpretive skills

When starting out on developing skills in this area it is probably best, if possible, to spend some time carrying out observation work prior to entering into interactions. In this way you can give yourself time to develop a sense of the individual's general style. This 'baseline' information will help you in your efforts to notice and interpret their responses once you do enter into an encounter. Observation work of this kind is useful whether or not the person communicates verbally as well as nonverbally.

In addition to the act of observing in itself, we also emphasize the value of recording your observations in some way. This may involve writing notes, talking into a tape recorder, or speaking to another person about what you see and hear. Externalizing your thoughts and impressions often has the effect of further raising awareness and increasing sensitivity to subtle aspects of behaviour. New thoughts arise and connections are made. Having done this, it is clearly of benefit to retain such things as notes for further reflection and reference. If this is done over a period of time you are likely to be struck by a process of development in your approach and understanding, and this is both useful for the people in your care and rewarding for you.

It is important here to mention again the distinction between observation and interpretation. As you become more skilled in observation and more used to reflecting on what you see and hear in an interpretive fashion, you run the risk of blurring the boundaries between what is observable in terms of behaviour and actions and what you make of it in your own mind. Try to find ways of reminding yourself of the distinction. One method for reinforcing this when writing notes is to have two columns marked 'observation' and 'interpretation'.

Since we have emphasized throughout this book the importance of nonverbal communication in working with people with dementia, and because of the need to counteract our inherent bias towards language, we start with consideration of skills development in this area. First of all, however, we should acknowledge that learning new skills is hard work. It takes a lot of conscious and effortful practice, but if this is maintained then the transition to smoother functioning will take place.

Everyday observations

1 Look around you while waiting for a bus, observe people in the canteen, turn the sound down on the television, and simply *look* at what you see. It may be easiest to start by making a point of studying one particular aspect of nonverbal communication first, and then moving on to others. Where verbal communication is concerned, when you have the opportunity to overhear conversations rather than focusing on the words themselves, try tuning into the qualities of voice, tone, volume and rhythm that accompany them. Notice how much you can learn about the speakers' states of mind, their attitudes and their relationship.

As you try out exercises of this kind, you can gradually try expanding your awareness to more and more features at once. Remind yourself of the observation/interpretation distinction here. Notice the boundary between what you see, hear and so on, and then what you make of what you are seeing. You can also progress to considering your own emotional responses to what you observe, but again be aware that this is adding another layer to the whole process.

2 From carrying out observational practice in situations in which you are uninvolved, you can then move on to trying out similar skills during inter-actions of your own. This will demand that you make space for awareness of nonverbal aspects of encounters alongside taking an active part in con-versations, but again with practice this will become smoother.

   Such situations also provide opportunities for you to try to heighten your awareness of your own style of communicating nonverbally. Think about the various aspects separately at first, then try to build up a more conscious sense of how you are coming across more holistically.

3 From here you can try to identify friends or colleagues who would be will-ing to carry out simple observation exercises providing feedback on the nonverbal dynamics of interactions. Playing both participant and observer roles will help to increase your skills and confidence.

   The most reliable way of capturing the details of interactions and being able to study them in detail is to use a video camera. Such technology can be cheap, accessible and easy to operate, and it allows repeated examination of sequences of behaviour (both or all parties). Clearly there are ethical dimensions to work of this kind (even if it does not involve clients or resi-dents), and agreements about the nature and scope of the exercise must be made explicit.

The sensitivity you can derive from exercises like these can be brought to bear and developed in the context of interaction with the person with dementia. It is very difficult, however, to be very much more specific about interpreting the actions of any one person in any one situation, both because of the variability in the nature of nonverbal communication, and also because these processes are not easily verbalized, not being available to normal awareness. What seems to be required is a heightened general openness and alertness, and an accept-ance that you cannot be consciously aware of everything which is going on.

Interpretation of language

In Chapter 4 we described the four main constituents of spoken language – the sounds of words, the words themselves, ways of combining words to convey ideas, and the social rules of language use. The effort of interpreting what the person says involves maintaining an awareness of a variety and combination of the changes in these areas. Is the person struggling to articu-late the sounds of the word they have in mind? If they are having difficulty finding a particular word, their efforts are likely to produce words which are related both in sound and meaning, or from a similar category, so that 'sister' becomes 'daughter', for example. An example of this from John's experience was when one woman who, referring to his tape recorder, used the word 'philharmonic'.[15]

Broken rules of syntax are generally fairly easy to interpret. When the observance of social rules has changed in some way it may take longer to get a sense of what is different, whether it is in the area of relevance, the time taken to speak, or the exchange of turn-taking. Again (as we noted in Chapter 4) the person may be operating in a different time-scale within the conversation, so you will need to look out for responses which although substantially delayed, still make a meaningful contribution to the dialogue.

In order for meanings which are not obvious to be grasped there is a need to bring to bear a quality, which is again hard to describe – an imaginative openness to what the person is saying, which strives for a balance between immediacy of attention and a rapidity of reflection. In all of the above, of course, you can also tune into the level of the nonverbal aspects of speech such as the tone of voice, volume, pitch and patterns of intonation and stress to discern the mood and import of what is being said. These can provide vital clues, as was described in relation to Jean Copeland, whom we introduced in Chapter 4.

The following account is an example of successful interpretation regarding words, and the way they are used, from the work of dementia trainer Sally Knocker:

> Maggie, a woman who had recently moved into a residential home against her own wishes, said to me 'There is no reason to camouflage me like this. It's about a lot, you know. I've been camouflaged.' Whilst camouflage was not an obvious word to use, it was a poignantly apt and meaningful metaphor. She felt that she was being hidden away and that her views and desires had been covered up. It may be more than coincidence that the word rhymes with sabotage, which also captures some of the sense she was trying to get across. It seemed to me that Maggie was making a statement about her current dilemma and I responded to this 'Do you feel that your wishes have not been considered enough?' and she said with clarity and relief, 'Yes, that's exactly it. Thank God you understand.'[16]

The following excerpt from Anthea McKinlay's book about her mother strikes us as an extraordinarily rich example of the depth and complexity which can characterize the words of people with dementia. Among other things it reminds us that in our eagerness to perceive conventional sense, we are at risk of overlooking subtle dimensions of meaning. As with all of her conversations, this one took place over the telephone. Her mother, Catherine, speaks first:

> I was looking at the wall for ages
>
> then I realised
>
> that there was an encyclopaedia hanging on it
>
> *an encyclopaedia? hanging on the wall?*
>
> yes
>
> *the huge book? hanging on the wall?*

yes

so I said to myself:

'well – that's doing no good hanging up there' –

so I went over and took it down,

and hung it up inside my head

and you've no idea the difference it's made

what kind of difference?

well, I'm learning all kinds of things that I didn't know before

like what? can you tell me something?

the acid and passive

do you mean the <u>active</u> and passive?

well, you could say active but I don't want to

why?

acid is stronger – it takes the surface off

is that important?

yes, very

why?

because then you can see what lies underneath . . .[17]

Commenting on the part she played in this exchange, Anthea says:

> My mother encouraged me to look beyond the surface of things, and to live from my deepest self. My questions in it are to draw out of her what she was meaning to communicate to me. In terms of her dementia, it was often my experience that without such questions she would 'stop' as if losing momentum and then would 'start up' again immediately following on from a question – when she could hear in my voice that what she was saying was very important to me and I wanted to understand. I was learning so much from her about how to listen and how to live.[18]

Issues in interpretation

As we have seen, ways of creating meaning out of our own words and actions and those of the person with dementia is a complex business. Some of it is available for observation and reflection, some of it is not. In the following sections we examine a few of the issues which arise.

Conscious and unconscious reasoning

We have in this chapter described two main approaches to interpretation. The first, conscious observation and interpretation, where there is a relatively clear and identifiable process underway, which can be described and justified to others. The other is the much less well understood, and less well respected faculty of intuition. How compatible are these approaches? To what extent can they be separated or combined? The reality for most of us most of the time must be that we call on both forms of interpretation, in a complex combination, and the very act of trying to ponder the distinction is likely to blur it further.

The process of developing skills in this sphere is similarly likely to be a combination of the implicit and explicit. We might be able to identify and describe some of the changes in our approach or understanding which have taken place over time, but be unable to give what seems to be anything like a complete account. Often we recognize changes in our outlook only by discovering evidence of it in an indirect way. So for example, when you go back over notes you wrote about something several months previously, you may be struck by the fact that you did not mention something which would seem obvious to you to consider now. Reading books like this may reveal a similar pattern – at one reading certain ideas stand out while others do not have any real resonance. Later, however, other subjects emerge as being of particular interest and significance.

Uncertainty

All kinds of interpretation involve uncertainty. In reality we can never be totally sure that we have understood things correctly, and our lives would be significantly disrupted if we tried. We have to get by using our best efforts to make sense of the complexity of ourselves, our relationships and the world around us. We learn to tolerate a degree of uncertainty, and most of the time things work out alright.

This also applies to our work with people with dementia. Sometimes, even when an individual's language and nonverbal communication has changed significantly, a feeling of conviction is possible. This is what Caroline Keegan was describing when she was quoted talking about 'a strong sense of what is being meant'.[19] However, perhaps more of the time we have to operate within a context of uncertainty, going with hunches, theories and intuitions. While in other interpersonal situations we have a range of ways of clarifying our impressions, for example by asking someone to repeat or expand on something they have said, or to supplement their nonverbal communication by verbal means, in encounters with people with dementia such means are not so readily available.

In John's experience, asking someone to repeat or clarify an utterance is rarely successful, and may actually serve to disrupt the flow of communication by drawing attention to ambiguities or difficulties. Nonverbal channels are even less amenable to discussion. We are obliged to proceed with much less certainty about the meaning of what is being said or enacted, and this can be uncomfortable. Some of us are better at handling this than others, but it does mean that communication is harder work since tolerating lack of clarity places extra demands on our information-processing systems.

Successful interpretation will depend, as in relation to other features of communication, on one's ability to generate ideas about what is being expressed by the person, to entertain hypotheses, modify their own behaviour in response to these, and to provide appropriate support for the individual who is struggling to express their ideas. There is the need to strive to achieve this difficult balance between identifying and pursuing plausible interpretations at the same time as maintaining an open and questioning attitude to what is happening.

Sometimes ideas about what someone was trying to express will only arise after the opportunity to develop an interaction is over. This is frustrating but inevitable. But no effort is wasted in this regard. You may have the chance to continue with the person in question, or pass on your idea to someone else who is involved.

Getting it wrong

We started out by discussing the fact that interpretation is an inherently risky activity. In trying to make sense of what we see and hear we court the possibility of distorting precious opportunities for the individual with dementia to express their views and needs. We may misunderstand particular words or phrases, miss the emphases and muddle up the emotional messages, and at times we may get the whole thing completely wrong. How should we cope with the fear or reality of these things happening?

The first point to make is that refraining from using skills of interpretation with people with dementia in response to fears about making mistakes is not an option. As we have seen, this is something we all do all the time in relation to all aspects of our lives. We cannot simply suspend this activity in relation to people with dementia, and proceed in a kind of pure state where no efforts are made to make sense of what we find and experience. Accepting the reality of errors (the vast majority of which will not have devastating consequences), but continually working on improving skills and awareness, seems the most rational response to this state of affairs.

It is also important to recognize that an inevitable aspect of learning new skills is that along with the developmental process there comes a greater awareness of the possibility of mistakes. Whereas prior to starting to develop knowledge and skills close attention would not have been paid to one's own behaviour and its effects, once a process of conscious learning and reflection has become established, errors suddenly acquire a new prominence and this can be very demoralizing. This sort of experience is actually part of a wider process which occurs in all sorts of areas of skills learning, and it is discussed at greater length in Chapter 14 on implications for care.

When you do not understand at all

Sometimes, despite your best efforts to identify patterns in a person's speech, you will find yourself unable to do so. Such situations present special challenges, and may give rise to feelings of anxiety or inadequacy. John has taken part in a great many conversations in which his understanding of the subject or subjects under discussion was severely lacking. The excerpt of his conversation with Jean Copeland from Chapter 4 is an example of this. However, in many instances the nonverbal signals accompanying the person's speech give strong indications of the nature of the messages being conveyed, and the type of response required. Although the exchange of meaning is not at the level of the precision of individual ideas, it nevertheless can constitute what seems to be a deep and affirming form of communication.

When understanding seems impossible, however, there is always recourse to humour. Here is John Bayley describing the part it played in his relationship with Iris Murdoch:

> Our mode of communication seems like underwater sonar, each bouncing pulsations off the other, and listening for an echo. The baffling moments at which I cannot understand what Iris is saying, or about whom or what – moments which can produce tears and anxieties, though never, thank goodness, the raging frustration typical of many Alzheimer's sufferers – can sometimes be dispelled by embarking on a joky parody of helplessness, and trying to make it mutual. Both of us at a loss for words.[20]

Implications for care

If the care of people with dementia were to be organized much more explicitly around the goal of promoting communication, through and alongside all other forms of activity, then the recognition that effort and energy must go into interpretation should follow. What might this mean in practice? For one thing the time it takes properly to reflect on interactions and any notes or transcripts arising from these needs to be recognized. Although this is an outlay in terms of resources, there are the gains staff make in terms of greater understanding of those in their care, a greater sense of meaning and satisfaction in the work, and heightened sensitivity to future interactions which is likely to follow from reflecting properly on previous ones.

The expectation that staff members should make efforts to think about the meaning of what is being offered to them needs to be communicated in various ways: in conversation with peers, supervisors and managers, and in the systems which exist for keeping records and communicating with other practitioners. The sharing of insights between staff members is a particularly important aspect of this; indeed it seems often to be the case that it is in the discussion of incidents with others that new ideas and perspectives in the search for meaning actually arise. Opportunities of this sort should also be geared towards helping staff, in a supportive way, to challenge their own negative assumptions about dementia as a condition and the effects of these on their dealings with individuals. This needs to be an ongoing process, with everyone recognizing the baggage they have accumulated which distorts perceptions and the possibilities for specific encounters.

Underlying all of this is the urgent need to boost the confidence and self-esteem of those who spend most time with people with dementia in undertaking this sort of work. Given sincerity and positive regard for the person, the frontline worker has most to offer as regards interpretation work, both in terms of what is being meant by an individual on any one occasion, and also the nature of the whole process itself.

Ethical implications

Our values

As we discussed at length in this chapter, we make sense of our experience with reference to a set of underlying beliefs. It is crucial to recognize here that beliefs about aspects of our lives which do not involve people (for example, the weather or the passage of time), are neutral in value terms, that is not relating to ideas about what is right or wrong. Where beliefs about people are concerned, however, they are almost always value-laden. Our ways of thinking about people are permeated by ideas about what is good or bad, admirable or blameworthy, in terms of their characteristics, attitudes and actions.

In addition to more specific beliefs and assumptions, we have images in our minds – stereotypes – buried deep in our ways of thinking, of what people, especially people who occupy certain roles, *should* be like. As we have already mentioned, we live in a culture which is deeply prejudiced against older people, and which has very narrow ideas about their characteristics. The more pervasive the prejudice, the narrower is the stereotype within which individuals can be considered acceptable. Within these restrictive ways of thinking, there are idealized images of what a 'good' or 'acceptable' older person should be. So for example, a common perception is that an older woman should be sweet, agreeable, and grateful for help given to her by others. If she displays these characteristics, she might be considered a 'nice old lady'. She certainly would not be described in this way if she were assertive, demanding and disgruntled. Ideas about dependency, vulnerability and differentness are closely woven into these images. We have similar prejudices about people who are ill and disabled and near death, and have corresponding expectations about what are good and bad ways to play out these roles.

In addition to those images which are handed to us to through the media, literature and so on, we have our own personalized images. These are based on our own experience, and that of those close to us, and they develop through our idiosyncratic ways of filtering and interpreting those which exist in the dominant culture. Thus someone who has experience of an older person being stoical and self-sacrificing will have a different reaction to the television portrayal of an older person who is dying, from someone, say, whose contact with older people has been characterized more by perceptions of dependency and vulnerability.

All this may seem to be very far from the business of communication with people with dementia. But it is actually crucial. Whenever we encounter an individual and begin to try to make sense of their actions and words, and the dispositions and motivations which underpin them, we do so through the filter of our notions of what they, or someone in their position, is or should be like. Because our ways of thinking about people and their behaviour are always value-laden, this process of interpretation is unavoidably value-laden too. We may tell ourselves that as professionals we can be above such a personal dimension, but this is, in our opinion, an example of self-deception. Our own very personal experiences, beliefs and needs are right there in the encounter. This is one example of how working with people with dementia demands the involvement of the whole of us.

Of course these processes are at work in all of our interpersonal dealings, they are the very stuff of our social existence. What makes them of particular significance where work with people with dementia is concerned, is that here we are dealing with persons whose identity and coherence in the eyes of many has been put in question by the presence of the condition, and who are relatively powerless. Whether we believe that their personhood is threatened by the dementia itself, or more by the way that those around them react to it, it is undeniable that the behaviour of such an individual is regarded as being importantly different. It is subjected to a more conscious process of interpretation, and that process of interpretation is more likely to include speculation, not only about the meaning of words or actions, but also about whether any meaning can be attached to them at all. And the fact of their relative powerlessness means that although we are all the time constructing and responding to our own internally driven images of others, those who are not compromised by a condition like dementia are more likely to be able to influence our perception of them, and attempt to correct perceived biases, than is the person with dementia.

All this means that in our encounters with people with dementia we are, through the processes of interpretation, at a much greater risk of distorting the identity of the other, allowing our own biases and needs to gain the upper hand. Speaking of how nurses make sense of the actions of people with dementia in their care, the Swedish nurse researcher Astrid Norberg says:

> It would be dangerous if caregivers were to impute meaning to the patient's cues in an uncontrolled manner. The patient would then become a creation of the caregiver, an object.[21]

Given that we cannot avoid the involvement of our own idiosyncratic ways of

thinking, and that there is a degree of distortion and prejudice in the belief systems of every one of us, how can we best minimize their effects? One answer would be that we must try to deepen our understanding of our own systems of values, and how they influence our day-to-day behaviour. The more aware we are, the greater are the chances that we will be able to identify biases and counteract their effects. Some of this heightened awareness comes through private reading and reflection, and we hope that the material in this book will help. But a powerful way of developing greater understanding comes through talking to others, sharing ideas and experiences, and testing out the extent to which one's own ways of understanding accord with those of others. Often it is only in the act of speaking about something that we realize that we actually believe it. As we shall explore in some depth in Chapter 10, writing is another powerful tool in this effort.

Divergences in values reveal themselves most sharply when difficulties arise or there is a need for a decision to be made. They are tested when we are faced with the choice of whether or not to support someone in making a decision that we ourselves feel to be a mistake. The extent of our commitment to upholding the personhood of the other is also put to the test when their choice conflicts directly with those of other people who are involved. At times people with dementia will say or do things we ourselves find distasteful, shocking or even disturbing. At such times it is especially important to seek out opportunities to reflect on what it was that was so personally affecting.

The following questions may be helpful in bringing our values into more conscious awareness:

- What, at the most basic level, do we value people for – their intellect, their ability to remember, their emotions, or their capacity to relate to others in positive ways?
- How committed are we to seeing people with dementia as being basically more similar to ourselves than different?
- How able are we to deal with the fact that the person with dementia may have values and habits which are very different from our own?
- How far can we support the person's right to make choices about their own life which differ from the ones we would make ourselves? How much uncertainty or anxiety are we prepared to experience ourselves in the course of doing so?
- How committed are we to supporting the person in taking part in their own emotional life, especially when those emotions are painful? To what extent do we perceive our own role as that of protector or even withholder of the opportunities for people to experience emotion?

If we are committed to encountering people as they actually are, whether or not they conform to our ideas about what is desirable or admirable, then this must rely on the creation of opportunities when people can express their own ideas and feelings and ways of seeing the world. This is the essence of good communication, and it is only through this kind of direct experience that our narrowness can be challenged and stretched. We are reminded here of the words of chaplain Debbie Everett (p. 38), who characterized people with dementia as 'magic mirrors' helping us to encounter ourselves at a deeper level.

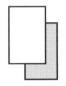 **Part 2:** Practicalities

7 Making contact: 'To get us into a normal situation'

In the next four chapters we explore practical approaches to interacting with people with dementia. Alongside material with a specifically practical emphasis we include discussion of issues and ideas to encourage you to reflect positively but critically on your own experience. In this way we hope to help you to gain confidence in using skills and knowledge, and find ways of enabling the people in your care to communicate more successfully. In this first chapter we examine ways of initiating relationships and commencing interactions, but we begin with some more general points.

Preliminary considerations

The way that an encounter between two people begins is important. Facial expression, tone of voice, body positioning and one's choice of words all combine to create a powerful initial impression which reaches into the rest of the interaction. Some people make us feel instantly at ease, others uneasy or even anxious. Sometimes an exchange establishes itself and unfolds in a relaxed way, others take time to find their rhythm, some feel sticky and awkward throughout. We have all had the experience of wishing that we could abandon a particular encounter and simply start again.

Sometimes no special thought is needed about when or how to speak to someone. At others we give a lot of consideration to the best time and circumstances in which to open a conversation. Where does communication with people figure in this? How, in Alice Jopling's words, can we find the best way 'to get us into a normal situation'?

Breaking into the world of the person with dementia

Although we are fundamentally social beings, each of us inhabits an internal world of thoughts and feelings, and a sphere of private actions. We have to integrate this inner world along with that of being and interacting with other human beings. Every interaction we enter into involves judgements and decisions about intrusion, and again this applies as much to people with dementia as to those without. Of this Laurel Rust, a care assistant, writes:

> Like all of us, the very old have codes of their own: sometimes you can find your way into them and sometimes you can't. I struggled with the question of if I was intruding. Does an 83 year old woman want to be comprehensible? Does she want me to follow her?[1]

It is another function of the power differential between ourselves and people with dementia that we are less likely to give consideration to the matter of whether our own behaviour could constitute an intrusion when an approach to a person with dementia is being contemplated than one to someone without the condition. It is as if we assume that the individual should be available to respond to our attention at any time. This matter is complicated by the fact that while other people are more likely to be able to give clear messages about whether they are open to an approach, the person with dementia may project more ambiguous messages.

So there is a dilemma here. We are advocating that people with dementia need far more opportunities for genuine communication than they commonly receive, but we are also saying that we need to be alert to the possibility of making an unwelcome intrusion into their world. How can you, on any individual occasion, know whether it is right to approach the person and attempt to initiate an interaction? There is, of course, no simple answer to this question. It is one we explore further in the material on ethical implications at the end of this chapter.

State of mind and expectations

Whenever we enter into an interpersonal encounter we have certain expectations about what will happen. For most encounters, the kind which make up the main part of our social dealings, we are not especially aware of our expectations. They have become habitual. For other sorts of encounters, for example asking another person out on a date, making a complaint or denying having committed a crime, we would be much more aware of what we hope or fear as an outcome.

In circumstances where one person is disabled and the act of communication itself is the goal, awareness of our expectations is likely to be heightened. Inevitably this will exert an influence on the way we think, feel and behave, whether to positive or negative effect. At the same time the degree of certainty about the nature and course of the encounter (compared to a more mundane situation) may be much reduced, and this greater uncertainty will influence our actions and responses. There is also the crucial matter of the expectations of the person with dementia. For the most part we can only hypothesize what these may be, but there is value in doing so, and we come on to this in a later section.

These are all exceedingly complex psychological phenomena, and while it is impossible to explore them in depth, they deserve some consideration. We therefore devote space here to considering what these may be and their potential effects on the interaction.

The desire to make contact for its own sake vs having a sense of duty

We could readily agree that being motivated by an inherent desire to connect with and affirm the personhood of another human being is better than being propelled by a sense of duty about attempting to communicate because it is expected by others. The reasons why any one individual is in contact with a person or persons with dementia will be hugely various, and we cannot enter into a discussion of the moral status of these. But we hope that the very fact that you are reading this book means that you have an interest in and a desire to enhance opportunities for communication, and suggest that even if you do not feel that you can lay claim at present to a passion for this goal (and if so, this is probably closely tied up with the number and extent of other demands on your time and energy), this is something that can develop in the course of practising the art of in-depth communication. The satisfaction and sense of meaning that successes bring become their own reward, and probably even more potent will be the positive effect that true connection has for the individual with dementia.

Preconceptions about the chances of success

As we discussed in Chapter 6, we inevitably carry into the encounter the baggage of our 'knowledge' (more accurately described as beliefs) of dementia in general, of the apparent effects of dementia on the ability of a person to communicate, and of the capacities and dispositions of the individual person. We remember our experiences of previous interactions, and are aware of the context (and sometimes the external purpose) of the encounter. It is not easy to put all of these aside and invest energy in approaching the interaction with a clean sheet, but we again suggest that this is a skill which can be developed, and brings real rewards.

It may be helpful to bear in mind the variable nature of dementia as a condition, and the heightened effects of the social and built environment on the functioning of the person. Familiarizing oneself with and recalling accounts of unexpected levels of ability in people with dementia (this book provides many examples) is useful. Reminding yourself that your own bearing and behaviour are likely to have a significant impact on the opportunity can also help you to try as hard as possible.

Possession of prior information about the individual

In situations when you are meeting a person for the first time, the question arises as to whether it is necessary or helpful to have information about them before engaging in interaction. Obviously where you are encountering the person through a referral system, information – whether verbal or written – comes first, and is given status commensurate with the values of our social and health care systems. However, when nothing is known prior to the first encounter, this can prove to be an advantage. We suggest that even in situations when some information has already been provided, there is merit in meeting the person before seeking further knowledge about them. Being in possession of the person's medical history tends to channel our view of them into the template of a cluster of symptoms rather than of a whole person. This can be true even of the kind of information which is detailed under headings like 'Social History' and 'Other', because our ways of training practitioners encourage succinct factual description and therefore inevitably the condensation of rich and complex experience into simplistic categories. Reading the medical and/or social care notes before being introduced to the person may seem like the rational and safest course of action, and going forth without the armoury of such information may seem unprofessional, but we advocate that these are values and practices which need to be challenged and experimented with in the service of empowering individuals with dementia.

Self-consciousness and authenticity

We have already talked (in Chapter 2 on personhood) about the importance of maintaining an image of ourselves as rational, competent and appropriate individuals, both in our own eyes and in the eyes of others. Social norms and specific rules of etiquette help us to navigate the complex waters of social interaction, and most of the time we get by without giving offence or suffering significant embarrassment. The occasions in all of our lives when things go wrong make wonderful anecdotes, and most of us never tire of hearing about these small misfortunes of others.

Where communication with people with dementia, or at least some of them, is concerned the issue of the definition of 'normal' behaviour can change. While certainly not wishing to suggest that all or even most individuals with the condition will engage in bizarre behaviour, it is undeniable that we can be presented with situations which are outside of the normal range in terms of conventional social interaction. These alterations in social behaviour may be relatively subtle, for example a greater or lesser amount of eye contact or a slightly slower rate of verbal response than is usually the case. Or they may be of a very much more noticeable nature. Their verbal responses may be of an unfamiliar kind which are difficult to understand, or there may be only occasional outward responses from the person at all. If the person's actions are of an unpredictable nature then their potentially challenging effect is likely to be heightened.

The mere thought of trying to interact with someone whose capabilities are uncertain and behaviour is unusual is enough to induce feelings of anxiety in most of us, and the idea of attempting to engage in such interaction in front of others, some of whom may not know or appreciate the motives for doing so, is certainly likely to trigger strong feelings of self-consciousness or even embarrassment. If the concept of personal authenticity is related to the degree of congruence between our inward feelings and our outward behaviour, then such a situation as this is likely to bring about a painful sense of being inauthentic. These feelings have to be acknowledged and worked through, both for our own well-being and that of the other person. One of the demands (and rewards) that working at enhancing communication with people with dementia brings is to challenge our values about what is normal or acceptable and to expand our repertoire of skills and intuitive sensitivities.

It is a platitude to say that practice makes perfect, but it really is true that the more you try out the skills we describe below the more natural and authentic they will feel. But you should expect it to feel strange at first. Hopefully you will have an experience of success (however defined) early on, and this will encourage you to continue trying. It is helpful to remind yourself frequently why you are doing this in the first place, and making up a sentence which you can repeat to yourself when in doubt will be useful. (An example is 'Most people with dementia are desperate for conversation and communication. Their needs are more important than my need to seem in control.') The more you can hold the reality of the personhood of the other and the purpose of the effort to the front of your mind, the less chance your fears about appearing incompetent or strange will have to hamper the encounter. As you concentrate on the details of the interaction and become absorbed in the responses of the other person, you will find that your feelings of self-consciousness will lessen or even disappear altogether for short periods at a time. By now your value system and repertoire of skills are undergoing change, and the sorts of behaviour that triggered feelings of embarrassment previously will take on a new sense of significance and power. Authenticity is restored in a richer and more diverse range. The time you spend in attempts to engage in genuine communication will undoubtedly help you to develop as a person yourself – a gift from the individual and a deep reward indeed.

Holding realistic expectations of the encounter

While real and in many ways astonishing gains can be made from investing effort in promoting interaction, it is important to be realistic in one's expectations. You will not change the life of the other by a single act of genuine communication. You may at first attempt go only some way towards clarifying where the particular challenges with an individual lie. But if you have managed that, and also laid the foundations for future relationship, then this is a major achievement. You will probably have made only provisional contact, but may with a mixture of positive intentions, skill and good fortune, have experienced one or two moments of memorable communion. We have to be content with small advances, and unexpected and occasional gains in this work.

The state of mind and expectations of the individual with dementia

Here we give consideration to possible or probable preconceptions and states of mind of the other person. The first thing to recognize is that for the vast majority of such people, there will be within their experience many instances of unsuccessful communication. The reasons for these will undoubtedly be complex and difficult to tease out. But this history of failure, and the likely emotional and behavioural effects – frustration, anger and even despair, and perhaps aggression or withdrawal – must be taken into account.

We know from research that when encounters between an older person in a care setting and staff take place normally they are most likely to be brief and instrumental (that is, in the service of some other goal, for example personal care).[2] They are likely to leave the person feeling outpaced (see Chapters 3 and 4 for a fuller discussion of this idea) and generally disempowered. It is important to bear in mind that this pattern of experience is a possibility when making the first approach.

Opportunities for in-depth communication which are tuned closely to the needs of the individual, and place the motivations of the other party firmly in a secondary role, are rare. We therefore cannot expect the person with dementia to adapt immediately to the prospect of having such an experience. Sometimes people with dementia appear only too eager to enter into relationship, but if, for another individual, the effort of communicating is a tiring one, then we should understand if they show signs of wariness about investing their energy in such an attempt. We can only imagine the emotional effects when others reach out in only the most superficial and hasty manner where there is a great need for substantive communication, and therefore we can understand the consequent withdrawal by the person into their own world.

We have dwelt upon discouragement here because it is such a common occurrence. Occasionally, however, one encounters someone who has had good conversational experiences recently, and this becomes immediately apparent by the ease with which they respond to your approaches and the relaxed body language which is visible from the outset. Occasionally, too, there is the person whose reaction is almost over-enthusiastic: on encountering John for the first time, one woman started shouting 'I love you!' across the room and miming an embrace. Here a quietly calming response seemed called for!

Some people seem well aware of the potential for normalization inherent in the communication process. Alice, whom we met in Chapter 1, was such a person and voiced this thought in the sentence we have adopted to form part of the title of this chapter.

To return to instances where lack of success in other encounters has set up an impediment to progress, one can take heart from the knowledge that in this first interaction, the foundations of future success can be laid. An example from John's experience is Judy, whose story is told on p. 107.

Getting started

We have attempted to be as practical as possible in what follows, but since we are discussing scenarios which are extremely complex, it is impossible to cover every eventuality.[3] It is therefore necessary for the reader to interpret our advice within the context of their own service or care setting.

Place of interaction

Generally speaking we should afford the individual privacy in this matter, as we would if dementia were not a factor. However, given the physical layout and facilities provided in many care settings, aspirations to complete privacy are often unrealistic. Having said that, it may be possible, given judicious arrangement of chairs and screens to create a sense of intimacy even if others are nearby. What is likely to prove unproductive is having others (relatives or staff) observing but not participating in the interaction. This 'goldfish bowl' scenario is insulting to the person with dementia and unlikely to encourage them to be forthcoming.

If most conversations are going to take place in a public area then you will have to get used to entering a roomful of people and making your initial contacts under the curious gaze of others. This can be an uncomfortable experience. If you do not know anyone in the room, who should you approach? John's usual practice is to find a vacant seat and then look around. It does not usually take long to catch someone's eye, and if the response is favourable you can then move closer. In some instances, when you know who you are going to speak to, it would be more tactful to ask someone to fetch the person so that you can meet them in privacy rather than have this happen with an audience.

You may have to get used to others taking a close interest in the early stages of the interaction; if this is uncomfortable you will have to make a decision about changing the location in some way. There is the possibility of interruptions from others who would also like to speak to you. Some firmness is needed in dealing with this scenario. Explaining that this time belongs to the person you have begun to talk to, and their time could come later or on another occasion is one way of responding. If the attentions of the third party become persistent you may have to transfer your interaction to another place.

It is a common feature of John's experience that being visibly engaged in communication in a public area heightens others' awareness of their need for genuine interpersonal contact so you should not be surprised if this occurs.

Although many people do prefer a quiet and private space in which to speak or otherwise interact, for some individuals time is more comfortably spent in a 'transitional' space such as a corridor or hallway. In John's experience many significant exchanges have taken place on the move, either inside or outside the building. This suits people for whom walking is an important activity, while talking in the more impersonal context of a corridor can create a feeling of relative safety or ease of escape for them if the situation becomes too intense.

Many people with dementia spend a great deal of time indoors, even when opportunities for being outside are within reach. For some people the effect of being outside of a building or in some other setting altogether may be dramatic. The following is an account from Trisha Kotai-Ewers, who works as a writer with people with dementia in Australia:[4]

> After lunch we sat in the sunshine. Grant's fluency increased. He spoke of being a volunteer and helping in the Centre. I was overcome with confusion. Could I have made a mistake? Was this really a new volunteer? For ten minutes while Grant spoke, I agonised about how I could explain my mistake to him. Suddenly his language lost cohesion.
>
> Several times during the following months I observed a similar improvement whenever we were outside. I was intrigued as to possible causes. Was it direct sunshine? Or the freedom of open space? Or more probably a combination of these, together with the relaxing effect of nature. Some time later sociologist, Elery Hamilton-Smith assured me that researchers have found that even a picture of natural scenes can relieve tension. Presumably, for Grant at least, one of the outcomes of this release was improved verbal communication. He confirmed this preference for sunshine when I visited him at a respite home one afternoon.
>
> 'This is probably the best time. I like doing things in the warmth and things.'[5]

Of course in the UK going outside is not a guarantee of experiencing sunshine and warmth! However, perhaps we underestimate the benefits for people with dementia of being outside buildings even when the weather is not particularly benevolent. The stimulation of fresh air and wind, even of being out in the rain, sleet or snow, is a normal part of life for most of us, and for those who have led outdoor lives – for occupational or leisure reasons – spending a great deal of time indoors may be a particular deprivation. So often we deny these aspects of life to those we perceive as being ill and in need of protection.

Going outside to spend time with someone can have the added benefit of being more private, and if there is a prospect of a series of interactions, the stimulation involved can become part of a distinctive context which may enhance memory.

When to make contact

There are many factors which bear on the issue of when conversations should best take place. Most of us have a daily rhythm of times of alertness and tiredness, and for people with dementia these variations can have a marked effect on their level of functioning. The difference in the ability to engage in an interaction between, say, late morning and early afternoon could be very significant. Obviously trying to notice when an individual seems most lively, and capitalizing on this as an opportunity for the demands of one to one communication is sensible. We appreciate that in busy service settings, however, it can be difficult to make the most of these times.

For others the patterns may be less predictable. A combination of factors may need to coincide to allow the person to communicate at their best level. We need to be watchful for the indicators, both in terms of body language and verbal ability, which mark the optimal times. These may include heightened openness to eye contact, smiling and greater than usual responsiveness to the physical environment. Maybe the person will begin to talk spontaneously or ask questions about family, friends or other people, their current circumstances and so on which demand a response in the moment. Such occasions may be relatively rare, and we need to be there for the individual at these times. We discuss further the issue of the organization of care in relation to communication in Chapter 14 on implications for care.

Some people need the focusing of a time set aside for communicating, others are more forthcoming when the conversations arise incidentally, for example during mealtimes or times set aside for personal care. Talk accompanying activity can act to take the emphasis off an individual's verbal ability, thus freeing them up to speak less self-consciously. One practitioner has identified bath-times as the best opportunity for the deepest exchange between her and a particular woman with dementia.

The role of nonverbal communication in establishing contact

In Chapter 3 we gave primacy to this aspect of communication, and it is never more important than in this crucial stage of relationship-building. First impressions count for so much, and if you are tentative in your approach, or over-confident in projecting yourself, this will be picked up instantly by the individual. Remember the resources you have at your disposal. Initially there is eye contact, with all the fellow-feeling that can be conveyed in a look. In terms of facial signals, an expression of relaxed openness will best invite a positive response.

The position you take up in relation to the other person is important: any stance adopted which exaggerates a power differential immediately threatens to outweigh any other efforts you may make to establish a mutual level of interaction, so it is helpful to make this a priority. Touch can convey a great deal if used with sensitivity. It can reassure and be non-threatening, and help the other person to loosen and venture a contribution. The tone of voice you employ can be as important as the words you use in setting the other person at their ease, and convincing them of your sincerity. We are aware that following this advice may result in what will appear to you or others as exaggerated emphases, but this often seems necessary to make a positive initial impact. As you proceed you can gradually adjust to a more normal-seeming level of intensity and also a balance with verbal dimensions of the interaction.

At the same time as projecting your own nonverbal messages you will need to be attending to those given out by the other person. All the aspects will have something to tell you, each nuance will give out a message for you to interpret. On the basis of what you observe you can make alterations to your own responses. In one sense it complicates matters to have to filter and interpret messages coming back at you, but if you look at the situation positively it is enormously helpful in sustaining the interaction to have this information to work on. Every piece of relationship-building is two-way from the start, and though the initial impetus may have to come from you, the likelihood is that you will quickly find yourself in a give and take situation in which the possibilities begin to unfold.

Starting off an interaction

For the purposes of what follows we have not attempted to separate verbal and nonverbal communication. In many ways it is an artificial distinction anyway, and we need to demonstrate their interdependence even in an account of an interaction with a strong verbal component. Assuming that the person with dementia does not approach you first (in which case you have been given a lead to follow), what is the best way to start? Observing rules of social etiquette we suggest that a conventional greeting and the offering of one's name should come first. It may be appropriate to offer a hand in some cases. One should then await a response. If it is positive it is appropriate to move straight on to the next stage which would be to ask the other person's name and say a little more about yourself (who you are and why you are there).

If no response is forthcoming it may be that the person is bewildered by the approach and needs more time to adjust. Maybe language is a problem for them, in which case facial expression and eye contact will be an aid to interpretation. Or the person may be rejecting your overture, in which case this too should be apparent through nonverbal means. If you are met with a blank you have to decide whether to withdraw at this stage or attempt a further approach; we would suggest the latter course of action as the person may need more time to come to a decision, and it would be a pity to deny them this opportunity out of excessive zeal to avoid intrusion. It is important also to bear in mind that the person with whom you are attempting communication may not be able to see or hear you very well, and you will need to make adjustments for this. Since the pace of the interaction has not yet been established you will need to allow extra time for the other person to respond.

If talk is going to be a feature of the encounter, you need now to switch the subject from you to that of the person with whom you are hoping to converse. It is probably best to aim not to talk about yourself at all except to answer questions. If there is enthusiasm shown for talking, and an ability to articulate thoughts and feelings demonstrated, you could say something like 'Would you like to have a talk just now?' If this is answered positively, you could continue with 'Would you like to tell me something about yourself?' or 'What would you like to talk about?'

Either of these questions gives a clear message to the other person that the focus is on them, and it gives permission for them to take the lead. However difficult they may find this role, by showing that you are interested primarily in them you have made a very important statement. If no verbal responses are offered you must look to any nonverbal signs of interest and pleasure. If these are present you can keep scanning the face and body for evidence of understanding and response, remaining quiet and letting the two-way nonverbal messages carry the meaning.

At this point whether you are communicating both verbally and nonverbally, or mainly nonverbally, you can consider whether a further token of relationship-building should be offered – for example whether to take hold of the other person's hand. This can have quite a powerful effect, sometimes releasing torrents of language in someone who until then has remained hesitant and sparing with words. If the person does not like this intimate gesture they are likely to withdraw their hand quickly. The offering of your hand conveys another important message: it indicates that you are happy for touch to play a part in the interaction. As we have discussed previously, many people with dementia have a highly developed tactile sense, and may wish to express a welcome to your approaches by touching your hand and face, and this may occur quite early in the relationship. It may be one of the things about which you feel self-conscious at first, but touch can be a fundamental part of an interaction and lead quickly to a deep level of engagement.

Occasionally an individual may be overwhelmed by your attentions, and even at the initial stage of making contact show a strong emotional reaction such as bursting into tears. A rapid judgement about how to deal with this is called for. It is helpful to consider that your presence as an interested and reassuring person may have triggered the release of griefs whose expression would otherwise have been suppressed. It could be that the person is expressing happiness or gratitude at what you are offering them. Either way one should resist the commonly held view that crying is an inherently undesirable behaviour which should be stopped as soon as possible. If crying continues, and the person is obviously in a distressed state you might consider going a stage further in terms of physical contact and offering an arm around their shoulder. This may well be interpreted as a gesture of solidarity and have a comforting effect.

Before you move into a further stage of developing the relationship, this may be the time to consider whether the other person is comfortable, both with the chair they are sitting in (if this is their choice) and in the environment in which the interaction is taking place. It is important if the conversation is to realize its potential for both parties to be at ease with each other psychologically and in themselves physically.

In all the above we have discussed processes as if you are meeting the person for the first time. Of course this may not be the case, but we believe that it is important to recognize that because of the nature of the condition you may have to go through a similar or telescoped version of what we have described on subsequent occasions. The same applies to much of the advice given in the succeeding chapters. Regarding the importance of greeting and leave taking, the following description comes from an activities organizer working in a nursing home:

> When I enter the unit for the first time in a day I will probably meet somebody. I will take them by the hand and take them for a walk, if that is what they choose to do, or sit down and talk to them. I would then greet every other resident on the unit individually in a similar manner. I wouldn't organize any activities until I'd spoken to everyone. Similarly when I was leaving I would go round everybody individually, and say goodbye, and give them some time if they asked for it. I allocate a substantial amount of time every day to these essential procedures of communication.

Interactions initiated by the person with dementia

We have been talking so far as if the person with dementia is always the passive recipient of an approach. This is not, of course, the case. In much of John's work, encounters were initiated by the other person. This has often come about through him being in the environment, perhaps sitting quietly in a public room, and in a variety of ways projecting an openness to being approached. The sorts of nonverbal channels described above are of service in this situation – open facial expression, smiling, eye contact (although of a less intense variety than that which is used once the encounter has begun). Some care workers have described other nonverbal means of communicating that they are available for interaction with clients or residents. One example of this is the slightly extended crooked arm, which is an invitation for someone to take it and walk with them.

At other times it is clear that the person with dementia has something to say, but attracting the attention of another may prove difficult. The following quote from a woman illustrates the importance of responding to this:

> *One day I wanted to get something off my chest. I had something to say. But each time I tried to speak to a person about it someone came in between. And the next day I couldn't remember what it was I wanted to say.*

Periodically John has come across people who are highly proactive, approaching him in the corridor or immediately on entering the building. Such encounters can sometimes develop rather too rapidly for comfort. A situation can arise where, for example, someone comes up to you in a corridor and immediately begins talking in an intimate manner about things which concern them. It may be impractical to respond adequately at the time, but assuming that you are free to converse, then the first move might be to steer the person to a place where a conversation could develop in comfort. If it proves impossible to settle them at once, then the interaction could commence on the move, with the hope that in course of time, equilibrium could be restored sufficiently as to permit a more relaxed outcome.

One day as John entered a day unit a man came hurrying towards him in a very agitated state. Immediately he posed a rather startling question: 'Who's in charge of the spare words?' After pausing to consider this, John realized that no one could have such a specific responsibility, but he offered 'Well, I'm a writer. Perhaps I could help.' They then sat down in a private corner and painfully teased out what was concerning the man. Eventually they established that it was a question that he wanted to ask the person in charge but he had not known how to articulate it. Together they wrote it down, and John accompanied him to the manager of the unit where the man read it out and received an answer.

A common factor influencing the willingness of staff to get involved in interactions with people with dementia is the fear that once the exchange is established it will be difficult to stop. General pressure of time and work creates a classic avoidance routine whereby a journey through a roomful of people or down a corridor is accompanied by the fervent hope that no one will ask for anything or seek personal contact. At times this scenario is unavoidable, but if it is a general pattern this means that something is awry, and needs to be addressed, probably at an organizational level. It is a practice which is likely to be associated with high levels of anxiety in service users.

The perception that an interaction will always take a long time and be difficult to end is unrealistic and does a disservice to the person with dementia. If care practice were organized more explicitly around the aim of keeping communication to the fore, then we would probably find that this has the effect of reducing the sense of pressure which comes from being focused on tasks, and having to keep people at a distance in order to complete them. Encounters do not have to be long in order to have an effect. Brief interactions, especially if they are well timed and tailored fully to the person's needs may be just as effective in enhancing well-being as longer ones. They may need to be more frequent, but if the person can become used to regular interactions, the anxiety which originally gave rise to the need for contact may subside.

One day when John had been working on a unit for some hours a woman made it plain that she wanted to speak to him. After a long period of circling around she at last stood before him.

'May I ask you a question?'
'Of course' he answered.
'Is there a moment between birth and death when one becomes more important than the other?'
There was a long pause.

'I'm sorry. I can't answer your question because it's too profound', said
John 'but thanks for sharing it with me.'
'That's all right, I just wanted you to know that that was what I was
thinking', the lady said and walked away.

The whole memorable interaction had lasted no more than 60 seconds.

Ethical implications

Intrusion

As we said earlier on in this chapter, situations which involve making an
approach to the person with dementia always call for judgement and sensitivity as regards the possibility of intrusion. But in addition to the practical
issues, it is important to give some consideration to what it is about our way
of thinking about dementia which gives rise to particular concerns about
intrusion. An important theme here is the idea that dementia is a condition
which puts a barrier between ourselves and those who live with it. The perception that people with dementia exist in a different dimension of experience
is one which we come across again and again. There is often something about
the way that people present which suggests that they are not fully present, and
the most ready explanation for this quality is that their separateness is inherent in their condition. In their book the occupational therapists Tessa Perrin
and Hazel May describe the world of the person with dementia as having
shrunk, meaning that more active approaches are required from others.[6]

The self-fulfilling prophecy can come into being here. We can easily create
conditions of isolation by reducing opportunities for ordinary contact and
conversation, and then label the way that the person responds to this as evidence of their dementia. We sometimes also conceptualize a degree of apparent withdrawal on the part of the person as a coping response, that the person
finds ways of escaping from a reality which is unpalatable or frightening. Here
we need to consider the possibility that a degree of withdrawal is not an
inevitable concomitant of the condition, but rather a response to surroundings which are stressful or over-demanding or the actions of others which are
seen as threatening to personhood.

Of course as with so many other aspects of understanding dementia, the
idea that people with dementia are somehow separate from us can function as
a justification for certain types of behaviour on our part. If we assume that the
person has withdrawn in order to cope with their difficulties, then we could
easily convince ourselves that to attempt to make contact with them and
involve them in activity would constitute a challenge to their way of coping.
Leaving them alone could then be seen as the most respectful strategy, while
the reality is that the person is desperately in need of contact. There can be a
perception that it is kinder to allow the person to drift in their own world, and
that by engaging with them we are forcing them to confront the changes
which have come about.

Arousing expectations

Whenever we encounter a new person we are uncertain as to what will tran-
spire, whether we will get on well together or whether there will be tension,
whether the relationship will develop into one that is significant or remain
superficial. These considerations apply as much to people with dementia as to
anyone else. Again, as a function of the power differential between people
with dementia and ourselves, and the fact that they are so often deprived of
the contact and affirmation they need to maintain their sense of identity,
there is a potential for harm through disappointed expectations.

In the context of developing approaches to in-depth communication, we
need to consider what it is that we are offering to someone in an opportunity
for contact. At the most practical level, how long might the interaction be? Is
it likely to be a one-off or is there the possibility of repeated contact? On a
deeper level, there are questions like: are we offering ourselves as someone who
will respect confidences, accept the expression of deep emotion, even be a partner on a journey? We may or may not be clear about these things ourselves, but
we also have to consider what the other person's understanding of the situation
might be. This is complicated by the fact that we cannot know at the outset
what will come of an initial approach, or what the person's preferences and
needs are. It would be unrealistic to expect oneself to have all of these contin-
gencies worked out in advance, indeed it would be rather strange if we did – a
degree of spontaneity and openness to possibilities are necessary for positive
relationships to develop. When an approach does seem to have been successful, however, receptiveness to the emerging and deepening rapport is essential,
but all of this raises questions about how far we are prepared to go, and to what
extent we have a responsibility to communicate the limits to the other person.

Alongside reasonable concerns about expectations, there is the possibility of
more specific worries. For example, will the other person develop expectations
of us that we cannot fulfil? Is the need so great that it will threaten to swallow
us up? Such fears are likely be a powerful inhibitor to the development of real
relationships. While it is only realistic to acknowledge that there is potential
for difficulty here, we should not automatically assume that people with
dementia are unable to understand that others have limitations. And if we are
open to the idea that they are able to give as well as take, our concerns about
being overwhelmed by unmet needs may be lessened. We discuss the issue of
how far we can extend ourselves by becoming involved in the experiences of
others in Chapter 15.

8 Developing the interaction: 'With you I am putting things together'

In this chapter we build on the advice given in Chapter 7, and examine in detail what qualities and strategies are necessary for sustaining and developing an interaction once it is underway. These ideas apply both to first encounters and subsequent ones. Although we will discuss a range of means of doing this, the crucial message here is that we must discover and deepen our ability to listen. We cannot emphasize this too strongly, as we are convinced that it is the single most significant contribution we can make to the act of communication and relationship building.

This point was memorably made by the woman we quoted on p. 177. She clearly perceived the significance of the activity in which she and John were engaged. At the time he was writing down what she said but she did not refer to this, as it was secondary to the act of listening. She revealed herself to be painfully aware of the consequences of poor listening. This, of course, is something that we can all feel at times, but for a person with dementia it must be especially disappointing, if not conducive of despair, to find this core aspect of the interaction is lacking. But what does true listening actually involve?

The need to stop talking

Perhaps the first thing which springs to mind when thinking about listening is that we must stop talking. We cannot talk and listen at the same time. But how easy is it simply to talk less? As we discussed in Chapter 4 on language, conventional rules of discourse include ideas about equity in a conversation – that both parties should talk for roughly the same amount of time. Although this way of thinking is deeply ingrained and expressed in our social behaviour, it is a habit which needs to be altered when attempting to establish communication with a person with dementia, certainly in the early stages of interaction, and perhaps throughout.

Of course listening involves much more than simply refraining from talking. There is a depth and quality of attention which must be brought to bear in order that two main purposes are served. The first is that not only must we listen, but also our demeanour must in a variety of ways *demonstrate* to the individual that this is, without any doubt, going on. We believe that it is often only when an individual reveals themselves to be truly present and open to the other that the person with dementia is enabled to share their deepest and most significant thoughts and feelings. The second reason is that highly concentrated and sensitive listening is often essential in order for one to get alongside and tune in to the person's style of communication sufficiently well in order to understand the messages they offer. Closely related to these practices is the experience and use of silence.

'Learning to sit in the silence'[1]

As with other aspects of interaction and conversation, we labour with strong cultural injunctions as regards silence. In our society, silence during conversation by and large means failure. Silence is awkward, embarrassing, it must be filled up. Talk, of any sort, seems preferable. These rules are powerful. If you doubt it, sit unoccupied in a room with another person, and neither of you speak. How does it feel? What do you want to do? Laugh? Leave? Pick up something to read? Busy yourself in some other way? Whatever it is, silence feels wrong. This is another way in which learning to communicate deeply with people with dementia demands that we learn a new set of rules.

In general, John's experience is that communication with people with dementia involves a great deal of silence, and sometimes silence which persists for considerable periods of time. In order to respond in the most helpful way, it is obviously necessary to develop sensitivity as to *why* silence is occurring. We examine some possible reasons below, but it is impossible to give fully detailed advice on how to decide what a silence means as each encounter is unique, and different individuals will express the possible states of mind in different ways. It is also important to bear in mind that there may be more than one reason for silence, and both parties may be silent for different reasons. Remaining alert and using one's general social sense should give you an idea, and if you continue to spend time with the same person, you will certainly become familiar with their style. Having developed an idea of what is underlying the silence it will be clear that different courses of action will then be appropriate.

Silence as evidence of thinking

In a situation where silence is occurring because thinking is occupying the energy and capacity available to the person with dementia, it is *vital* that you allow the process to take its time, and do not interrupt in any way. We have already discussed the fact that for whatever reasons (psychosocial or organic or both) dementia seems to bring about a series of obstacles to thought and expression, and that much greater effort and concentration is required to marshal resources in the service of thinking, reasoning and communicating. Having established a relationship in which the person with dementia is encouraged to share their ideas and experiences it would be crass in the extreme then to trample on their delicate strivings with questions, comments and statements of our own. (We deal later with the issue of asking questions in an interaction.) At these times we need to remind ourselves that our holding back from filling the silence is an essential part of the process of allowing the other person to breathe mentally and gather themselves to make a contribution if they wish. It may be helpful to repeat to oneself the words of the person with dementia quoted earlier: 'the stillness of silence, that listens and lasts' (p. 80).

Unfortunately this sort of breaking in on silence must happen over and over again. We can only imagine the feelings of frustration and dismay induced in the person with dementia by the careless destruction of a rare and precious opportunity to share something important with another human being. As we have said before, perhaps for many people the decline in verbal expression over the course of the condition is as much the result of the effects of repeated disappointment in this way, as the outcome of direct damage to the brain. Further, the reality is that opportunities for real contact being lost is not the result of deliberate effort to hamper communication, but rather a clumsy failure to perceive the significance of a situation, and the pressure to maintain a façade of normality in conversation. Surely we would do well to learn to sit in the silence with many of our day-to-day communication partners, and not just those with dementia, but here is an urgent need indeed.

A word here about an alternative scenario. Having allowed the person with dementia time to reflect and shape their thoughts (and not destroyed them with a verbal intervention), it may be that the individual chooses not to share the outcome of this process – that their silence, on this matter at least, is held, and perhaps permanently. The private nature of this makes it impossible for us to know exactly what has happened, and there is no overt demonstration of meaning having been achieved. But the experience and results of having been given permission to follow their thoughts through, in the silent presence of an empathic and empowering listener, may be profoundly valued. We like to collect evidence of the effects of our actions, but we cannot always have it.

Silence as evidence of lack of engagement

When silence seems to be reflective of a lack of the necessary sense of connection, then obviously this will call for a different course of action. A decision may be required about whether it is worth investing time and energy in striving for a greater depth or whether to steer the interaction to a close. This will depend on many factors. However it works out, it is important not to chalk this outcome up as a reflection of some permanent state of affairs. It may have been that this was not the right time or place for an interaction. You or the person with dementia may have been affected by a feeling of tiredness or preoccupation with other matters. There may have been emotional factors affecting the encounter which were attached to some other situation or relationship. On many occasions and with many people, John has had the experience of failing to establish a strong link at one time, only to have a highly successful encounter at another.

Silence as evidence of disengagement

As well as the sort of scenarios where real contact has not been achieved at all, there are situations where subsequent to a period of meaningful connection, the person with dementia lapses into silence which may be indicative of tiredness. We know that deep communication demands the expenditure of considerable energy on both sides, but especially so for the person who is having to struggle with significant barriers. Silence may mean that the encounter is over. We talk more about this crucial phase of an interaction in Chapter 9.

Silence during nonverbal communication

Of course we may continue listening and there may be nothing at the end of our wait. If the main part of the interaction is based in nonverbal communication, then we should not expect words to figure prominently as well. We are again reminded that, despite our cultural worship of words, speech is not essential to relationship. It is perfectly possible to be with a person, without movement even, perhaps holding hands or maintaining meaningful eye contact. Indeed, such experiences sometimes convince us that words can actually get in the way of communication. They can function as a convenient means of filling up gaps in time without having to think or feel deeply. Denied this temptation we may be released to get on with the real business of experiencing togetherness. We are reminded here of the quote from Michael Ignatieff on p. 52.

Silence as evidence of difficulty with language

The man we introduced in Chapter 7 who asked John 'Who's in charge of the spare words?' seemed to be expressing his frustration at not being able to exercise sufficient command of language in order to formulate what he wanted to say. We know that because John was able to help him to phrase the question he wanted to ask a member of staff. Not everyone with dementia might feel able to admit to such a lack, or even find the words to explain their need. In these instances silences may occur. It is just one of the possibilities we need to be aware of in making a judgement about the cause of a silence. Once we are sure that problems with language are inhibiting a response it may be appropriate to make a gentle offer of assistance. Even if this is unsuccessful, at least we can offer empathic support in being with the person in difficulty.

Silence as part of activity

In considering conversation we have said that engaging in activity with the person with dementia can often stimulate talk. It is as if taking the emphasis off language makes it easier for the person to venture into words. But the opposite may also occur. Doing something practical may let the individual 'off the hook' verbally, relieve them of the burden of engaging in meaningful dialogue. Some activities, in any case, demand concentration of an intensity that precludes talk. Where a person with dementia is experiencing loss of skills successful performance of a task may already involve greater application than they can command. Silence in these cases may have nothing to do with lack of communication skills or the desire to use them. There is more on the subject of communication and activity later in this chapter.

Silence as an effect of strong emotion

As we discussed in Chapter 3 on nonverbal communication, it sometimes happens that the experience of strong emotion inhibits our ability to speak. The word 'choked' is a highly appropriate word we might use to describe such a situation. It may be that because of the particular problems they face, combined with a heightened experience of emotion, this is a predicament more frequently encountered by people with dementia than the rest of us. In many such instances offering comfort and reassurance through nonverbal means will be a helpful response, and through this it may be possible for the person to reach a sufficient resolution of the emotion to continue. The subject of powerful feelings arising during an encounter is also dealt with later in this chapter.

One further consideration on the subject of silence is our own concern that refraining from talking may signal a lack of interest in the other individual and their feelings, especially if neither eye contact nor touch forms part of the interaction. While acknowledging the well-intentioned motivation of this worry, we should not underestimate the simple power of being with a person in distress. The fact that you are physically present with them (and providing that your own body language is not expressing signs of distraction), and you are not filling the silence with inconsequential talk, this provides a forceful message of support and respect.

Clearly silence during communication is another illustration of the complex and subtle nature of the challenge we have accepted in enhancing our relationships with people with dementia. We end with the words of Danuta Lipinska, who is a counsellor working with people who have been recently diagnosed:

> I encourage us all as we seek to listen to the 'voice', but of equal importance to the silence. Those moments between the lines where we actively and attentively share the silence are the spaces where the penny drops, the light goes on, the shoe fits – making sense of self, and our world. It becomes part of our 'bearing witness', the process of being alongside, on each unknowable journey.[2]

What follows continues the theme of interaction which does not rely on words.

Nonverbal communication

This remains important at all stages of the interaction, and is a powerful force for connection. We discuss the major aspects of nonverbal communication under separate headings.

Eye contact

In order to support the development of the interaction, we need to be carefully observing and registering the intensity of eye contact, the size of the pupils, the frequency of eye movements, the degree to which a gaze is held or the number of occasions it rests elsewhere. The consistency of one's own gaze, at the risk of appearing prying, is of primary importance. We have to get over the message of our commitment to this interaction and the eyes are our most powerful messengers.

Facial expression

It is possible to communicate friendly interest and ongoing effort of attention and concentration in a variety of ways. A generally intent expression will convey this disposition, and your facial reactions to particular meanings will reassure the person that you are fully present to them.

Voice

As we have emphasized before, apart from what you actually say the voice is a potent means of reaching the other person. On the subject of its expressiveness, the academic John Hull (who is blind) says:

> The crucial thing in any new acquaintance is the sound of the voice. I am continuing to learn more and more about the amazing power of the

human voice to reveal the person. With the people I know very well, I find that all of the emotion which would normally be expressed in the face is there in the voice: the tiredness, the anxiety, the suppressed excitement and so on. My impressions based on the voice seem to be just as accurate as those of sighted people.[3]

Touch

The hands, for example in gesture or in touch, may be used to reinforce the main message where appropriate. Sometimes the person with dementia will use their hands to explore and enter *your* world. A first tentative examination of your hand or face can lead to a bolder grasp, stroking and even firmer pressure as if to reinforce other aspects of the interaction. You will need to make a decision on how to respond. It is impossible to give advice that will be applicable in every instance, but we believe that if you are fully absorbed in the interaction you can trust to that sense of rightness which permeates a fully alert and respectful mutuality.

Posture and body movements

As the interaction develops, the way we use our bodies, too, conveys a great deal. If you are stiff and formal in your movements this may carry the message that you are apprehensive, forcing yourself into a situation you would rather not be in, or at the very least, are uncomfortable with because you do not know what is expected of you. Whereas if you are confident in your course of action this will lead to smoothness in your movements. Spontaneity is essential in every relationship, and you can work towards achieving relaxation within your resolve, which demonstrates to the other person that you are someone who knows what they are doing and in whom they can place their trust. Every movement you make carries a message as potent as any words you can utter. Again, as we discussed in Chapter 7, it is likely that when you are setting out you may experience feelings of awkwardness. However, with more practice this will lessen, and you will find your own style.

Similarly you can tell a great deal about the state of mind of the person with dementia by noticing their movements, whether they are awkward or easy in them, whether they seem comfortable with their body. Jane Crisp gives a good illustration of this:

> I know that I am in for a difficult visit if I sense that my mother's body is stiff rather than relaxed; when she is really worked up she crackles with an almost demonic energy, pushing herself vigorously along in her wheelchair or planting her feet on the ground and refusing to be pushed. Carers rapidly learn to read these signs, since ignoring them can result in a forceful clout from hands or feet. If I stay with my mother when she is agitated, I have to work at keeping myself relaxed; otherwise my tenseness will make the situation worse.[4]

Mirroring

The important practice of mirroring was introduced in Chapter 3 on nonverbal communication. It can really come into its own at this second stage of relationship-building. While some forms of mirroring can be particularly absorbing and exclusive, this approach may also be used in a humorous or light-hearted spirit, and can take its place in an exchange which involves verbal dialogue as well. As with other matters of judgement, it is difficult to give advice as to when such an approach might be best used. At times you may engage in mirroring without realizing that you are doing so. It is only one of many strategies which can be utilized, but we believe that it is a special one.

Pacing

The matter of the pace of an interaction has already been introduced in Chapters 3 and 4 on nonverbal communication and language, and also in Chapter 7 on beginning an encounter. Some further considerations pertaining to the development phase need now to be explored. It may be that once the interaction has passed through the early stages (and this applies as much to subsequent encounters as to first-time ones) and has become established, there will be an alteration in the pace.

This could come predominantly from you, especially if you feel that you have achieved a degree of rapport and are keen to develop it. A sense of enthusiasm and involvement in the encounter may be expressed by a stepping up of the speed at which you talk and communicate nonverbally. As part of this, your expectations of how quickly the person with dementia should be responding will heighten. Although this is a natural pattern in many interactions and indicative of success, for many people this acceleration will not be helpful. It may take a longer time for the person to achieve a greater fluency and speed of response, or it may not happen at all. If, however, you observe the pace being influenced by the other person, it will be safer to reciprocate. As usual, a high degree of sensitivity and awareness is demanded.

Of course the opposite may take place, and you may become aware of a slowing down of responses as the interaction develops. This could happen for a variety of reasons. It may be that the person is taking their time to think or would prefer the exchange to proceed nonverbally. Tiredness may be the most important factor in this, and again your judgement in how to respond most helpfully will be called upon.

There are particular challenges inherent in maintaining concentration when someone is speaking very slowly. Our minds get used to processing information at a certain rate, and when the incoming flow does not match this, the risk of our attention wandering and other ideas or thoughts floating into awareness is considerable. You need to acknowledge to yourself that this is a difficult area – the nature of thinking is such that our thoughts do not conform easily to attempts at control. Like everything else coping with this is a skill which needs to be practised. Some forms of meditation recommend that during efforts to maintain a quality of mental blankness, thoughts which arise should be acknowledged and then gently laid aside. There is little point in berating oneself. Another strategy is to focus underutilized attention on your own and the other person's nonverbal communication. This is such a complex activity that it should absorb you, and have the benefit of honing your skills in this area too.

Going with the flow

If talk is likely to be a major feature of the exchange, how is this best encouraged? Our general maxim is again that this should be controlled as much as possible by the individual with dementia. In John's experience, people who want to talk do not require much direction, and often following the kind of general opener described in Chapter 7, the ball is rolling. The way this then develops is often fascinating, and may call upon skills of supportiveness, empathy and occasionally mind-reading!

The ebb and flow of talk is a natural characteristic of all our conversations. Topics are taken up and dropped, enthusiasms surge and interest flags in complex patterns. Although it may not be particularly noticeable in the normal course of things, ordinary talk is full of hesitations, overlapping talk, diversions, irrelevancies, subject-changes, lost trails and content-free 'padding'. Sentences are very often repetitive, ungrammatical, incomplete and ambiguous. Eavesdropping aside, the main way in which we are exposed to the conversations of others (in which we are not involved ourselves) are those we hear on television, and this gives us a misleading impression of the nature of normal conversation. Scripted exchanges do not reflect the messiness of real dialogue. If they did, viewers would quickly become irritated and switch channels. Even 'real people' TV is edited so that the maximum meaning is conveyed in minimum time. Given that our own conversation is so ragged, we should not be surprised to encounter these features in the talk of people with dementia. But it is a fact that when we do, we are liable to interpret them as symptoms of the condition, and respond to them in an artificial manner.

There can also be talk which does not seem to have a coherent focus or which seems to move from subject to subject without obvious links. Again, this may be devalued as being meaningless. As we saw in Chapter 5 on memory, altered memory functioning may well be pertinent here. Talk which could be dismissed as 'rambling' may very well be connected by meaningful links which are not signalled or explained (see the discussion of pragmatics in Chapter 4).

Although many conversations with people with dementia have sequences with conventional connections, for many people the above characteristics of speech do develop, and in a way which increasingly interferes with the conveyance of meaning. Given sensitive and encouraging listening, these features can almost always be accommodated without any awkwardness or embarrassment. With some people and in some situations, it may be quite possible for things to proceed without it having to become clear that you are not following the connections between topics. But a challenge may arise when changes of direction which are sudden or puzzling occur in the sorts of conversations where frequent responses are expected from you. It can be difficult to know what to pick up on and in what manner. Responding helpfully in these circumstances is a matter of intuition, quick thinking and luck. Sometimes it will work out, sometimes it will not. The following excerpt is an example of a successful guess (and is from a much longer conversation with other similar exchanges):

1 *Edith:* *Some places are very interesting.*
2 *John:*   They are.
3 *Edith:* *Yes.*
4 *John:*   Where do you like particularly?
5 *Edith:* *In Italy.*
6 *John:*   Ah. Right. You've been there a lot?
7 *Edith:* *Um? . . . We're very fond of St Andrews.*
8 *John:*   Right.
9 *Edith:* *And you get very little . . . small . . . small min . . . minmat.*
10 *John:*   Mmm.
11 *Edith:* *And you can tray . . . that . . . that you purt, you purted and . . .*
             you didn't put your feet in.
12 *John:*   Right. No. Well the sea can be a bit cold at St Andrews, can't it?
13 *Edith:* *Exactly. Exactly. Yes.*
14 *John:*   It's got lovely sand, but once you go in the water it's a bit chilly.
15 *Edith:* *Oh well very very nearly being chilled . . . pretty good for it. Yes.*

From the beginning of this piece of dialogue Edith Frame is setting the agenda in terms of what she wants to talk about. In line 4 John supplies a question which supports her in this role. She mentions Italy, and again John asks her a question which will enable her to continue, but suddenly there is a switch to the subject of St Andrews (a seaside town in Scotland). John's short response perhaps conveys his surprise at this move, but the flow is unaffected. Edith then continues but her speech becomes less fluent. She appears to be struggling either with finding a word or getting a sound right. John's response in line 10 is correspondingly open and non-committal. Edith continues with her attempts to express her thoughts, and eventually manages a more conventional sequence. There is then the sense that it is John's turn to speak. Despite some feelings of confusion on his part during Edith's more hesitant speech the last few words have provided a clue as to what Edith might have been getting at – St Andrews and not putting 'your feet in' – the sea! His statement about the temperature of the water draws a very positive response from Edith, and it therefore appears that he has been following her thoughts successfully. This excerpt is concluded with the sense of them both being in the same place, and is therefore affirming.

Jean Copeland, whom we met in Chapter 4, provides an example of a situation in which it is much harder to work out from the language alone, how to respond. In much of the conversation John plainly does not know what to make of what he is being told. He is reduced to asking straight questions of a conventional kind, without any certainty that they are receiving answers, or agreeing with what has been said because that seems the appropriate emotional response. If at any time Jean had asked him a question he would have been floored. However, at no time in a conversation lasting nearly half an hour was John in any real doubt about how to fulfil his role. This is particularly surprising because Jean talked at a breakneck pace. However, she spoke with such fluency and enthusiasm, in a tone of great warmth and enjoyment of the process, that he was carried along by a tide of togetherness. Real contact was being made. This may be an extreme example but it demonstrates that at these times it is more important to draw on your skills of responding to the emotional message, and let the intellectual interpretation of what is being said take care of itself. What is still vital is the demonstration of close attention, interest and empathy.

Incomplete utterances

A commonly encountered feature of the speech of people with dementia is the incomplete utterance. This can take the form of a relatively confident and clear beginning to a sentence, followed either by an abrupt cessation or a gradual loss of momentum. It is as if the person has lost their way, perhaps forgetting the end of the sentence in the effort of articulating the beginning. Sometimes this is accompanied by an overt expression of frustration, sometimes the person seems less aware that their thoughts remain unshared.

We have all had the experience of forgetting what we were going to say, and while the underlying problem here may be different from those affecting the person with dementia, it provides the basis for empathizing with them. Of course, the usual pattern in this situation is for the thought to pop back into our minds, sometimes within seconds, sometimes taking longer. This may not occur for the person with dementia, or if it does memory problems may prevent them from making an explicit connection between the original difficulty and the new information.

Choosing a way to respond in these situations depends on a variety of factors. If you know the person, you may already have learned that patient waiting sometimes results in them being able to reach the end of the utterance. If you sense that they are still trying to articulate the original thought, a carefully timed prompt, that is repeating the beginning of the sentence, may help them to go a little further. This will also demonstrate that you have been listening closely, and may encourage them to feel that their effort is worthwhile. At other times, you may feel that although the person has not completed their sentence or expressed their main thought, they have actually moved on in terms of what they are thinking about, and prompting them to go back to a previous thought may prove counterproductive. Subtle nonverbal clues such as gaze, eye and head movements, and muscle tension particularly around the eyes should provide enough information for you to develop a sense of which strategy to take.

The most difficult situation in relation to incomplete utterances is when the individual seems unable to fully express any thought, and is constantly encountering frustration and distress as a result. For any communication partner this is also a painful process, and there is a danger that one's own discomfort and tension with the situation will feed back and amplify difficulties for the person with dementia. In these situations, it may be that a gentle and sensitive suggestion to change the focus of the interaction away from pure conversation may be helpful. In some instances this will not prove the right way forward, but for some a shift of attention may have an immediately relieving effect, and an indirect consequence of allowing thoughts and utterances to take shape.

Another strategy is to suggest possible endings to the sentences to the individual, and monitor verbal and nonverbal cues to judge their accuracy. The likelihood of this approach being helpful will probably depend on the specificity of what is being discussed. If the subject matter is reasonably restricted, the better your chances of coming up with likely suggestions for the rest of the thought. There is the danger, of course, that verbal interventions from yourself will exacerbate confusion and difficulty, and again close monitoring and interpretation of responses from the person should help you to identify whether this is happening.

Asking questions

When you are puzzled by what someone has said, the natural reaction is to ask them about it. Similarly if you have misheard a remark the obvious thing is to ask the person to repeat it. In John's experience with people with dementia these strategies are rarely effective. He has found that most people act as if they have not heard the question. It is as if the effort to articulate the next sentence is occupying all their attention, and what they have just said is already a thing of the past. Where the struggle to say anything is slow and painful it would seem insensitive to draw attention to ambiguities in the speech of the other person by querying meanings.

Having said this, we are reminded of the exchange which took place between Anthea McKinlay and her mother (pp. 135–6) in which questions played an essential part in the success of the dialogue. In this case, however, because the conversation took place over the telephone, utterances of her own were Anthea's only way of conveying to her mother that she was present and listening keenly.

As usual there cannot be any categorical advice in this area. In some situations questions may constitute a valuable contribution, in others we should simply be grateful for the communication we receive, and make use of all the verbal and nonverbal clues we are given in order to make as much sense of it as we can.

Communication during other activity

Although we have been highlighting the importance of giving primacy to the business of communication, as was mentioned earlier it is also true that for some people and at some times an exclusive focus on talking or pure interaction is not helpful. There are situations in which we all find that talking comes more easily alongside and woven into another activity. We have all found ourselves looking at things or fiddling with objects while struggling with words. This may arise because of emotional difficulty or other psychological factors.

In John's experience, there have been many highly significant and successful conversations which have shared time with an occupation such as walking or looking at pictures, handling an object or watching events or other people. If anxiety is a factor in communication, the activity may serve to induce relaxation and thereby enhance the interaction. It may provide distraction at times when finding words or sustaining contact is more difficult. Or it may supply topic ideas for someone who would like to be in conversation, but struggles with what to say.

As usual it is ideal if the person with dementia can be encouraged to express a preference in this matter, but there may be times when you sense that the individual would like you to suggest something, and if this is done in a sensitive manner which promotes choice then it can help things along. If you have taken the lead it is especially important to be alert to signals from the person regarding their feelings about the activity.

For some people who spend long periods of time engaged in certain activities like walking or touching objects, the only chance of establishing contact will be to share their actions. If an approach by you seems to be welcomed, an intimate partnership can develop, even if this does not involve actually talking or engaging in a great deal of touch or eye contact.

Dealing with strong emotion

Sometimes a person, perceiving that you are someone in whom they can place their trust, will express themselves in an emotional manner. Such a development may come about gradually, or the conversation might suddenly take a turn into very personal territory. The expression of strong feelings may accompany such disclosure. An example is a woman who said to John:

> *I'm on the edge wi' it. It's just this feeling that's come inside o' me. When we were waitin' to get in, it's just a funny thing, it's not a shouting thing. Why do they come like that?*
>
> *It's your head first, then your heart, then your legs – you seem to feel everything. I feel it even in my hands, you ken? It's like you're on a roundabout, only it's inside o' you.*

It was clear that she was experiencing a flux of emotions, and it was important for him to listen and accept what she was saying. What would probably have been unhelpful in this situation would have been for him to try to persuade her that everything was alright, and that she should ignore what was going on inside her.

Another woman said:

> *God so loved the world, but He doesn't love me. I used to be happy, but now I'm angry with Him because I am still here.*

She went on to express a whole complex of emotions, sadness and anger being the most prominent. Where, as here, the feelings appear to stem from her perception of her predicament as irreversible, there is little that can be done to ameliorate matters. However, to stay with someone in this position, offering such support as you can by means of words or touch may help the acute feelings of grief to pass, enabling the person to move on to other matters. Telling the individual not to be upset or cry, and making attempts to steer the person onto less painful subjects would seem demeaning. Remember (as we discussed in Chapter 3) crying or an outpouring of this kind can be a great relief, and you may be performing an important service to the individual by encouraging this expression. The same applies when crying or other emotional release has no identifiable cause. The principle of 'being with' the person operates over a whole range of situations and states of mind whether we understand what lies behind them or not.

Here is another woman expressing her state of mind vividly to John:

> *Oh dear, I do feel rotten. Why do I feel like this? I'm seeing spots before my eyes. Can you see them? Well they're there. Just because you can't see them that's not to say they're not there. Oh dear, I do feel awful. What should I do? I'm seeing spots before my eyes. I don't like them. I don't like all these lights jumping about, jumping all over the place. Oh dear, I do feel funny. I don't mean funny funny. I mean funny. I feel funny. You can't help me, can you?*

Although the exact quality of her experience remained unclear, her distress and need were palpable, and she makes a direct appeal for help and relief. On this occasion John was unable to answer her questions or remove that which was upsetting her. There have been many other encounters with similar characteristics. We have ample evidence that painful feelings and troubling thoughts and memories are very real to individuals with dementia, and that requests for help, understanding and comfort are heartfelt. But for a variety of reasons, whether related to John's inability to understand or it being beyond his power to meet the person's needs, he felt fundamentally unable to assist. In these situations, general comfort and reassurance are all that are available, but the interaction may still end with the person feeling distressed and searching for help.

Not understanding

One dilemma which arises very directly in the course of communication work is the question of whether it is right to tell the person when you cannot understand what they are saying. When someone is expressing themselves confidently, and appears to be enjoying the contact, is it ever right to stop them and confess that you do not know what they are talking about? This is a situation that John has encountered many times. It would certainly feel wrong to do so. Even if the linguistic content is not meaningful, there is often a very strong sense of understanding at an emotional level. Although at times it may feel uncomfortable to create the impression that you know what someone is talking about when you do not, it is necessary to consider the likely consequences of an alternative course of action. Telling someone that you actually do not understand will call attention to their difficulties in such a way that could damage their confidence. At least while the person is talking there is an open channel, and the possibility that you will be able to get to the point where understanding is possible is there.

As the encounter develops you will not know how much in the way of specific ideas the person is going to be able to communicate. Sometimes it happens that once they have got 'warmed up' to speaking, the expression of meaning becomes easier, and you certainly wouldn't want to stop someone before they got to that point. In any case, once you have got going, and you have taken steps to encourage them to share whatever they want to, you are unlikely to sense a point at which it would be suitable to state your lack of comprehension. In any case, if we accept that much of what is being exchanged is at an emotional level, then as long as you feel that you are connecting with the person in this way, there is no dishonesty.

In some circumstances it may be necessary to admit to lack of understanding and to engage in the kind of process where you are more openly acknowledging the difficulty of exchanging ideas. Another approach is to feed back directly what you have understood, and in so doing you will let them know at what level you are in tune with them. An example is saying something like 'I'm not sure of the exact details of what you are saying, but I am picking up that you are very angry about something.'

The presence of others

Our main interest is in the possibilities inherent in the one-to-one situation, but sometimes other people (staff or relatives) may become involved, and occasionally other people with dementia may interrupt or join in when things are well underway. We certainly would not wish to claim that the presence of a third person cannot under any circumstances bring stimulus and variety to a conversation, but what can be stated categorically is that it alters the dynamics of an interaction, sometimes very markedly.

Some disturbances of a carefully built-up pace with the focus squarely on the person with dementia can be disastrous, as when a care assistant questioned the basis of John's work by stating dogmatically in the presence of the person: 'There must be some mistake – Mrs Jones has nothing to say for herself'. Similar statements may be made by others, who assert that efforts at communication are wasted on account of the person's inability to engage with and sustain an inter-action, that they have 'gone away'. Where the possibility of such an inter-vention can be foreseen, then time spent explaining beforehand to the individual(s) involved the delicate nature of the task you are engaged in could be well spent. If it is a relative you could ask them to wait for a while with min-imal explanation, and then offer a fuller account of your reasons at a later time.

In a situation where another person with dementia makes moves to enter into an ongoing conversation or otherwise intervenes, it may well be that they see attention of a kind that they would like for themselves being given to another. You could explain that this is a private conversation, but that if there is a possibility of spending time with them later, you could offer this.

In general, we recommend that you make every attempt to preserve the character of the one-to-one situation because of the unique benefits it can bring to the person.

Talking about yourself

We now have a few things to say about the matter of bringing oneself and one's own concerns into the conversation but this important subject will be dealt with at greater length in the section on ethical implications at the end of Chapter 12. We have already made it clear that, by and large, the focus of the interaction must be on the person with dementia and not upon ourselves. It is not, however, an absolute rule and once a relationship is established there may be times when answering questions about oneself or even offering un-solicited pieces of information is right and helpful, and makes a significant contribution towards affirming the person with dementia. But we have to pro-ceed with caution in this area. Each relationship will unfold at its own pace, and we should aim for the other person to influence it as much as possible. Also, each individual will vary as to the degree of curiosity shown about you.

We shall end this chapter as we began it with consideration of the all-import-ant subject of listening. 'You are words' said the woman we referred to at the outset, and she surely meant that we are judged by the language which we choose to employ. Another woman, highly enthusiastic about the conversa-tion in which she was engaged, said to John:

> *You're learning a lot, you say, but I'm learning so much* from you: *to listen and look so intently and to speak so calmly. Your English is so perfect, but mine is no longer perfect: with you I am putting things together.*

And here is a man who seems to stress the equality of the relationship, the per-ception that he has of being accepted for who he is so that he does not have to make a special effort to live up to a standard to which he cannot attain:

> *You're coming in straightaway, man-to-man, and I can talk to you. But if it's others, I have trouble with my mouth. I can't say a thing, I can't ask them anything. They mean trouble to me.*

Ethical implications

Bringing things to light

It would not be correct to imply that every encounter with a person with dementia involves the discussion of highly personal matters, but in John's experience such material is often at least touched upon. We all have painful issues in our lives, memories and feelings which, under normal circumstances, we tend to leave alone. We do not seek out situations which will stir them up, knowing that to do so will precipitate emotional pain and perhaps practical disruption to our lives. We may choose to do so only if there is a particular need to address the difficulties, and would normally take care over how we went about it, perhaps enlisting the support of a skilled and responsible person whom we trust to help us.

What about people with dementia in this regard? They too have psychological landmines, and need ways of coping with these. For some it may be that features of their dementia make old ways of coping with problems more difficult. Or circumstances in their present lives may act to expose old hurts and fears in ways of which others are completely unaware. One example is a person who has a history of sexual abuse or assault which is brought sharply back into awareness by the need for intimate care.

The kinds of approaches described here have the potential to bring deeply buried issues to light, and stimulate certain sorts of needs. Of course in an ideal world, people with dementia would have access to as much personal contact as they require, and it would be available in whatever form was most suitable for them – verbal, nonverbal, based in shared activity, fun or whatever. But the reality is that many people are, and may for a long time have been, starved of real, open-ended contact with others. The accumulated needs and hurts from the deprivation may be very powerful, meaning that when opportunities for genuine communication are presented, the resulting flow of profound thoughts and feelings may take both the speaker and the listener by surprise. Some of John's experiences have had this feel about them.

We also have to ask ourselves questions about whether offering the kinds of opportunities for in-depth communication we have been describing might have the effect of tapping into people's vulnerabilities in such a way as to put them at risk of further hurt. This issue is related to that of the continuity of what we seek to provide, and the danger of arousing expectations which cannot be met, as was discussed in the ethical implications section of Chapter 7.

We have all had the experience of talking frankly about ourselves on a given occasion, only to decide later that we have said too much and regret what was shared. Sometimes alcohol plays a part in such scenarios, or it may be that other features of the situation influenced our behaviour, or we may feel that the person who was the recipient of the disclosure exerted pressure in some way. A painful sense of exposure can be engendered by such experiences.

Again, these are things we need to think about in relation to people with dementia. Because they are so often deprived of opportunities for personal contact, there may be a sense of urgency to utilize those that do arise in a more intense way, meaning that things move much more quickly than is usual. Here there is a delicate balance to be struck between supporting someone's right to reveal what they choose to and helping them to protect themselves. One woman John knew springs to mind in this context; she is mentioned in Chapter 10 on writing. At the time of composing her narrative she gave the impression of being comfortable telling the story to John. But when he visited her again to share the text with her, she rejected it completely and denied that it was her own. Could it be that she had had second thoughts about whether her story was for sharing, and was exercising her right of control over the intimate details of her life? If so, it was just as well that an opportunity for her to react to the text and express feelings about the earlier conversation was provided.

There is also a risk that in our eagerness to demonstrate our availability to the individual we steer them towards talking about particularly personal issues. Receiving a confidence from someone can be flattering, and if we are at all inclined to gauge the success of an approach by the extent of personal disclosure, then again there is a temptation to move into what may be controversial or painful areas.

Another ethical dimension which relates to the subject of bringing things to light is that sometimes people tell us things which have implications in the here and now, and which pose a challenge to confidentiality. Such instances are not likely to be frequent, but when they do arise they can be very difficult. An example would be being told something which suggested that a vulnerable person, such as a child or another older person, was at risk in some way, for example of abuse.

Finally, it is important to acknowledge that as well as there being the potential of strong emotional responses in the person with dementia, there is also the potential of reactions in ourselves too. Whenever we are open to another individual, there is the possibility that something which is said will touch upon an issue of our own which is painful or unresolved, or which will change our way of understanding personally significant matters. While this need not always have negative effects, it is nevertheless true that there is an element of unpredictability and this is one of the ways in which we must be prepared for the work to change us.

9 | **Endings:** 'With regard to silence, I think it should be observed'

It may seem strange to devote an entire chapter to the act of ending an interaction, but we all know how important this phase of a significant encounter can be. No matter how enjoyable or stimulating a time we have had with someone, if the manner of the parting is wrong it can take something important away from the overall feeling of the experience. Given the particular nature of the demands involved in achieving true communication with people with dementia, and the deprived nature of many of the interpersonal contacts they have, this part of an encounter can become a very delicate and complex operation which requires considerable skill and sensitivity.

General points

It is easy for us to make the mistake of investing all our energy in the beginning and ongoing phase of an interaction, and overlook the importance of ending it in such a way as to try to ensure that its benefits remain with the person, and that they are helped to make the most of subsequent opportunities. A general point about all of the varieties of ending an encounter described here is that this phase needs to be given sufficient time. So often we

use up all of our time in the actual interacting, overlooking that a good parting is a process rather than an event. There is also the fact that because of the
sorts of difficulties experienced by the person in terms of verbal expression, a
rushed ending may increase the obstacles in articulating something important which has a summarizing or concluding function. In John's experience
many of the particularly memorable or significant things said to him by
people with dementia came towards the end of an interaction, perhaps
because it had taken time for them to become accustomed to the situation or
because the individual perceived the need to express their thoughts before
the end of the encounter. It would be a great pity for both parties to miss out
on this because of poor planning or a failure to appreciate the significance of
this phase.

Of course, we should also recognize that people vary in the way they are
used to ending with others. Some people seem to need this part of a conversation to be strung out, perhaps in quite a ritualistic way. They may have been
used to having long chats with neighbours or friends who had similar habits
in having three-quarters of a conversation punctuated by frequent references
to having to go, followed by further forays into talk. Some people prefer swift,
decisive endings which are intimated only briefly. There will be variations
within individuals according to mood, the person they are talking to, the purpose of the conversation, and the general characteristics of the situation. As
ever the same kind of variation will be found in people with dementia, and we
must be ready to adapt to this.

Another reason why it is important to give consideration to the matter of
endings is that the manner of the ending of an encounter, and the sorts of feelings we have about it, have a way of reaching forward into the whole of an
interaction and quite radically affecting its quality. We have all had experiences of meeting someone, starting to talk, and almost immediately being preoccupied with thoughts about how we are going to get away. This may occur
most markedly when there is a rush on or when we know that the person with
whom we are engaged is difficult to detach from. If these sorts of feelings arise
in relation to a person with dementia (something we discussed in Chapter 7),
it is very unlikely that the opportunity for real communication will be realized. Developing a sense of confidence as regards endings, and preventing anxiety from pervading the entire encounter is vital. This takes practice and trust,
both in yourself and in the person with whom you are engaged.

Another point which applies to all of the following is that when we are dealing with people who have dementia, the fact that many may operate on a
different time-scale from ourselves needs to be borne in mind. This may mean
that at least some of the effects or meaning of an encounter will be appreciated only after a delay. By this time you may be long gone, and if others
around the person do not know what has happened (in whatever level of
detail), the risk is that the individual will be unsupported. On account of
memory problems it may even be necessary for others to help the person to
piece together why they are feeling the way they are by reminding them of the
earlier interaction.

We shall tackle the subject by discussing in turn the possible ways interactions can end.

Happy encounters, reluctant endings

Sometimes an interaction seems so meaningful to the person with dementia (and therefore to both parties) that the prospect of ending it is unwelcome. Even considerations of tiredness can be swept away by the sheer intensity and enjoyment of the proceedings. But beyond a certain point, it is usually a mistake to believe that more is always better. Here is a woman (whom we have quoted elsewhere) deeply caught up in the process:

I'm tired, but I don't want to fall asleep because I'm thriving!

However stimulating and productive, such a conversation does have to be brought to an end before total exhaustion sets in, and on that occasion this was accomplished with the promise of continuation the following day, which was fortunate. This scenario demonstrates that we need to develop sensitivity to when a person is becoming fatigued, and this will usually be through vigilance for subtle nonverbal signals such as signs of tiredness around the eyes, postural change, and changes in the quality of the voice.

Endings initiated by ourselves

There are many possible reasons for needing to bring an interaction to an end. There may be someone else waiting to speak, or a task which needs to be undertaken, or the end of a piece of work or shift has come. Alternatively, it may be that you have become tired after a period of intense concentration, and know that you can no longer give full attention to the person. This is perfectly understandable. In terms of explaining the actual reasons for going, it is best to be straightforward. After all, most people will understand that things cannot go on for ever. Attempts at subterfuge are likely to be seen through, and it would be a pity to undermine the benefits of the interaction in this way.

Whatever the specific reason, there are considerate ways of going about ending your time with the person. A gradual disengagement is preferable since an abrupt departure may be hurtful to the person with dementia, as well as unhelpful for the reasons described above. As a way of preparing for the ending you could indicate to the person that you will have to leave in a few minutes. This provides some time for them to gather their thoughts before you actually go. Reinforcing the verbal cue with nonverbal cues such as sitting towards the front of your chair or looking at your watch may be helpful. Most people are highly sensitive to these sorts of messages.

In terms of handling the actual parting, common considerations of courtesy apply, so that it would be polite to begin by thanking the other person for talking to you, and commenting on what you have enjoyed or appreciated about the time you have spent together. You should also leave time for them to thank *you* for your effort as this often occurs. If it is likely that you will see the person again, you can say that you are looking forward to this, and give some indication of when you could come back. If you have been using a notebook or tape recorder, it will be necessary for you to indicate the arrangements for providing feedback, if this is appropriate. Sometimes people ask for their words to be read (or played) back to them then and there; if you have the time this should be done.

If you are hoping for there to be a series of interactions with the person, it is worth giving some thought to developing a routine for ending which is distinctive so that the person has the best chance of getting used to the final phase of the time you have together. Part of such a routine could also include a specific reference to the fact that you will come back, and providing something like a card you can give them with your name and when you will return. It would be helpful if either you or others around the individual can make a point of reminding them during the intervening period, and especially immediately prior to the next occasion. All this obviously requires some planning, but carrying things through in this way is respectful to the individual, and also helps you both to make the most of the time you have spent together.

If you have no plans to see the person again it is only fair to say so, and not to set up expectations in their mind which will not be fulfilled. When an encounter has gone well, and if the person expresses a hope that you will come again, it may feel quite difficult to do this. But it is better to explain the situation, and allow them to express their regret and sadness, and for you to offer yours, than to fudge the issue. It is certainly not right to assure the person that you will be back, assuming that because they have memory problems they will forget your promise.

Endings initiated by the person with dementia

It would be crass to suppose that the responsibility for ending an encounter will always fall on you. Some interactions will be brought to an end by the person with dementia, and through a variety of means. It might be done in a very deliberate and measured way, as with Bob (whom we shall meet in Chapter 10 and whose words gave the title to this one). He always used to bring things to a close by saying 'With regard to silence, I think it should be observed.' On other occasions the message may be just as unambiguous, but less gracious, as with Alice (introduced in Chapter 1) who, you will recall, once effected John's departure by calling to a care assistant in an exasperated manner 'Take this man away. I'm tired of answering his questionnaires'! On another occasion John was temporarily excluded from a three-way conversation when the man he was attempting to interview (and this, unlike the situation with Alice or almost anyone else, did involve him asking the man specific questions), picked up his dressing gown and threw it over John's head with the words 'Let's shut John up, shall we?' He was later (after approximately ten minutes) allowed back into the exchange, but the man had made his feelings only too clear!

Here is a woman confronting not her past but her future in a brave attempt to come to terms with it. She chose to end the conversation with these words:

> *I'll be dead soon. Yes, really. Nothing to ask for now. One year, and a half a year, at the most. My mother's down . . . down that street, you know, whatever they call it. But I'll not be going there, I'll be going <u>down there</u>, down the long . . . you know, into the ground.*

Some people may curtail an encounter by getting up and walking away, or starting to talk to someone else. It may be that emotional factors or memory problems play a part in these situations. Or the person may express a feeling of tiredness, indeed in some instances in John's experience people actually fall asleep.

A more difficult sort of ending is that in which the person with dementia is struggling so much with feelings of frustration and anger at their inability to access memories or give clear expression to what they want to say, that they feel they have to bring the interaction to an end in order to avoid further upset. This is clearly not the most desirable kind of ending, but given the nature of the condition it does happen. Taking time to offer comfort and acknowledgement of the difficulty, and the kind of feelings it engenders is important. You would not wish to add to the person's distress by appearing to be fazed or embarrassed by such a situation. If possible, extending the offer of coming back at another time might offset the distress associated with failure. Sometimes the person may prefer to be left alone at this point, but if they are willing and it is feasible, you could agree that you will spend a little longer together, but not attempt more conversation. Going for a short walk or joining in another activity are possibilities in this regard. Anything which avoids the person feeling that you are withdrawing your commitment mainly in response either to their difficulties or their expression of distress is important. It may even be that taking the pressure off verbal communication in this way will actually help them to relax to the point of being able to give expression to thoughts and feelings.

Again on the theme of emotional distress, sometimes in the course of in-depth communication memories may be accessed which cause the person to become tearful. Different people have different feelings about crying in front of another. For some, it seems acceptable. It is certainly our view that the act of crying itself is not necessarily to be regarded as a negative aspect of an interaction. For others, however, such a development would lead to embarrassment, which in turn would necessitate a withdrawal from company. In such circumstances, if you are not in a position to see that they are in a safe place while feeling so vulnerable, and check on them later, it is obviously important to let someone else know what has happened.

Staying with the subject of strong emotion, it occasionally happens that a person becomes so distressed that a decision needs to be taken by you about whether it is wise to continue. Again, we emphasize that it would be very unfortunate by leaving abruptly giving the impression that the expression of strong feelings is unacceptable, but if the person seems to be becoming overwhelmed and needs some support from outside to handle their feelings, it is sometimes right to suggest that a break from talking might be desirable. It may be that a change of scene or activity, without actually leaving the person, is sufficient to help them to regain a necessary degree of control.

Ambiguous endings

Some interactions are characterized by endings which although seeming to be initiated by the other person, are less clear-cut than others. Here is the last part of a conversation John had with Elaine, in which powerful emotions had been expressed concerning the deaths of those close to her:

John: Life's a bit of a sad thing, isn't it?
Elaine: *It is, yes. There's so many people that needs to be . . .*
helpful, to be helpful.
John: Yes. People are helpful to you?
Elaine: *Always . . . it's only small things, isn't it? If you'll excuse*
me, I'd better get up.
John: Mmm.
Elaine: *. . . for a moment.*
John: Okay.
Elaine: *Well, I can come back, as a car . . . as a cars'll . . . maybe*
it's because I've done such a lot, I'm just showing . . .
John: Yes.
Elaine: *I've done . . . saving the children, I've taken to school and*
that by this . . . just about . . . this but I've got whatever you
say but . . .
John: Are you going to come back again?
Elaine: *Well's . . . I can . . . I'd like to if just . . .*
John: If you're going to walk round for a few minutes, and
you . . . and come back?
Elaine: *Well, I don't think . . . not gone into that sort of thing, but I*
don't, I don't really . . . excuse me . . .
John: Yes.
Elaine: *I'm not sure what it was but it was right, yes.*
John: All right. Thank you, Elaine . . .
Elaine: *Sorry, I have to . . .*
John: Yes.

We do not know whether Elaine's reticence over the actual ending was related to her having had an emotionally charged conversation, or whether this was her natural style. Politeness was probably also a factor. Perhaps she really wanted to get away but, out of consideration for John's feelings, may have felt that to express this directly was rude. In situations where things are ambiguous in this way, nonverbal cues are likely to provide important indicators of the person's disposition.

Whatever was going on here, it is an illustration of the fact that at times we will need to exercise judgement over what it is that the person needs to do, and how they feel most comfortable in communicating those needs.

Ending interactions which the person with dementia wants to continue

Perhaps the most difficult type of ending is the one in which you have to go, but the person with dementia very much wants you to stay with them. This may be expressed, perhaps strongly and emotionally by the other person, or it may be a much more masked wish. Either way it can be a painful, even wrenching situation. The desire of the person can arise from a variety of factors. They may, sadly, have very little in the way of real human contact, and simply need more. It may be that having got started in managing to communicate thoughts and feelings, they realize that there is more to say and feel somewhat desperate at the prospect that they are going to lose the all-important link with another person before serious things have been said. The need may be heightened by awareness that, due to the fluctuating nature of the condition, opportunities to express themselves are few and far between. In such a situation it is obviously necessary to go as far as possible towards extending the time available. As we have said before, trying to make sure that there is someone else who knows what has happened and who can offer comfort and support is extremely important. We return to this scenario in the discussion of ethical issues at the end of this chapter.

Endings initiated by others

Sometimes interactions are curtailed by the arrival of relatives or friends of the person, or another visitor with a particular reason for seeing them. It may be possible if you are still deeply involved in the interaction to negotiate a short extension of time, but often visitors are in a hurry with plans to be away at a certain time, so you may find yourself in the position of having an ending imposed on you. You can express your regrets and arrange another time if that is possible.

In Chapter 8 we raised the possibility of an interruption by another person or persons with dementia, and there we advised the steering of the third party or parties away so that the current interaction can proceed. If a real disturbance has been caused, and the concentration of the person you are engaged with has been broken by this, it may be better to bring the encounter to an end, and try again on another occasion.

Endings caused by routine events

In service settings, many of which have their time punctuated by regular events, an artificial time limit may be imposed on interactions. The person may be aware of this and insist on keeping to the timetable. You have no control over these events, and must be prepared for them. If you are yourself a staff member then you may be able to bend the rules somewhat to accommodate an extension to the conversation if things are going well. Otherwise you will need to apologize and explain that the ending was not of your choice.

Ending interactions which have reached a natural conclusion

This is obviously a less challenging situation overall. It may be that there has been a long silence or diminution in nonverbal interaction, or a gradual tailing off in the momentum of the conversation. Or it could be that the person with dementia has reached the end of a story or seems satisfied with the amount of talking they have done. Even when this phase of the interaction seems to have taken care of itself, it is still important to offer the same sorts of concluding steps as described above. The extent to which these are welcomed or needed has to be judged on an individual basis.

Ending interactions that have not been successful

Some interactions may never get off the ground. It may be that there were longstanding factors impinging on the encounter which proved to be barriers. Examples include another condition such as depression or a sensory disability such as deafness. The person may be taking medication which dulls their responses so much that concentration is impeded. Or the problems may have been more transitory in nature. Tiredness, discomfort or the effects of recent emotional distress may have interfered with the opportunity to establish rapport. Or the person may have been having an off-day, as we all do, for reasons which are unclear.

It is also important to consider factors which pertain to yourself. Were you not feeling your best? Were you preoccupied with another matter or daunted by the effort involved in extending yourself to the other person? When things do not work out, it is too easy to pin the blame on the person with dementia when deficits of sympathy, awareness and adaptability lie in ourselves. This can be hard to accept, but it is one of the challenges that working with people with dementia poses us: it tests our powers of empathy and understanding, and all of us will be found wanting at some time or another.

In a sense it may be easier to end a conversation that has hardly begun, but since it may be difficult to judge whether the interaction is just taking time to establish itself or whether it has no real potential at all this can be delicate. Exactly when do you throw in the towel? Should you wait for the person with dementia, by some word or action, to terminate the encounter, or should you take the lead? It is impossible to give clear guidance on this. Again, attending to the nonverbal cues will help you to decide.

Here is an example of a woman providing a very clear explanation of her refusal to accept an invitation to conversation. Each time John approached her she couched her response in similar terms:

> *You have hurt me. You have hurt me deeply. Because you will go away . . . I don't want to talk to you. I don't want to see you again. Because you will go away.*

We must be mindful of others who do not have this degree of foresight, and embark on relationship innocently unaware of the disappointment that may await them; perhaps a deep sense of loss which could suddenly flow into them when we take our leave. As we said at the outset of these practical chapters, we make a moral choice when we break into the world of someone with dementia, and the responsibility we bear comes home to us particularly keenly in negotiating the timing and manner of our departure from them.

Not managing to establish and maintain positive contact can be very dispiriting, but it is not realistic to expect success every time. However, we should also recognize that as well as your feelings of disappointment, there are likely to be reactions to the lack of success in the person with dementia. Given the poverty of opportunities many people with the condition suffer, your invitation to make contact may be the only one that has arisen in a long time. We cannot make easy assumptions about how the individual may interpret this outcome, but however it may have been understood, the offer of consolation to the person is important. It may be easier to do this nonverbally by taking their hand. Finding the right words is difficult, but perhaps you could say that you are sorry you have not been very helpful and perhaps you could try again another time. Or maybe you could comment that neither of you seemed in the right frame of mind on this occasion. As mentioned above, continuing to spend some time together in silence or asking the person whether they would like to do something else or joining in any other activity which is available may be helpful. Or it may be that they would prefer to be alone.

When we take all the variables into consideration we may, of course, still be faced with the conclusion that the necessary chemistry for developing a positive and enjoyable relationship is lacking. No one can expect to be able to achieve rapport with everyone, and this applies as much to people with dementia as to those without. This is something we discussed in the section on ethical implications in Chapter 2.

On the more positive side, you can remind yourself that no interaction is a total failure; it may be that the other person has gained something of which you are not aware, and there is in any case something to learn from every attempt. Reflecting on these, making notes about experiences or speaking to someone else may reveal valuable pointers for increasing your chances of success the next time. If you suspect that an influence such as depression or deafness is contributing to communication difficulties, then it is vital either to follow this up yourself or to pass on the information to someone who is in a position to do so. It is simply not acceptable for treatable problems, or ones that can at least be alleviated, to go unattended. As with other situations, it is desirable, if appropriate, to let a member of staff know how things have worked out.

Again (as was mentioned earlier), it is also important to bear in mind that the factors which underpin successful communication can change rapidly. It has been John's experience that mood and attention in someone with dementia can alter radically within a short period of time. A person who in the morning seems withdrawn and unresponsive by the afternoon may welcome the chance of a conversation and prove extremely forthcoming. Never let an unfortunate experience prevent you from making further attempts.

Your own feelings on leaving

We have talked a great deal here about the feelings of the other person when an interaction comes to an end, but we must also recognize that given the amount of energy and commitment you have brought to the enterprise, it would be surprising if there were not feelings present for you. These may range over a great spectrum of emotion, depending on what has happened, what has been said, and how things were left. As we shall discuss further in Chapter 10, reflecting on the experience and perhaps writing notes about it are very important. Seeking support from another person, whether or not you share the details of an encounter, is also a valuable strategy. The main thing is not to underestimate the impact of the experience, and proceed too directly to the next since this is likely to lead to your feeling overwhelmed and confused about what has been happening. Valuing and taking care of yourself is part of honouring the personhood of people with dementia.

Ethical implications

The sorts of ethical issues we discussed in relation to earlier phases of an interaction will have a bearing on its ending as well, but there are also matters which pertain specifically to this part of an encounter. Our feelings on leaving the person will depend to a large extent on how the interaction itself has unfolded. In most instances, the act of taking one's leave will not raise particular problems, but when this is complicated in some way it can be very difficult, even poignant.

A very delicate situation arises when the person with dementia does not want you to go, or expresses a strong desire for you to come back again when you know it is not possible for you to do so. At such times there may be a strong temptation to assure them that you will return, assuming while you do that the individual will, on account of their memory problems, forget this undertaking. You may be further tempted to tell yourself that this is the kindest thing to do, sparing the person the need to confront disappointment. The

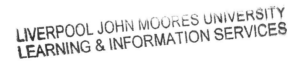

reality is, of course, that we do such things to protect ourselves, and it cannot be right to deceive someone in this way. As we discussed in Chapter 5 on memory, our understanding of the way that memory works in dementia is at best partial, particularly in the area of emotional memory. This seems to point to the conclusion that honesty is called for, along with attention to the person's need to express feelings and be supported in doing so.

There is little else that can be said in a situation such as this other than that it is difficult and painful, but that sad partings are a part of life that most of us will experience and people with dementia are no different.

Aside from considerations about whether you are going to be able to spend more time together, there can be difficult issues around the act of leaving someone behind when you go away, especially if you know that they are unhappy in their situation. The fact of being able to walk away and return to the life which is more usually your own highlights the gulf between your situation and that of the other person. These are often the times when our efforts to make sense of the complexity of life operate at their deepest, and we can value such experiences for these promptings. We may wonder why it should be that one's own life simply seems more rich and satisfying than that of the other person, and this may even give rise to feelings of guilt. In these circumstances we can remind ourselves that most people with dementia would discourage this, and urge us instead to use our energies to do something useful to improve their situation.

Finally, it is important to acknowledge that despite our best intentions and efforts to engage with people, it is sometimes a profound relief to get away and return to a more usual level of intensity in interactions. While this situation too may bring about feelings of guilt, such a reaction is understandable.

10 | **Writing:** 'It's a good idea, this writing it down'

So far we have been concentrating on spoken and nonverbal encounters as they arise and develop in the present moment. Here we extend the discussion to ways of capturing aspects of them through writing and recording also referred to here as 'externalizing'. This is an important subject because despite the pivotal role of our thoughts and feelings in our day-to-day lives, they often remain fleeting and unexaminable. Writing is a way of overcoming this. There is something objective about seeing one's words written down. It puts them into a different time-frame, lends them a certain permanency. It also places them in a different context: they are no longer swimming around in one's head like fish; they have been 'caught', and laid out for inspection alongside other 'catches' of one's own and other people.

The following remark was made by the philosopher Graham Wallas:

How do I know what I think until I see what I say?[1]

The practice of externalizing one's thoughts and feelings does seem to facilitate the process of reflecting, ordering and developing them. It helps us to examine them more closely, enabling a heightened level of reflection and making of connections. There may also be benefits to memory, both in the sense that writing something helps to fix it in the memory, and also that the writing itself constitutes a kind of external memory.

The development of writing was a great advance for civilization: at last it was possible for ideas to be recorded and transmitted in a reliable manner. It also allowed human thought and experience to escape from the tyranny of the present moment. Instead of being imprisoned in 'now', we can time travel to the thoughts of other people in other centuries, and also to our own thoughts at earlier stages of our lives.

Diary and journal writing have a long history, but in recent years they have become especially popular. Imaginative literature is full of examples of individuals exploring and evaluating their experiences by writing them down. During the 1980s and 1990s there has grown up in Britain a movement which promotes the use of creative writing for personal development.[2] Herman Hesse, the German novelist, describes such writing as:

> a long, diverse and winding path, whose goal it would be to express the personality, the 'I' of the artist, so completely, so minutely in all its branchings . . . that this 'I' would in the end be as it were unreeled and finished.[3]

This is obviously a largely unrealizable goal, nevertheless behind it lies the view that self-exploration through language can be a revelatory process.

Why undertake writing with people with dementia?

We hope we have already demonstrated that many people with dementia are capable of expressing thoughts and feelings verbally, and that this is something which demands to be acknowledged both for their sake and for ours. Writing down their thoughts constitutes another dimension of communication. We now go on to identify a variety of specific functions which we believe writing can fulfil. By this we mean that the actual writing should be undertaken by you, rather than the person with dementia.

● *Writing demonstrates that the encounter is being taken seriously*

Writing confers importance on the utterance, and thereby on the person who does the uttering. We have made the point a number of times already that one of the ways in which people with dementia tend to be disadvantaged is in the lack of attention paid to what they have to say. Proper listening is a way to counteract this, but writing their words down reinforces it powerfully. One woman said to John:

> *It's been very exciting doing this. It makes me feel important.*

● *Writing helps the person to reflect on their own thoughts*

As we said earlier, writing involves the process of externalizing. One man said:

> *What I say is not important, but it can be stated and looked at.*

Those words 'looked at' seem significant. The visual nature of writing may help in the process of collecting and organizing thoughts – observing continuities and discontinuities, resemblances and dissimilarities. It is a form of pattern-making; you are building up a picture which it is hoped will have some coherence. People with dementia especially need that structure, that clarification. They also need to be able to exercise control in some areas of their lives, and maybe seeing their words assembled on the page assists that process. It may even be that the process of having thoughts written down can help the person to sort out their priorities in terms of what is most important to them, to focus on those aspects of their experience which contribute most to their central sense of meaning. One woman said:

> I'd like to do away with old age. But you've got to live with every day. Yet this talking about it helps get things straight and off your mind.

Very significantly, the woman (who was first quoted on p. 80) who said:

> I'm talking, talking, talking all the time. I didn't know if you would understand, with you living on the other side.

also added:

> But with this writing you might find out what's what.

Writing may promote fluency

For some people having their utterances written down may actually help to promote fluency. As we have already discussed, for people with dementia it seems that the act of speaking aloud, of sharing feelings and ideas with another person who is properly listening and is truly alongside the speaker, provides an essential stimulus. Seeing their words being written down is a concrete demonstration of their being caught and held, while the person continues the labour of bringing more ideas to birth.

Writing can become an integral part of an interaction

In earlier chapters we explored the idea of various forms of mutuality in interaction. We think that with some people and in some situations the process of writing can enter into this. Writing down someone's words captures a quality of 'at-onceness'. It also resembles the practice of mirroring of which we spoke first in Chapter 3. There is the sense of reflecting back to the person what belongs to them. The writing becomes an integral element of the communication, a part of the dance. Writing may also supply a sense of rhythm to the activity of talking. The pacing involved could provide cues which give shape to the discourse, almost like musical motifs in a composition.

Writing can reinforce identity

Related to the above point about mirroring, it may be that the act of writing the words of the person has the effect of reinforcing their sense of who they are. One woman, before receiving a transcript, was already expressing her enthusiasm for the project:

> *Lovely, them notebooks, aren't they? Let me see your book. I've done that, haven't I? And I've liked it. Absolutely fantastic! Just shows what I am!*

A piece of writing can become a prized possession

A piece of writing can become an artefact upon which the person with dementia confers value. It becomes a personal possession they have unexpectedly acquired. Some people keep it and show it to others. Some have multiple copies made and insist on others taking them away. In this way the piece can become a kind of gift.

Writing supports memory

Clearly people with dementia have difficulties with memory, and writing can function as a way of offsetting problems in this area. Seeing words being written and the sense of occasion which goes with this may help the person to lay down a stronger memory of the experience. Also the writing is a form of external memory. It becomes an element of continuity in circumstances where this is often lacking. Without it important occasions of intimacy might largely be lost since one cannot rely upon memory to provide accurate details of subtle moments when understanding is transmitted. As one man said:

> *It's a good idea, this writing it down. It's got a nice bit of merit. It's tantamount to saying that you're speaking from your memory all the while.*

Writing provides a record for subsequent interpretation

We have already discussed the fact that for many people language use becomes increasingly difficult, with words and sentences beginning to take unconventional forms. In these circumstances understanding and interpreting meaning is a challenge. Writing down what people say can provide an opportunity for further reflection which does not rely on the fragility of memory. One woman seemed very clear about this:

> *I'm glad you're writing this down, because when I say it to myself, it's gone.*

A text could be used to build on in subsequent conversations or interactions

Once a text has been transcribed and, if necessary, edited (we say more about this process later) it can be shared with the person with dementia (again, more later). Just as the original process of writing may have helped the person to articulate and develop their thoughts, the subsequent stage of sharing the written text may stimulate more reflection, with the person providing a commentary on the original. Just as a series of interactions can be the building-blocks for a structure of relationship, so a series of writings can spark off new subject-matter or deepen exploration of topics already uncovered.

A text can sometimes be shared with others

Where permission has been granted (and again we discuss this issue later), there is the further potential benefit of sharing texts with relatives and other staff. Through this kind of sharing there are opportunities for others to gain insights about the person, and their life and concerns. In John's experience others are often deeply surprised at the complexity and profundity of what the person has managed to express, having assumed that the dementia had robbed them of such capacity. Sharing with others may also aid interpretation. They may be able to throw light on idiosyncrasies of language or provide facts which make sense of obscurities in relationship or chronology.

The practice of writing down and sharing the words of people with dementia also enables relatives and staff to build up a bank of information which can be used to put a life into context. Anything that counteracts the tendency for people to see those with the condition in two-dimensional terms is surely to be encouraged.

Practical aspects

We hope that we have convinced you that in theory writing down the words of people with dementia is not only of interest but can also be a valuable tool in the search for understanding. We now come to a detailed account of what is involved in the practice. We shall cover both writing and tape-recording at the time of the conversation and transcribing at a later time.

Asking permission to write or record

It is a basic tenet of our approach that permission should be obtained from a person before engaging in an interaction, and the same applies to writing and recording. (The matter of what amounts to permission, and how we know whether this has been granted is a highly complex one, and must be a matter for judgement at the time and checking and monitoring throughout the process.) These requests are best not presented together, however, as it might prove confusing to the person. In any case, it may well be that making a record of a conversation is neither necessary nor desirable in all cases and you need to have the freedom to make that decision. If having established contact, you do decide that writing or recording would be beneficial, you will need to exercise further judgement about when and in what way to raise the matter. John usually says something like 'What you say is very interesting. I would like to write it down/tape record it. Is that all right with you?' If the person does not seem happy with this proposal, you have to decide whether to let the matter drop there, or to explore further their reasons. It may be that the person has misunderstood or requires explanation, and if this can be clarified would be happy to continue. If you do proceed without writing or recording, however, the person should not sense any diminution in your commitment to the interaction.

The writing itself

You will need a notebook and a pen or pencil which you should be comfortable with as you may have to write very quickly. You could try leaning the notebook on your knee or on the table or the arm of a chair. It is best if the person can see that you are writing, and also what you are writing if they choose. Achieving a comfortable and practical position for this, which is also compatible with the other suggestions for physical positioning in the course of communication work, can be quite a challenge. At times you may come away feeling quite tired. But it is important that the practice has a shared quality, which is as open to the other person as possible. You certainly do not want it to appear that you are making notes about them. Writing down their words is an intimate act, and needs to be a transparently honest one.

Probably the most complex aspect of writing down what people say is concentrating upon the activity while at the same time paying attention to all those areas of communication outlined in Chapters 7–9. Because of the difficulty of formulating in conventional language what you sometimes hear, you certainly have to have your wits about you in putting signs on the paper which will make sense later. Shorthand would speed the process up, but unfortunately much of the language of people with dementia does not conform to its rules. It can be very frustrating to hear one thing, and while one is grappling with how to write that down, to be presented with the next baffling sentence. Should you concentrate on getting the first part right, and attempt a poor approximation of the second, or miss the second part out altogether, thereby breaking the continuity of the discourse? There is no foolproof answer here. The text will never be totally accurate. It may catch the general flavour of an utterance, or be more accurate in specific places. Either way it is far better than nothing.

Recording

A solution to the challenges of writing down what people say is to use a tape recorder. There are again, of course, issues about obtaining permission from the person for this practice. Any device which is unfamiliar may distress the person, and occasion uncharacteristic reactions which invalidate the whole procedure. In John's experience some people respond adversely to the idea of being recorded but are positively enthusiastic about having their words written down. Somehow the sight of a notebook is reassuring, even affirming, presumably because the whole operation is visibly under control.

The tape recorder should be shown to the person, and its purpose and use explained, and demonstrated if this would be helpful. If the person is agreeable to it being used, it should be placed somewhere its presence is not obtrusive, but also without it being in any way hidden. The fact that it is visible can then prompt the person to ask about it again or raise any concerns they have about the process. You will need a small machine, but one which is sensitive enough to catch mumbles, sighs and whispers which might play an essential part in conveying meaning.

When you first attempt recording you will probably have to overcome feelings of self-consciousness, but you can remind yourself that the person with dementia and the interaction are the most important things, and that the matter of recording and later producing a transcript are secondary. Being there for the person is what counts. When you come to replay a tape you will need to come to terms with hearing your own voice, but time and practice work wonders in reducing the dismay that this experience can occasion.

In a research project undertaken by Kate, exploring ways for staff to encourage people with dementia to express their views of services, practitioners were supported in making audio recordings of their conversations with service users.[4] Most were nervous initially, but once they got started they found the practice so revealing that they became enthusiasts for it.

Caroline Keegan, a mental health nurse in a hospital long-stay ward, gives the following account of using a tape recorder as part of her work:

> Every day I listen to my colleagues relating things which residents have said which may sound bizarre yet they get a strong sense of what is being meant, but as nurses we are all too shy of expressing our ideas, other than to each other, in case our interpretations are ridiculed for being too subjective.
>
> I felt that these 'hunches' which we all experience were too important to ignore, so I committed conversations which I had with residents to paper, so that they could be properly scrutinised. Using a tape-recorder initially for accuracy, this became a natural process which did not detract from my delivering normal nursing care as all my 'data' was gathered while helping residents to get washed and dressed, serving them breakfast, during tea-time etc.
>
> For me the results have been truly illuminating. Putting their words on paper has allowed me to listen to what is being said at a more profound level, and gradually I feel that this process is helping me to break down communication barriers between myself and the residents with whom I work.[5]

Challenges of writing

Writing down what a person says while they are speaking can be difficult. These include situations where the syntax is fragmented, or the vocabulary is a mixture of the known and unknown. Sometimes the person makes a sound which could be interpreted in different ways, and perhaps with important implications for the meaning of what has been said.

Another set of issues is raised by any dialect in which the person speaks. If you are unfamiliar with a particular localized vocabulary and accent it becomes difficult to discriminate between words which belong to that dialect and have a specific meaning, and those which may be invented or be approximations of standard words. In those instances where you do understand the meanings of dialect words, you are faced with a choice of whether to 'translate' them into standard English for the benefit of others who might read the text, or leave them as they are. Our view is that the latter course is preferable, since it seems important to keep all aspects of the language of a person with dementia intact so that it may be examined as a whole. The fact that a person expresses themselves in a particular way is an integral part of their identity, and we need to observe all aspects if we are to make respect for personhood a reality.

Some of these difficulties are alleviated by using a tape recorder since this frees you to concentrate on the interaction itself, and allows you to transcribe later at your own speed. You can also rehear over and over again difficult passages until you arrive at a version which satisfies you. However, some of the same problems (unfamiliar words, ambiguous sounds) arise in transcribing from tapes in the same way as when you are writing during an interaction.

Another decision you will have to make is whether to include your own words in a transcript. There cannot be a golden rule here. Clearly if the interaction takes the form of an even-handed conversation it will be necessary to include this element to make sense of what the other person is saying. But it is John's experience that many attempts at conversation take the form of a monologue interspersed with his own occasional words of encouragement. It can be irritating to read a piece of dialogue where one partner's contribution is reduced to regular yeses and noes and ums and uhuhs. In these cases it may seem reasonable to present the words of the person with dementia as uninterrupted speech.

In all of these circumstances you will have to settle for a text which is imperfect. But you should not be too downhearted about this. A reasonable shot is better than no attempt at all, and there is the satisfaction gained from the interaction for both of you, and indeed from your attempts to write it down. Although writing is a real challenge, it can bring special rewards to you, the transcriber. To do this work effectively requires very close concentration, and as a result of this discipline it may be that your skills as a listener on subsequent occasions will actually improve, with your attention becoming more acute and your awareness deepened. These are benefits which can also enhance other relationships in your life.

Capturing nonverbal aspects of conversation

A transcript can convey only the words of a conversation, none of its nonverbal nuances. So much is missing of the meaning of what someone says if you do not have details of the various aspects of the voice, the expression of the face, the movements of the body and so on. Where a significant event occurs, for example someone walking away and then resuming the interaction, or becoming tearful, then these should obviously be noted. It may be that as part of the skills development you undergo in writing you will be able to design your own code for recording the nonverbal aspects of an interaction. But however good you become at making notes, you will have to accept the fact that what you produce can only be a partial account of a complex human activity.

Sharing of texts

A text is there for you to look at, remember the details of a conversation, and analyse for meaning, but it may, as we have argued, also have considerable potential as a stimulus to further conversation with the person, as an artefact for them to value, and as a document which can provide information and insight to others – relatives, care staff and even a wider audience. How should you go about attempting these activities?

Sharing a text with the person themselves

This is the prime sharing activity, and no other should be attempted before this process has occurred. Because of memory loss and fluctuations in mood and attention span, among other factors, however, it may prove difficult if not impossible. The person may reject your approach on the second occasion, or not remember you or the activity which resulted in the text. Or they may remember you and the occasion, but not recognize the words as their own. This does not, of course, invalidate the text but undermines the possibility of sharing it.

When sharing does occur, you will still have to choose the timing of the occasion carefully if the maximum value is to be derived from it. You will need to explain clearly what it is and how it came about. A decision has to be made about whether the person is able to read the text for themselves or whether they will need to have it read to them. Even when every step has been taken to make the occasion positive and affirming, there is still a degree of unpredictability.

Not everyone is as robust as the man who said 'Hand the bloody thing back to me and I'll be your corrector.' It has been John's experience that, although he always makes the transcript available, some people show little or no interest, and some are actively hostile to the idea. Some do not recognize their words. One man actually screwed the text up and swallowed it! One man, despite the innocuous nature of the material, was seriously concerned that it might find its way into the pages of the *News of the World*, although it contained no elements that could conceivably have appealed to the readers of that newspaper. When a recording has been made, some people ask for it to be played back to them and either find the sound of their voice upsetting or do not recognize it.

One woman made a long tape which was transcribed. When presented with the text, she rejected it as not being her life story and the voice as not being her own. She demanded that the transcript be destroyed and the tape wiped clean. In this instance, however, John suspects that she was alarmed that she had revealed more about herself than she felt comfortable with. The transcript represented many hours' work, and this story serves as a reminder that there are serious time implications involved in using a tape recorder: the time has to be added to that already spent on the interaction itself. The sharing of a text can be a very positive experience, however. One person who was clearly delighted with what she had managed to say, gathered up as many staff as were on duty at the time and proudly declaimed it over and over again.

Asking permission to share it with others

Some, probably most, texts will not be suitable for sharing. The expression of intimate feelings or the disclosure of personal details or experiences is material which, in most circumstances, should rightly stay private. Where sharing does seem a possibility, however, the first principle must be that the person with dementia is familiar with the text that might be shared. Although you have transcribed it, the piece of writing belongs fundamentally to them, and they can do with it whatever they choose, from actually sharing it with others themselves or destroying it. But in most circumstances you can certainly suggest the idea of sharing it if this is not forthcoming from the person. You need to be very clear about what you are proposing: is the piece to be shown to one other person (who?), or a group of people (name them), or offered to a wider group (talk about anonymity)? Reasons for suggesting sharing the text should also be given. If it is proposed that a relative is involved, you could suggest that they would be proud of what has been achieved. If it might be shown to staff, you could suggest that they would find it interesting to find out more about the individual. If the material, or an extract from it, might be published, you could stress the sharing of the achievement or the information aspect or both. Remember Alice's words in Chapter 1:

> *Anything you can tell people about how things are for me is important.*

It would be a mistake to think that people with dementia are necessarily unable to appreciate the implications of what is proposed. One woman handed a text to John with the injunction:

> *Publish it!*

In some instances it may seem appropriate to obtain written permission from the person and perhaps from relatives before sharing the piece of writing. In others a clear affirmative from the person may be sufficient. Whichever procedure you adopt, you must satisfy yourself that the person understands what they have agreed to. This matter is revisited later in this chapter.

Sharing with relatives and others

Relatives, in John's experience, give mixed receptions to the practice. Some are highly enthusiastic, and read and re read the transcripts, treating them as evidence of the continued coherence of their loved one. Some seem set against the possibility of their relative still having a meaningful contribution to make; as if it were easier to assume that communication had ceased altogether than to face all the uncertainties of a less dogmatic position.

We need to realize that seeing the words of your loved one written down and absorbing the messages they contain can be a deeply, even at times overwhelming, emotional experience. It can go to the heart of longstanding relationships, with all their complexities, and have a direct bearing on the process of adjustment occasioned by the dementia. The following story illustrates the rawness of feelings which can be uncovered.

A woman on one unit, with great difficulty but determination, composed her story with John's assistance, and asked specially that it be presented to her husband. When John did so, in her presence, he screwed the paper up and threw it across the room, with the words 'I don't need you to prove to me that my wife is mad.'

The moral would appear to be that writings come in all shapes and sizes and take their place in a variety of psychological and social contexts. It is necessary to exercise discretion in the ways in which we make them available to people. It is important to remember that a written document carries an authority greater than the spoken word. It is as if it is in some way 'official'. It also has a permanence. It could be read by people who understand little of the circumstances of its composition and have little awareness of the principle of confidentiality. So transcripts must be kept in a secure place and only those authorized to do so should be given access to them. A woman speaking to John summed up the situation well:

> You're like this: snip, snip, snip – picking up every little bit that's dropped from the lips. Well, don't be leaving it around!

Editing

We return to the matter of 'editing' referred to earlier. Really all we have in mind by the use of this term is going through a text, particularly one that has been made at speed, and making sure that everything is clearly written; this is best done as soon after the interaction as possible while things remain fresh in your mind. It also gives you the opportunity for second thoughts about words or expressions at which you made a stab at the time but which on reflection might have been interpreted differently. We are strongly of the view that a transcript should be as accurate as you can possibly make it. This includes indicating pauses, fluffed attempts at words and sentences, and sounds which are on the borderline of language. We owe it to the person to treat their attempts to communicate with as much seriousness as we would anyone without the condition.

Another meaning of the term 'editing' which is certainly relevant to the activity we are engaged in is where certain portions of a text are highlighted, even to the extent of being removed from context. It would be unrealistic to pretend that all the parts of some texts are of equal interest. Judicious cutting can prove helpful by isolating passages for special consideration. Some of the passages quoted in this book are of that kind. We are not, of course, advocating the altering of vocabulary or the modifying of the structure of sentences in an attempt to 'improve' the original, in accordance with some hunch or theory of our own about what was being communicated. And the original full text would always be retained to be consulted wherever necessary. Writer Trisha Kotai-Ewers has a similar approach to the material she gathers:

> Increasingly I work with a complete section of the transcript. However, often I look for themes. In a 45 minute conversation with Rae, she kept returning to the theme of being in the dark. When I collected these references they made an almost two-page piece.[6]

Creating poems

There have been some attempts made to shape the words of some people with the condition into poems on account of a perceived natural symbolic content (see Chapter 4 for a consideration of this characteristic). John has probably been the writer who has most consistently attempted this.[7] The following is an example:

An eye-shot in summer

A little eyesight in the middle,
some of it retained for a purpose.

I can see a sleeve of purple
And then there is yellow in the sky.

The trees are good and dry,
young and basking.

It's a wonderful setting,
this whole melting scene.

Is it opening or seizing?
The view – it's got the ring of expand.

All the woman's remarks in the interaction were about the visual world and the way she observes it. There were comments on the landscape outside the window, on the lounge in which they sat, and on the process of seeing. Of these three subjects there were more observations on the landscape than on the other two, so John took four of these and introduced them with a comment on the nature of seeing. The poem is held together not just by its subject matter, but by the consistently imaginative use of language: 'eye-shot', 'basking', 'melting', 'seizing' and 'the ring of expand'. Of course a great deal of editing has been done, but this is usually the way with art – many practitioners speak of the process as a paring away of material until an essence is revealed. This seems to us perfectly acceptable so long as nothing is added, and we bear in mind that what we have at the end is a selective rendering of the original utterance.

People doing their own writing

It has been John's experience in nursing homes that very few of the people he works with retain the ability to write for themselves. Here is one man talking about this subject:

> I don't write and put anything down because I've gone off writing at the same time. Yes I am. And I find that very awkward too. I find it difficult, so I've gradually given it up. Not for good, I'm not planning that, but if I don't come across writing I don't, so to speak.

However, there are examples of people with dementia keeping journals and even writing books. In Kim Zabbia's book, mother and daughter both chronicle the course of the condition.[8] The last entry of the mother, Lou Howes, is a reflection upon losing the ability both to read and write:

> I have a problem in my writing and my reading. I am trying to see if it will be easier to read if it was a dark black pen. It is hard. I have realized that I cannot read my own writing. I thought that if I could not read it, nobody else could read it. I really don't have to write. I could live the rest of my life not writing, but I would be very sad.[9]

After diagnosis Robert Davis embarked on the major task of writing a whole book about his experience of travelling into dementia.[10] He was fighting his cognitive and linguistic losses from the start:

> Last September as I began to outline thoughts for this book, I was able to write them out. Although many words were missing and many sentences unclear, Betty, my wife for twenty-nine years, was able to decipher my intent and type it into my computer. Then together we read and discussed until I felt sure my feelings were recorded. Chapters 1, 8, 9 and 10 were completed this way. By January I could no longer type a complete thought or keep my head together to write out very much, so I rented a dictaphone and wrenched Chapters 3, 4, and 5 this way. Chapter 7 became so disjointed that we had to take the paragraphs of my description of the physical aspects and let Betty re-write them. Chapter 6 and the Epilogue are Betty's alone. She also has a mammoth job to condense my running on and on and repeating myself.[11]

We are aware that these last two quotations stress negative aspects of people with dementia doing their own writing. It is in fact a deeply meaningful process for those who are able to engage in it, conferring insight and purposefulness on the authors, but it is not to be embarked upon lightly. Both Lou Howes and Robert Davis had support, and we need to ensure that this is in place before encouraging anyone to attempt something so demanding.

Carers and relatives keeping journals

An alternative to the person writing for him or herself, might be for a carer or relative to keep a journal for someone with dementia. Early in Beth Shirley Brough's book, her friend Reg urges her to put pen to paper. Reg speaks first:[12]

> Will you write about us? Tell them. Tell them about us?
> Would you like that?
> Would I ever! But, but, more importantly – *they'd* like it. They'd like to know.[13]

And thus was born a book which was a sustained, and perhaps sustaining, enterprise for them both. It seems that Reg's view of the project might have differed from Beth's. He appears to have been seeing it in terms of relationship, and while this subject is clearly deeply important to her too, aspects of her writing are an account of the progress of the condition as well. Alice in Chapter 1 was aware of the enterprise she and John were engaged in, and of its difficulties, describing them as '*a far fetch*'.

Many carers and relatives find the process of reflection is facilitated by keeping a personal record of the experience in which they are caught up. It could be not only valuable as a record, but also empowering: a stay against those feelings of helplessness which can so easily overtake them. They might then go to write about other aspects of their lives. Self-reflection through writing, as we have already stated, is a potent medium.

What people say about the writing

Comments on the process abound in John's work. Some are enthusiastic:

> *You'll be able to look at what you've got and decide: one good, one bad or one hell of a nuisance!*

> *I saw this done, what you're doing. It's good. I done it meself in the past.*

> *When you said you did what you are doing I thought perhaps you might be able to do something for me. Do you do much of that which you are doing now with different people? What you are doing I could try to sing to.*

Occasionally a person expresses serious doubts, as in the following examples:

> *You shouldn't really be writing this down. It's against the law of the jungle.*

> *I'm not sure about this . . . that you're doing. They may think it funny, all this*

notebook thing, but it's not funny at all. It isn't as though we had a source of going to look at it. Not that I would want to see it.

What I want to know is: what is this doing for <u>you</u>? You'll have me filleted then!

Obviously in these latter instances the practice ceased at once.

We end this section with extracts from John's journal, which constitute a more extended illustration of the important role played by the written word in an interaction:

16th November

This is the first time that I have worked with Bob Frampton. I have seen him many times before and noted his bearing: many of his actions are unusual, and in most people's minds would be suggestive of a very severe level of disability.

He talks fluently but ramblingly. He seems fully aware of the nature of what is taking place and seems to attach considerable importance to it. This is shown by the way he sits up straight on a table, looking composed and apparently thinking of the next thing to say. He answers my questions directly. His language is wide-ranging: occasionally he uses long words, sometimes invents them, often showing great imagination in the juxtaposition of words and ideas. After an intensive one-and-a-half hours in which I cover seven foolscap pages he brings the session to an end as follows:

> Where's my assistant? Oi! I've got one who's a raw tennis player. That lad I brought home from the patriarch is quick as lightning. I've got a marvellous young lady who looks after me. Is she authentic? What is a learned man? – they don't always know about cutting nails and cutting corn. Do you like jockeys and bottles? I do: I once won a pound and I take a drink. It's a quiet night outside— not a cut nor a quarrel. Early in the War mother used to say 'Do you want a country or an armageddon?' Father said 'Neither.' It got a bit heavy after that. We're hoping to go to Lexicon at about half-time, I wouldn't wonder. I never liked things over-askew.
> With regard to silence, I think it should be observed.

In the afternoon, after I have written out the text more clearly and taken it back to him, Bob sits up on the table in the same alert fashion and appears fully in command of the situation. He leans across and takes the notepad carefully, almost reverentially from me.

He turns over the pages of the text, but I get the impression that he is unable to read it. Eventually he finds a blank but lined page. 'Please cross this out' he says, pointing to a particular line. I do so. 'Thank you. You may continue' he says, leaving the table and immediately resuming his usual demeanor.

17th November
When I enter the lounge Bob is already sitting on the table waiting for me. 'Shall I divulge some things into you?' he asks. He again signifies the end of the session with the words:

'With regard to silence, I think it should be observed.'

In a chapter so full of problems and provisos we want to leave you with a positive image of the practice at its best. Many people with dementia are fascinated by the process of writing, craning over to see what John is putting down on the paper, taking and scanning the notebook, and asking for passages to be read back to them. They often appear moved by what they have achieved. One woman said:

I'm quite impressed. There's a tear rushing out of this eye.

Ethical implications

Confidentiality

We have already alluded to this subject in the main part of the chapter, and should acknowledge that this issue not only applies to writing, but also has more broad significance. Rules of confidentiality are, or should be, part of all health and social care, but the particular ways in which the principle is interpreted and acted upon may vary substantially within and between services. It is a complex problem in any case, but there are many ways in which our subject raises issues around confidentiality. Since the majority of these will arise in care settings, the main emphasis here is on situations where questions about whether it is right to share information about an individual with others arise in the context of those others knowing who is being spoken about.

Care settings are complex systems in which many people may be involved with any one individual with dementia, and in varying capacities. This gives rise to questions about who gets to know what and why. Decisions about this cannot be made simply on the basis of status (for example, untrained staff should know less than trained staff, and domestic staff nothing at all), since the kinds of relationships that clients and residents make with members of staff do not follow these classifications: it is often said that people who go into hospital, for example, will say more about themselves to the cleaner than to the nurse in charge. On the other hand, it cannot be respectful to the person to distribute highly personal information within a staff group without any consideration of privacy.

These issues come alive most acutely when a member of staff is in receipt of an important disclosure by a person with dementia, which seems to them to have relevance in the wider context of their care, but which the person does not wish to be shared with anyone else. This constitutes an acute dilemma, and puts the staff member in question in a very uncomfortable situation. Talking to the person with dementia about their reasons for wishing to share the information and reassuring them about any fears that it will be advertised widely may be sufficient to resolve the dilemma. In extreme cases, however, one may feel compelled to break confidentiality, to proceed without the person's sanction. In such instances we may dampen uncomfortable feelings by reassuring ourselves that we are acting in the person's best interests and that they are no longer capable of making such judgements. This, as we have seen, is often part of a much wider way of thinking about people with dementia, and one which needs to be challenged if we are to avoid simplistic and complacent decisions.

There is the potential for further complexity even where it seems that permission has been granted to share with another (or others) the gist or details of an interaction, and this relates to realistic concerns about whether someone does understand the nature of the issues. We are often in the position of not being sure of someone's grasp of a situation or request. Further, since dementia is a variable condition, this can cast doubt on even the most apparently authoritative sanction given. One day's 'yes' can turn into another day's 'no'.

Let us admit that this is a minefield, and always being sure of having done the right thing is probably an impossibility. Part of the answer to these questions must be, again, improvements in the way that we communicate with people and greater sensitivity to how we interpret their responses. If this is combined with genuine respect and concern for the privacy of the person, we are unlikely to go too far wrong.

Ownership of texts and recordings

The other matter we consider here does have particular relevance to writing and recording work, and it is the issue of ownership: specifically to whom a text or a recording belongs once it has been made. It is likely that in any enterprise of this sort, the outcome should most accurately be considered the result of a combined effort, in just the same way as any conversation or nonverbal interaction is a product of the involvement of more than one party.

This is a complex question even when a text or recording is recognized by the person with dementia as having come from them, but it is even more challenging in situations where the individual either seems simply not to remember it, or even actively rejects it. The question here is: to what extent does the notion of ownership entail the knowledge of ownership?

We are back in the realm of philosophy here, but without becoming overinvolved with this level, we need to consider where we stand on issues like this, and what follows from our judgements.

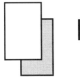

Part 3: Themes

11 | **Narrative:** 'I want to make up my story for myself'

Here the novelist Isabel Allende, sitting by the bed of her daughter, Paula, who is in a coma, describes what she is setting out to do:

> When you wake up we will have months, maybe years, to piece together the broken fragments of your past; better yet, we can invent memories that fit your fantasies. For the time being, I will tell you about myself and the other members of this family we both belong to, but don't ask me to be precise, because inevitably errors will creep in. I have forgotten a lot, and some of the facts are twisted. There are places, dates, and names I don't remember; on the other hand, I never forget a good story. Sitting here by your side, watching the screen with the luminous lines measuring your heartbeats, I try to use my grandmother's magic to communicate with you. If she were here she could carry my messages to you and help me hold you in this world. Have you begun some strange trek through the sand dunes of the unconscious? What good are all these words if you can't hear me? Or these pages you may never read? My life is created as I narrate, and my memory grows stronger with writing; what I do not put in words on a page will be erased by time.[1]

There is something elemental about stories. We encounter them first in childhood when they bring magic, adventure and an array of new ideas, emotions and characters into our lives. Through stories we have the opportunity to test out our reactions and ideas, and to learn to identify with others or distance ourselves from them. Stories invite us to develop the faculty of imagination, which can be an unending source of enrichment of a life. They help the child to explore the world, but in a safe way, before actually having to go out into it.

Our attachment to stories does not diminish as we become adults. Adult forms of stories abound around us – jokes, anecdotes, soap operas, novels, films, biographies, historical accounts, the details of the lives of those we are close to. Sometimes stories are short and simple, sometimes complex and unfolding with twists and ironies. Sometimes stories stay very much within a conventional frame; in others, such as fantasy or science fiction, the manipulation of reality is an integral part.

Just as stories fulfil important functions for children, they have a variety of roles for adults. Through stories we learn about ourselves, others and the world itself. We develop our ideas about what is basic and unchanging, and what transforms itself through time and events. It is often by hearing a story about something that we first feel the stirrings of an interest or passion. By listening and contributing to stories we develop aspects of ourselves which otherwise might remain unstimulated. We use stories to escape from the banalities and pressures of our lives, and by engaging with characters in soap operas, serials and novels we can participate in a fuller emotional life than our own circumstances engender.

Narrative and identity

The idea of the story underpins our most intimate relationship with our own experiences. How do you see your life – as a series of discrete events with only the most tenuous links between them? Or as a continuously developing story with episodes and chapters, with characters and themes moving in and out, with a central core of meaning? Surely the latter, for how could we bear it if this were not the case? The world bombards us with so many different experiences and we, as authors of our own stories, create the pattern that seems to make the most sense.

There is therefore an intimate relationship between our individual sense of who we are – our identity – and the stories which give shape to our lives. We have already explored the need to make sense of events, to find meaning within the complexity of our lives. This goes on in a very private, personal way in our own minds, woven into our thoughts, feelings and ideas, and is intricately bound up with our sense of identity. We need to keep telling ourselves our story, revisiting and reworking its themes and strands, turning points and recurrences. We sift and evaluate our experiences, deciding what is important, what is peripheral, which events and people have made the crucial contributions to our lives. Stories help us to look at things in different ways and from different points of view. In this way, the storytelling impulse is not only a central means of creating and consolidating the sense of who we are now, but also who we would like to be in the future. The story is perpetually fuelled by new experiences: it will never be told in full. The neurologist Oliver Sacks puts it this way:

> We have, each of us, a life story, an inner narrative – whose continuity, whose sense, *is* our lives. It might be said that each of us constructs and lives a 'narrative', and that this narrative *is* us, our identities.[2]

There is always an element of selectivity in the stories we create. They take shape according to our perceptions, needs and in the service of the desired self. A story must be told from a point of view, and that point of view will always influence its content and slant.

Those whose stories we do not hear or know – the 'unstoried' – are people who suffer a particular form of invisibility. Having, shaping and telling one's own story is a powerful way to be 'real', as the woman whose words form part of the title of this chapter seemed to know so well.

Narrative and relationships

Stories not only have a personal, individual significance. We use them in a social way. Much of our cultural inheritance exists in the form of stories – myths, fairy tales, historical accounts. In oral societies everyone told and relied on such stories. As well as storytelling within communities, there was a role for the itinerant tale-teller as well, moving between villages and towns and helping disparate groups to gain perspective on their culture. There are still societies which rely on this way of passing information, but of course these are increasingly rare. Stories, therefore, are a means of telling others about ourselves, and learning about them in return. We can also tell stories about times from earlier in our lives, thus extending our awareness backwards in time. They play an important role at the level of relationships, families, communities and whole societies, transferring information and values, and helping to maintain social cohesion.

Because the telling of a story is an inherently social act, the very situation provides a framework for people to relate to each other, to test out reactions, to affirm and enjoy one another's qualities. The listener is not a passive recipient, but an active contributor shaping the telling with their responses, both verbal and nonverbal. One story often stimulates another, and a series of stories can be a wonderful kind of conversation where new ways of seeing and understanding are created. Through this process people can move from the telling of stories to the kind of shared experiences which lead to new ones.

The role of stories in learning

Our society is awash with information. We are bombarded with it from all sides. Much of it is irrelevant to our lives and concerns, but some of it is important. How do we notice and remember it? Most of us find it easier to assimilate facts and ideas through a fictionalized account rather than confronting them in a raw state. Of course, not only are the facts made more palatable by this method, but also they are being processed, absorbed and contextualized by their assumption of a narrative form. It is as if our minds and memories are adapted to acquire information through stories. We all have our own personal examples of learning in a lasting way through listening to narratives of various sorts, stories we revisit often and are sure we will never forget.

Stories and decisions

We live complex lives in which we are frequently called upon to make choices, many of which have a moral dimension. In these situations we have a need to entertain different perspectives on the possibilities, to clarify our thoughts and feelings, and to generate alternative versions of the future which assist in the consideration of the consequences of our decisions and actions. Remembering and reflecting on stories we have already heard, the stories which provide an ongoing framework for our lives, and creating our own new ones, are ways of doing these things. The philosopher Alasdair MacIntyre says:

> I can only answer the question 'What am I to do?' if I can answer the prior question 'Of what story or stories do I find myself a part?'[3]

Nonverbal stories

When one thinks of storytelling, one naturally thinks of language, but this is in part just a reflection of our highly verbalized culture. What about the possibility of stories without words? The neurologist Antonio Damasio is convinced that nonverbal storytelling is a significant means of self-communication and describes the process as follows:

> Wordless storytelling is natural. The imagetic representation of sequences of brain events, which occurs in brains simpler than ours, is the stuff of which stories are made. A natural preverbal occurrence of storytelling may well be the reason why we ended up creating drama and eventually books, and why a good part of humanity is currently hooked on movie theaters and television screens. Movies are the closest external representation of the prevailing storytelling that goes on in our minds.[4]

Other nonverbal media which have the potential to convey stories include pictures, cartoons, dance and mime. When most people could not read, pictures were their main source of information.

The heightened need for stories

We hope we have established that we all have a need for narrative in our lives, and that this is present in an ongoing way. At certain times the need is even more intense. Growing older is such a time. The sheer amount of accumulated experience is greatest, and significant changes begin to occur at this stage of life. The individual has an even deeper need to make sense of their experience, to arrive at an understanding of events and to prepare for the future. At such a time a person's sense of identity may also be under attack through physical or emotional change, and a shift in the attitudes of others.

Experiences of illness and loss are also likely to heighten the need for sense-making through stories, and if the individual is confronted with the prospect of death, then this can impart an added urgency to the process of remembering, assembling and evaluating. Marie de Hennezel, a French psychologist working in a hospice, puts it this way:

> To tell the story of one's life before one dies. The telling of it is an act, and for anyone whose autonomy is so often diminished, this act takes on its full importance. There is a need to give shape to one's life and to show this shape, which gives it its meaning, to someone else. Once the telling of it has been accomplished, the person seems able to let go, and to die.[5]

Narrative and dementia

If storytelling is especially important for people who have a wealth of accumulated experience, are confronting change and loss, and are at risk of being devalued and dismissed by others, then people with dementia must be greatly in need of the positive potential of stories.[6]

This is a condition which seems to attack a person's sense of coherence, making them doubt where they are, where they have been, and even, in some instances, who they are. In this way they are 'losing the plot'. When a person feels threatened by changes in perception, linguistic ability, circumstance and so on, surely this acts to intensify the need to revisit and evaluate the past. The autobiographical impulse is a crucial means for maintaining this sense of identity.

However, alongside the need for the power of storytelling, features of the condition may make it more difficult. This is the challenge which people with dementia may face: an urgent need to create stories which satisfy them and help them to communicate themselves and their concerns to others, while at the same time struggling with memory and language problems which interfere with the process. The psychoanalyst Donald Spence appreciates the challenge in what he writes here:

> We are all the time constructing narratives about our past and our future; and that the core of our identity is really a narrative thread that gives meaning to our life, provided – and this is the big if – that it is never broken. Break the thread and you will see the opposite side of the story. Talk to patients in a fugue state, to patients with Korsakoff's syndrome or Alzheimer's disease, and you will sense the terror behind not knowing who you are, what happened yesterday, and what will happen tomorrow. Part of my sense of self depends upon my being able to go backward and forward in time and weave a story about who I am, how I got that way, and where I am going, a story that is continuously nourishing and self-sustaining. Take that away from me and I am significantly less.[7]

Examples of narrative

In the course of communication work it has been John's experience that storytelling in its various forms can surface at any time. Here are three brief instances.

Annabel Lane came up to him and said 'Always be true to your heart.' He responded with the question 'Have you always done that Annabel?' She replied 'Once. That's something to think about.' She sat down and appeared to go into a reverie, as if she was recalling the experience. This small exchange seemed to have stimulated the inner telling of a story, which perhaps did not need or was not ready to be shared.

Nesta was always ready to talk and had a fund of mostly sad stories. One day she said 'If you have a dream you forget about it, don't you? But I can't forget about this life that I've been through – it's with me always.' This reminds us that some stories would rather be forgotten.

Willie was a man who radiated bonhomie. He was usually to be found smiling and had a quip for everyone. Nevertheless he had his reflective moments, as in this example.

> Willie came into the room, took my hand and we stood looking out the window. There was no one else present. 'Sometimes I think about running away' he said. 'Right up through the meadow to the cliff. It's reasonably steep. Always keep myself trim to keep ahead of you. There's no change in this place.'
>
> After a pause he went on, 'Well, I'll be on my road out or they'll be getting the guns out.' But he didn't move. He continued 'I was known as Wee Willie. They used to take me down to the baths. I was a fast swimmer. I swam in all the teams. Especially the Boys' Brigade. They used to have trouble getting me out. Mum used to say 'We'll finish up bringing you back as a fish!'' Then after another pause he said 'Well, I'm still on a tether, so I'll have to be getting back.'

Willie tells two little stories from his life which he seems to wish to share through his relationship with John. They are far in character from the jokey banter which he usually enjoys. Both stories end with a reference to returning to his normal self and circumstances. It could be that taking time out for story-telling like this can be a way for someone to relieve tension and assert deeper values. This is particularly important where institutional life is concerned, for the relentless social milieu can inhibit reflection.

The following text is a more extended example of narrative in process taken from John's work.

Lily Anderson

Lily was extremely eager to tell him her story. She presented as a lively, enthusiastic person. Her narrative all came out in a rush, hence the lack of paragraphing. Any attempt to break the text up would destroy the sense of its headlong nature:

1 *I was in my teens when Joe went into the army. I was at home from choice.*
2 *I didn't want to go abroad. And I had to keep the business going. It was*
3 *his insurance agency. I was a certain amount of help to him. It's personal*
4 *ownership that keeps a business going . . . My, I didn't know I was a*
5 *Gabble-Gob! . . . I was born somewhere in Parliament Road, Liverpool. My*
6 *father was in the army. My mother was an Irish lady. It's a long time since*
7 *I was in Ireland . . . I'll give you a title for this – 'The Gift of the Gab! It's*
8 *all about people that have good talking experience and ability. I wouldn't*
9 *say that I had it – that would be conceit. I call myself 'Little Lily'. Don't*
10 *bring the worst out in me or it'll be bad for both of us! What's your name?*
11 *[sees my badge] Killick! That's an exclusive name! . . . 'The Gasp of the Gib'*
12 *– that would be a better title! . . . I had one sister, Elaine, younger than*
13 *myself. We went to St Henry's, then St Brigid's at lessons. I was better at*
14 *playing with the bat and ball. My interior physical world was good . . . I*
15 *never thought I'd be able to sit down and babble like this about my*
16 *educational times. My father didn't see the point of me being pushed into*
17 *study, the dear boy . . . You're not rushing me, I know that I want to do*
18 *this, I'm not a bairn, and I want to make up my story for myself . . . I*
19 *followed into the catering trade because that was the locality's business.*
20 *Cadena's in the first place. My mother was in catering, it was open to most*
21 *people there if you had some ability . . . My colleagues'll be having a good*
22 *laugh at me gibbering on like this, they'll say we've got a right one here!*
23 *. . . I was a tomboy when I was young, a natural thing. So I played with*
24 *boys. Boys liked me, and that probably had quite a lot to do with it. You*
25 *see, this is my dirty background coming out! I get worse for knowing, don't*
26 *I? Mother used to say 'It's cheek you've got not personality. Plus*
27 *impudence.' Joe and I, I don't think we courted for long, because we lived*
28 *at a close distance. We probably got married at the little church near at*
29 *hand to the college. I can't quite remember – that's old age and poverty*

30 *coming to the fore! . . . I'm a star in the breaking! . . .We had time together*
31 *after the War, Joseph and I. He's a good lad and sportsman – cricket and*
32 *football mainly. We're still connected, but we're a bit muddled up. It seems*
33 *an odd thing but I haven't got a lot of memory in that quarter. And yet*
34 *he's very familiar to me . . . Well, tempus is fugiting. And I'm 40, I think.*
35 *We just had the one son, Alan. That was after the War – wartime put an*
36 *end to that kind of activity. He lives here, this is his home. I'm here on a*
37 *visit. I can visualise the place I came from: it was 192 Western Road. I'm*
38 *not aware there's anyone else living here but there's a lot of cottages, aren't*
39 *there? . . . Is that it? Well, you're in the chair, for want of a better word*
40 *. . . I don't know whose home this is. I think it really must be mine. After*
41 *all, I can't see anyone just going off and leaving a room like this, can you?*
42 *You and I, John, we speak the same language, only you speak it straight*
43 *and I speak it upside down!*

The first thing that strikes one about this piece is its vitality. Here is a person who is in no way broken by the condition that has come upon her. Indeed she proclaims her pride in her individuality – 'I'm a star in the breaking!' (line 30). She does not want any help in formulating her narrative – 'I want to make up my story for myself' (line 18). She keeps breaking off to make comments about her own performance, and she also invents witty and self-deprecating titles for the piece – 'The Gasp of the Gib!' (line 11) – and reiterates her commitment to what is taking place. She packs a lot of detail about her life into this passage, and she spoke with a highly authoritative tone.

Lily also shows considerable awareness of John's role – 'It's all about people that have good talking experience and ability' (line 7). She declines to include herself in their company, but through modesty not failing powers. She sees John as in charge of the session – 'you're in the chair' (line 39), though it does not inhibit her perceptibly. She does refer to memory problems –'I can't quite remember – that's old age and poverty coming to the fore!' (lines 29–30) – but turns it into a joke. It is her perception that she has difficulties with language, and contrasts the 'upside down' nature of her speech with his 'straight' speaking (line 42). In fact she demonstrates awareness and clarity of reminiscence as well as considerable command of vocabulary and tone.

This adds up to a very convincing demonstration of self-possession, but some people might say that it also raises questions about accuracy. Some of the details of what Lily claims can easily be checked – her age (line 34), and whether her son lives with her (line 36) – and here she is obviously mistaken. She is also confused about where she is living. So perhaps we are here faced with a piece full of verve and wit but which may be unreliable as a factual record (it could be significant that she refers to the process using the words 'make up my story'.) Of course there is a sense in which any life story has invented elements because a narrative is always an interpretation of events rather than a straight and full account of them, but what we have here may go further than that.

Does it matter? This is a fundamental question in relation to the stories of people with dementia. In the profoundest sense, we suggest, it does not. Lily's narrative, with its sweep and interpolations, its juxtaposing of past and present, its memories and reflections, is more like a stream of consciousness in which the individual's present mode of operation is laid bare. We are privileged to gain access to her mind, and for a few minutes to see things as she sees them. Such a window into another's world is worth a dozen correct chronologies.

Aspects of narrative

The stories people with dementia tell, and the way that they tell them, have much to teach us about how they understand and experience the world, their condition, and how other people's attitudes and behaviour affect them. In the following sections we explore some of the major themes.

Stories and identity

What part can stories play in affirming and reinforcing a person's identity? We have already acknowledged that one of the ways we develop a sense of who we are, how similar or different from others, is through the telling and hearing of stories, our own and other people's. In the course of our inner life and in our relationships with others we all use stories to project and reinforce our self-image. As we discussed earlier, telling certain sorts of stories, and in certain ways, projects the message 'This is who I am!' For people with dementia, whose personhood has been under threat for a sustained period, this role of stories is especially crucial. They tell stories about their past as a way of saying 'I wasn't always like this' and about their present in order to say 'I can still do things.' Sometimes such stories have a whiff of exaggeration about them, as if the person feels that a slightly embellished form will have a greater impact. We may feel that the content of the story is not based in fact at all, but a sympathetic interpretation will allow for the idea that the person may be talking in terms of dreams or unfulfilled aspirations.

The following text appears to be an example of this. Oliver James, who told the story to John did so with a humorous demeanour, and an awareness of the difficulty a listener might have in swallowing it!

> *I'm a bit of a comedian, and I'll tell you why. I go to a certain place just up the town. And there's a man lying on the floor dead naked. And there's another bloke standing over him. And I see they're both well-built types. I go away and come back five minutes later and the naked bloke's been stabbed three times through the bloody heart! So I tell the police and they catch him. They're pleased with me, I can tell you. If you told anyone that story they wouldn't believe you!*

Structure of stories

Most stories have a fairly conventional structure – the classic beginning-middle-end format, with the description of a situation, the introduction of characters, some kind of problem or dilemma, the thickening of the plot, and finally the resolution. We get used to having stories take such a form; it helps us to understand their messages and implications, and aids our recall of them.

Despite their crucial importance to people with dementia, it is often observed that the stories they tell take a different form. There may not be a conventional ending with a resolution of all the issues it raised. Characters may appear or disappear without explanation, or the whole thing may tail off without any kind of conclusion. These changes may derive from memory difficulties, or the mixing up or linking of stories with elements in common or similar emotional themes. Altered experience of time or the possibility that the person is operating within a different situational frame (for example, believing themselves to be at work or in a family setting) also have parts to play. Jane Crisp has defined the essentials of narrative most cogently as follows:

> We can think of these fragments of past and recent memories and the present environment as being the mental equivalent of pieces of patchwork, scraps of fabric which are all that survive from previous garments – some of them garments once worn by us and others given to us by others. All these fragments are freed from their original context and organised into a new whole around a central person – the teller – to a pattern provided by the basic structures of narrative. Thus, at a time when memory is being eroded and one's sense of who and where one [is] is falling apart, narrative provides a means of bringing the fragments together and constructing an active identity for the narrator. And the very environment around oneself, by becoming the setting for these 'life' events, becomes invested with personal meanings that support that sense of identity, of belonging.[8]

Style of delivery

It has been John's experience that some people, once given the opportunity to talk, literally cannot stop. It is as if the ideas, incidents, feelings have been dammed up and just pour out. Some individuals who approach him are already telling themselves the stories, continue while with him, and carry on after he leaves. Other people need more encouragement, almost as if they are asking to be given permission to tell their story. Once this has been achieved, the sense of pleasure and meaning it stimulates is radiantly clear. Some people appear to be engaged in internal monologues (and dialogues) to which others are not permitted access at all. If dementia in some way acts to distance a person from the stories which give meaning and shape to their lives, the act of communication could be thought of as a way to help people to reconnect with them, whether or not this means that they go on to share stories or they remain within a private sphere.

As the quote earlier from Antonio Damasio highlights, we should not assume that stories are always purely verbal in nature. As well as the internal film sequence-type story, there is also a great deal of nonverbal communication inherent in the verbal delivery of a story. Qualities of the voice of the narrator – tone, pitch, volume – and also the rhythm and rate at which the words are delivered figure in this. Actions, gestures, facial expression and eye contact greatly add to the impact. The use of space or objects as props may amplify its message. Where people with dementia are concerned, such cues often provide vital help in understanding the meaning of the story, its significance to the person, and the reasons why it is being told at any particular time.

Veracity

One manifestation of our hypercognitive culture is a concern with information and its status. The idea that truth is achieved through striving for the accuracy of details and facts reflects deep values, and is intimately connected with a scientific approach which seeks understanding through investigating ever smaller units. Narrative partakes of a different level of truth-seeking. The truth or meaning of a story consists in something less tangible, something which appeals much more to the imagination and an engagement with the self. We are reminded here of the words of Lauren Slater (quoted in Chapter 5 on memory, p. 106), when she describes how she has used storytelling as a way of constructing a view of events which evaded encapsulation and understanding in more conventional ways. Perhaps when they tell stories this is what people with dementia are doing, both on account of the obstacles to the conventional amassing and ordering of information which their condition presents, but also because through the very loosening of the constraints of rationality, other patterns and constructions take on a vitality and saliency which compel the telling. If this is so, we owe them our very respectful attention.

The relationship between memory and narrative is certainly a complex and intriguing one, and dementia seems to throw its perplexities into relief. John Bayley reflects upon this in relation to the reminiscences with which he regales Iris. One story concerns some birds they saw on a holiday in Wales:

> As I create, or recreate, those birds for Iris I wonder what is going on in her head. Is she cognisant of an invention, a fairy tale, instead of a memory? For a writer of her scale and depth the power of creation seems so much more important than memory, almost as if it could now continue independent of it. And yet the one seems to depend on the other. So what are we remembering when we invent?[9]

Here Beth Shirley Brough speculates on her friend Reg's understanding of his own stories.

> Does he know the tales he is telling are tales of inner experience rather than descriptions of outer happenings?[10]

This reminds us to be wary of assuming that the person with dementia has no awareness of the status of this kind of activity.

Emotion

We have already discussed the relationship between memory and emotion, within the context of the idea that the inner life of people with dementia may be emotionally fuller than those of us who are accustomed to operating in a more intellectual way. If this is true then there may be a very important role for stories – helping the person to explore and give expression to these aspects of their personhood. They may also provide an essential way for people to work through and cope with their emotional experiences.

When a person is in a certain mood, stories which are congruent with that mood are likely to come to mind. Being able either to remember inwardly or to tell the relevant stories to someone else who affirms both the act of telling the story, and the emotional messages it embodies, may be a way for the individual to work through the mood, and to integrate it with other aspects of themselves, and their lives. Of this Beth Shirley Brough says:

> The intensity of these feelings had only been expressed dimly before the barrier between the conscious and the unconscious was diminished by Alzheimer's.[11]

Listening to the stories of people with dementia with a more explicit focus on the emotional content than on the ideas and connections between ideas could be a helpful way of approaching this.

Stories with a specific message

When we have a point to make we do not always express our feelings and thoughts to each other directly. It may feel too risky and threatening to make a bald statement. This is especially likely to be so for people who are relatively powerless. An alternative way of communicating is to tell a story, and let others interpret our meaning and respond accordingly. For a person with dementia to say that they are angry because they feel that they have been treated badly would be difficult for many, but an alternative would be to tell a story about someone who was angry for the same reason. In order to pick up on the communicative import of such stories we need to tune into what the person might be trying to tell us indirectly.

Altered subjective reality

Quite often people with dementia tell stories in which it seems that the perspective from which the story is being told is another time in their lives. They may speak as if they were a young adult, with small children and parents to support, or about being at work or out in the wider world. We mentioned the phenomenon of altered subjective age in Chapter 2 on personhood, and this is explored in more depth in Chapter 12 on relationships. But it is relevant here because it seems to figure in storytelling as well.

A striking vividness is often noticeable in such stories. The person may seem actually to be reliving the experiences he or she is describing. We wonder whether stories about experiences which are especially meaningful to the person take on such an intensity in the telling that they precipitate an episode of altered subjective age, and this in turn further reinforces the reality of the story. Or it may be that the person has undergone an alteration in felt age, and this prompts them to remember and tell certain stories. This sort of forcefulness may also be a function of the person's compromised memory, so that material which remains accessible has a greater vitality for the fact of other memories being lost or unreachable. Linda Grant says of her mother:

> Why had she never told me this before? And why now? Or was it that as tracts of memory vanished, those that remained were highlighted in sharper relief, like a single tree in a barren landscape after the soil has been eroded and the forest has died?[12]

The possibility that people with dementia actually experience time differently is also pertinent here.

We can also wonder about the person's degree of awareness of what is happening at these times. We may assume from their bearing and words that they are basically confused about where and when they are in their lives, but this may not be the case. It may just be that they have entered into a particularly vivid state of recollection, and if such a state is characterized by a sense of cohesion and solidity which is normally lacking, then it is understandable that the person would strive to maintain the frame of the story. Indeed this may be what is happening when a person becomes stuck with a certain story, as we discuss next. The ethical implications of this kind of thing are discussed later in this chapter.

Repetitive storytelling

Some people tell their story again and again, perhaps to anyone who will listen. The tale may be repeated in unvarying detail or there may be some alteration from telling to telling. Sometimes it will be elicited at particular times of day or in specific circumstances, sometimes it will arise at anytime and during any activity. What might underpin such a tendency? We should think about the content and possible meaning of the story, even if it seems very simple or inconsequential. What might be the significance to the person with dementia? What is the emotional tone of the story, and if there are variations in the content or style of telling, what might be the reasons for these? Could it be that the person can recall so little of their experience that one story is offered whenever something personal is called for? If this is the case we need to think about the scope for helping the person to communicate more fully about themselves and their lives. Approaches such as life-story work and personalized reminiscence may be appropriate in such circumstances.

For those around a person who frequently repeats a story there is a special set of challenges. No matter how hard you try, listening to someone say the same thing over and over again is highly wearing. It may seem impossible to muster up a fresh reaction, especially when you are tired or irritable, and you may wonder whether there is justification for pointing out that this story is an old one. Again there may be scope for helping the person to share more of themselves.

Fantasy and imagination

Earlier in the chapter we introduced the possibility, described by the neurologist Antonio Damasio, that nonverbal stories play an essential part in our inner lives. The ability to create images and ideas – imagination – is one of those rather shadowy aspects of mental life which has largely been ignored in the modern study of psychology. It has remained more the domain of artists and writers. Yet whether we engage in elaborate reconstructions of our lives and circumstances, or the use of fantasy is more limited to the manipulation of reality, imagination is an important facet of our inner life. We escape into it when our surroundings are unstimulating or unpalatable, and there we can have things on our own terms. Perhaps it is an essential refuge from the cold water reality of our day to day lives.

It is a highly personal domain. Even if we were inclined to share its contents with others, we would find it difficult. A verbal description is usually so inadequate and most of us lack the skills to depict our ideas in any other form. As we have mentioned, however, some people with dementia show artistic and expressive skills which have not been in evidence earlier in life. Could we routinely extend our understanding of dementia as an opportunity for people's lives to be enriched by a heightened level of imaginative experience? The drama therapist Paula Crimmens describes how during a storymaking session with some individuals with dementia, one woman, Dolly, whose behaviour was normally either withdrawn or aggressive, entered into the story:

> We were doing the story of Atalanta who as a baby is abandoned by her parents in the forest to die. I was playing Atalanta and was crouched on the floor trying to make the sound of a baby wailing. Suddenly I felt a hand stroking my hair and heard a voice, very low and soothing, telling me she was going to look after me. It was Dolly.[13]

Where language is concerned, we have already discussed the fact that sometimes the stories of people with dementia seem unconventional in their form and content, and show striking features of metaphor and allusion. Could it be that people with dementia are much freer in bringing the domain of imagination into their stories? If the use of imagination is related to circumstances which are inhospitable, then certainly people with dementia must have great need of it. Here is a man engaged in what seems to be an exercise of imaginative comparison regarding some of the people with whom he shares the unit:

Him's the Big Samaritan, as the fella said.
Him's the Lone Ranger, that's about his height.

My late father knew that fella: worked in Nooney's the Undertaker's.
He done them for years. Then he went quick enough himself.

The whole issue of the role of imagination in storytelling, communication and relationships is highly complex and poorly defined. We can only point out here that when stories are being told an element of imagination may be informing the narrative. This relates directly to our next subject.

Dreams

The experience of waking up having had an especially vivid dream, and feeling that the mood or details of the dream remain with us throughout the day is familiar to us all. But however powerful it was we retain an awareness of the fact that the experience belongs to another dimension, and has not actually occurred. What might be the experience of people with dementia in this regard? Could it be that the boundary between dream experiences and waking ones becomes much more permeable? We wonder whether the following text could be evidence of this kind of confusion:

I'll tell you, I've had a terrible night. It was a birthday party where it
happened. It must have been put in my tea or something. I know when I drank
the cup I was all dizzy. It must have been the partner did this to me.

I was sitting up in bed and holding my head. I knew I was drunk and I had
to stay there till I was sober.

When I woke up my son was there. 'Come on', he says 'I'll give you a bath.'
And he bathed me and dressed me. He put me in the only clothes we could find
in my wardrobe.

You canna believe it. You must believe it. Because it's true. And I don't tell
anything but the truth.

I'm telling you, all the troubles is inside.

Connie Keys clearly had a great need to tell this story, but did not appear to gain much relief from the telling. She went on repeating it to anyone who would listen throughout a whole day. If, as may well have been the case, it was a nightmare that she was recounting, this leads us to speculate: if waking hours for some people with dementia are filled with confusion which might be considered to have a nightmarish quality, how are they to discriminate between these and the hours in which bad dreams may actually occur?

On a lighter note, and to conclude this part the chapter, sometimes it is possible to take the essence of a series of narratives from the one person, and make a life story out of it, retaining their own words. This can be very satisfying for the person and of great interest to relatives and staff. The best definition of life-history work we have ever heard came from a woman with dementia who, summing up the process, said:

You climb to the top of the family tree and look at the vista from there.

Implications for care

There are lots of ways in which we can help people with dementia to use stories to express themselves and remain in satisfying relationships with others. The most general of these is for us to adopt a fresh attitude towards the stories we hear all the time. Listening with renewed attention to the details of what is present, as well as what is missing, and giving greater weight to nonverbal communication are important. Given that the telling of a story is a social act, the chances are that the person will respond to your effort, and in this way the whole experience can be enhanced.

We surround ourselves with objects which are associated with stories, indeed often the value we place on them is mingled with their stories. One way to help people with dementia tell stories is to demonstrate interest in the objects they have and seem to value. This may include jewellery and items of clothing. Photos are gifts to storytelling.

Other possibilities are related to the recognition of a heightened role of emotion in the lives of people with dementia. The importance of stories in helping people to cope with this cannot be overestimated. People need to have permission to relate stories with a wide range of emotional dimensions, and facilitating a range of emotional atmospheres, again through storytelling, may help them to explore and deal with their emotions. This is likely to involve both verbal and nonverbal actions from ourselves. In terms of verbal support this could take the form of reflecting back one's understanding of the emotional messages – not in a dogmatic way, but rather in the style of checking out. Also a form of mirroring of emotional messages could be practised nonverbally – acting out the emotions.

We have talked so far only about the practice of people with dementia telling their own stories. But we have also said that listening to stories is a basic human activity. What about the possibilities inherent in the practice of telling people stories, and using such an activity as a basis for enhanced communication? The story could either take a fixed form, being read out or told from memory by a member of staff (or another). The content of the story would have to be chosen with the individual or individuals involved in mind, and it may be appropriate to choose material which is known to relate to concerns or interests of the listeners. It could be that during the reading there are pauses when people are invited to comment on the narrative or describe their feelings and reactions. Or it could be that time is set aside at the end for discussion.

Another possibility is that the story has an element of openness or is purely improvisatory in nature, with listeners being invited to supply details and characters.[14] Pictures or objects may help the person in this.

Ethical implications

In this chapter we have been exploring the many positive possibilities for storytelling in the lives of people with dementia. What might be the ethical implications of these practices? Like anything else which has the power to help, there are pitfalls.

Impact of narrative on personal identity

The first we discuss here relates to the potential of stories to flatten or constrain our understanding of a person as well as to amplify and deepen it. As we have described in the main body of this chapter, we use stories as a shorthand way to encapsulate truths about ourselves, other people and life generally. The best kind of effect of such practices is to lead us on to deeper levels of understanding, enabling us to ask more penetrating questions about how things are, and to seek ways of integrating apparently contradictory truths. An alternative effect, however, is that stories are seen as being sufficient in themselves to achieve understanding, that an account of an incident becomes a replacement for the reality and the meaning of an experience. We may also forget that however many of a person's stories we know, there will be many aspects of their life which are unstoried, and that these aspects remain unstoried for a variety of complex reasons. We have to strike a balance between the need we all have to feel that we know someone, and the fact that there will always remain much that we do not or cannot know.

In addition to the risk that we reduce the complexities of human beings to a few stories, and given that we all make sense of what we encounter according to the filter of our own beliefs and needs, there is the possibility that we will respond selectively, either to particular stories or to particular elements of stories in such a way that they reinforce our stereotypes rather than challenge them. Our own stories can then become mixed up with those of the other person. The Swedish researchers Goran Holst and colleagues have written about narrative processes used by nurses in the care of people with severe degrees of dementia;[15] this is what they are warning of when they write:

> There is a risk, however, of 'storyotyping' rather than restorying, of making the image of the patient become 'flat', two-dimensional, and easily predicatable instead of 'round', multi-dimensional, complex and unpredictable.[16]

and:

> if the interpretations are based on fragmentary knowledge about the patient's life and the nurse creates a story of the patient based on guesses and/or through his/her own lifestory. Such stories may tell more about the nurse's life than about the patient's.[17]

As we have discussed previously, two important ways of counteracting such a tendency are first, for us to be providing as many opportunities as possible for people with dementia to tell us their stories, and in the ways they choose; and second, for us to increase our understanding of how our own experiences have shaped us and disposed us to respond to others.

Altered subjective reality

Another ethical issue which arises in the context of a consideration of the role of storytelling is that where the person who is telling the story seems to be experiencing an altered frame of reality, for example through altered subjective age or through the interpretation of current circumstances in terms of past experience. Given that we have been advocating that responding fully and affirmingly to people's stories is desirable, this raises questions about the extent to which we should enter into such scenarios. There is a distinction to be drawn between responding to someone's subjective experiences and actually embroidering them. These questions become most acute when it is clear that the person's story involves a manipulation of important realities, for example that someone who is actually dead is spoken about as if they are alive. Accepting and entering into the story may then seem to amount to a collusion in a distorted way of seeing things.

As Beth Shirley Brough's question on p. 221 (about whether Reg himself believes his stories) reminds us, however, in many instances the extent to which the person is engaging in what literary critics call a 'willing suspension of disbelief' is unclear. In some senses this only increases our potential discomfort: could there not be consequences in terms of how much the other person trusts us if we appear to be believing in something which the storyteller knows to be untrue and, further, knows that we know it too?

Trauma

The final issue we raise here concerns our responses to stories of a distressing or traumatic nature. In Chapter 5 on memory we drew attention to the possibility of the individual with dementia having experienced severe or traumatic events (whether in the distant or recent past), and the ways in which the aftermath of these is expressed. One of these ways is through stories, either told directly from the point of view of the person with dementia or else couched in less personal, perhaps almost fantasy-like, terms. Sometimes such stories will start out in such a way as to make their character clear from the start, but it has been known for an apparently innocuous tale to turn gradually or rapidly into one which makes our muscles tense and our hearts beat faster. It can be difficult to know how to respond to these, especially if framed in third person terms. In such a situation, it is probably safest to frame one's responses in this way too, so that instead of saying 'You must have found that very frightening', the phrasing could be 'I imagine that person must have found that very frightening'.

The sort of scenario which presents the most acute challenges is that where we suspect that what is being spoken about belongs to the present rather than the past. It may be that experiences, such as ongoing abuse (whether directed towards the person with dementia or another individual), will first be disclosed as a story which is ostensibly about someone else or another period in the person's life. This may be the only way the person can safely broach the subject, and an exceedingly sensitive response is called for. In our concern for the person and feeling of responsibility for intervening, we may feel tempted to confront them with direct questions. This may work, but there is also the risk that the person will retreat and feel too anxious to reveal any more. One would then be left with uncertainty and the sense that further disclosure is unlikely. There can be no hard and fast rules here. Our responses must be guided by all of our knowledge, sensitivity and intuition.

There are many questions in what we raise here, but one thing which *is* certain is that if we approach the storytelling situation with all of these concerns to the forefront of our minds, its potential for magic, transportation and deeper understanding will evaporate completely. We have both to be guided by our ethical principles and concerns and, at least for a time, a little careless of them.

12 Relationships: 'I like us being with us'

On 16 August 2000 the following account appeared as part of a report by John Gittings in the *Guardian* newspaper:

> North and South Korea were yesterday engulfed in an emotional national renunion as two groups of divided relatives met after 50 years apart. But there was more grief than joy as hundreds of fathers and daughters, sons and mothers, brothers and sisters – even husbands and wives – relived the agonies of separation.
>
> The North Koreans were smiling as they filed into Seoul's convention centre, but within seconds there were sobs, shouts of anguish, and appeals to the memory of dead parents. Relatives rubbed faces of those who had returned, as if to convince themselves they really existed.
>
> A northerner stroked his brother's forehead; a southern mother buried her head in her son's chest; another northerner writhed on the floor before his 91-year-old father, whose eyes showed no sign of recognition.

This may have been an exceptional occasion but it serves to illustrate in the most dramatic terms the importance of relationships in our lives.

In many ways this whole book is about relationships involving people with dementia, and how we can support and deepen them. We have already discussed at length ideas about how personhood is maintained through communication within them, and the subject of relationships is a recurrent theme in the words of people with dementia. Our aim here is to explore further their variety and complexity, and how dementia may affect them. We need urgently to learn more about how to support and enhance existing relationships and foster the development of new ones in the context of the condition.

Varieties of relationships

We are all part of a complex web of relationships, with each one standing as a unique example of how human beings relate to each other. No two human relationships are the same, and no relationship stays the same over time. Take the individual complexity of people, add it together, mix it up in convoluted ways, often over long periods of time, and you begin to approach the baffling nature of relationships. They are full of contradictions. At the same time we want to be similar to others, to have basic things in common, and yet also be different, unique and have this recognized and upheld by others. We need each other, and want others to need us, yet often we long to be free and unencumbered by others' needs and demands. Emotionally we experience deep ambivalence towards each other, and this complexity is intensified by our knowledge of our interdependence.

Our primary relationships are with members of our family, and within this category, parental relationships are the most basic. Of course not everyone has had relationships with parents (biological or adoptive), but this is the norm. Then there are relationships with siblings, then for most people as life goes on, with children, siblings' children, grandchildren and so on. Marital or partner relationships are obviously a major part of life for most people. Historically the norm has been for people to commit themselves in early adulthood to another person, and remain permanently with that person in a public and socially sanctioned relationship. Since the late 1940s or so, this pattern has changed radically. With the prevalence of marital upheaval, many people now have more than one marital or partner relationship over the course of their lives, with all the complexity and richness of involvement with ex-spouses, stepchildren and others which that can entail. In our marriage and family-centred society, however, it is easy to forget that this has not been the experience of everyone; increasingly, remaining single and childfree is the choice of many.

Friendship relationships are also deeply important to most of us, all the more so, in contrast to family ones, for being chosen rather than given. Much has been written through the ages on the subject of friendship and its place in human life. In considering the nature of friendship Aristotle said:

> Friendship is essentially a partnership. Also a friend is a second self, so that our consciousness of a friend's existence, when given reality by intercourse with him, makes us more fully conscious of our own existence.[1]

Friendships can have their basis in a variety of spheres. Some are mostly about shared activity and interests, some about chat and fun, some about deep emotional sharing and support. Some relationships arise through work and other activities, and while limited to that sphere of our lives, may nevertheless carry great significance, particularly as they help us to construct and maintain an image of ourselves as useful, competent and contributing to the life of our community. We construe friendship in different ways at different times of our lives and according to our circumstances and outlook, and have varying expectations of our friends in accordance with their situations and resources. We also value relationships which are less personal, but nevertheless bring fun, gossip and contact of a lighter nature than we may have with other more significant people. All in all, different sorts of relationships bring out and develop different aspects of our characters, and we need this variety to reflect the many aspects of our personhood.

Our experience of relationships, then, is one of great complexity and variety. The constellation of which we are part is an ever-changing, interrelated network within which our sense of ourselves – who we are, what we are like, what we do – is at once constructed, maintained, developed, undermined, fractured or even destroyed. We cannot overestimate the depth of how much our relationships shape our experience of what it is to be a person.

The essential ingredients of relationship

In Chapter 2 on personhood we discussed the fact that as persons we have moral status, and returned to the subject of our values in Chapter 6 on interpretation. We revisit this theme in acknowledging that in addition to all their other sources of complexity, relating to others is a domain of our lives which is highly value-laden. From the most superficial kind of contact we have with others, to the deepest and most precious relationships we enjoy, we have strong feelings about how people should behave. This has a profound effect on our experience of relationships.

The nature of love

The idea of love is one we stretch a great deal. Its use ranges from our day-to-day talk about things we like and appreciate to what we consider the most significant aspects of our lives – the spiritual or religious dimension of our beings, and certainly our relationships with others. Popular culture would have us believe that love is mainly a feeling – a warm, glowing, dizzy feeling. This state of mind is presented as the ideal, the way to be with others, the notion of perfect romantic love. But how realistic is it? The psychologist M. Scott Peck explores the distinction between the rather chaotic feeling of being 'in love', and that of the business of ordinary day-to-day loving, which is best characterized as a commitment: a kind of work, and certainly not continually suffused with feelings of delight and personal significance.[2]

Most love is of the latter type. When we love someone we are committed to them, in principle regarding their feelings and needs as being of at least equal significance to our own. A basic positive regard could be seen as fundamental, but invariably these feelings are mixed up with others like anger, jealousy, resentment and so on. Indeed relationships are the arena in which we experience most of the emotion, and in its strongest and most complex form, in our lives.

Similarity and difference

It is the domain of social psychologists to study the subject of attraction – why we like some people and dislike others, and how we identify and form bonds with those who go on to be significant in our lives.[3] For any one person the factors governing this fascinating area touch on our whole history of relationships, including those we had when very young. The way we interpret and respond to the behaviour of others is allied to the way we see ourselves and our values about how people should behave. The extent to which we seek out others whose views and habits differ from our own is also a major factor. We often enjoy another's company for their qualities of differentness. This is part of the way we learn about ourselves, the shape and nature of our own characters. But issues of similarity and difference can also constitute a great challenge to the experience and viability of relationships. This bears on the matter of change. As we have seen, we all change, in large and small ways, as time goes by, and if relationships are to survive they must adjust, shifting their emphases and rhythms. The situation is typically complex.

Self-love

The subject of love in relation to the self needs also to be acknowledged. It is said that one cannot properly love another person unless one loves oneself, but this often seems an impossible maxim to live by. Most of us do not experience a deep well of self-love, and many of our cultural and religious values appear to demand a disregard for the needs of the self and a downplaying of one's own positive qualities. However, as we first mentioned in Chapter 2 on personhood, a basic respect and regard for oneself is a necessary ingredient for a well-balanced life and successful relationships.

Reciprocity and interdependence

Complex patterns of dependence and interdependence also figure in our relationships, and this is related to something we assume is a fundamental part of a relationship, reciprocity. Relationships are based on give and take, which involves all sorts of things, from money, objects, time, practical help, emotional support, understanding, through to the more numinous love. Or perhaps love is made up of all these things. We need different things from one another, and these needs vary with many other factors in our lives. Healthy relationships seem to be characterized by balances in dependence and interdependence, with both parties offering and taking in reasonable equilibrium.

Of course the balance can always change if circumstances change, and the occurrence of illness or disability in one party poses a major challenge to these patterns. How well a relationship will adjust to such a development will depend on many factors. Clearly dementia is a condition which has vast implications for issues of dependence and interdependence within relationships.

Social roles

Part of the complexity of our interpersonal lives derives from the fact that each of us has multiple 'parts' or 'roles' to play.[4] A 50-year-old woman may, for example, be a grandmother, mother, wife, daughter, sister, granddaughter, friend, worker and neighbour all at the same time. Having roles gives structure to our time, and for most of us a large part of the sense of meaning we have in life derives from them. In this regard, having roles which are valued by ourselves and recognized by others constitutes an important part of our individual self-image and self-esteem. The roles we take on and fulfil in the different areas of our lives exist in an intricate constellation, with some overlapping, others remaining separate. For much of the time we relate to others from within specific roles, and see others in terms of theirs. The extent to which we see and interact with others separately from the roles in which we encounter them, is complex. This has implications for the depth and quality of relationships, and whether they play a part in personal development or remain at a superficial level.

The reality of change

Change over time, sometimes gradual, sometimes sudden, is a fact of our lives. The roles we have in relation to others shift both through the choices we make and with events beyond our control. Losing a major role, for example through having to withdraw from work or the death of a spouse, can be a deep challenge, forcing one to reflect on one's most basic values. The loss of roles which can accompany ageing and the development of conditions like dementia, and the impact of this both upon the individual and their relationships, are major issues which the dementia world is just beginning to address. We return to this subject later in the chapter.

Older people and relationships

Our understanding of the subject of older people and their relationships tends to be shallow and stereotyped. This derives, at least in part, from the ageism inherent in our society. Perhaps because younger people tend to relate to their elders mainly through family relationships, our minds spring automatically to the perception that older people's relationships revolve mainly around family, where involvement with contemporaries coexists alongside what may be considered the more desirable option of spending time with younger members of the family, particularly grandchildren.

Older people's attitudes towards the balance of family and nonfamily relationships has been the focus of some sociological research,[5] and the value that older people attach to friendships outwith the family and the crucial role of these in maintaining health and promoting well-being has been highlighted.

Dementia and relationships

Historically, dementia has been seen as having a basically destructive effect on relationships, and therefore the subject has been given little attention. The role of psychological and social factors (particularly the behaviour and attitudes of those around the person) in the maintenance of existing relationships and the development of new ones in the context of dementia has hardly been addressed at all. We have now to adopt an attitude of openness and find ways of learning from people themselves about their experiences of relationships, and what support they need from us to maintain them.

So what happens to relationships when dementia comes into the equation? The most fundamental thing to acknowledge is that people with dementia have a basic need to remain within a network of relationships, and that being able to do so is an essential part of supporting the person's identity. Helping the individual to do so is a fundamental aim of good care, and this of course relies on good communication.

In John's experience, people have a great deal to say on the subject of relationships. We present here some texts which illustrate a variety of points.

Maggie Green

Maggie was a small twinkling woman whose beam could draw you across a room. She indicated that she wanted to speak as soon as she saw John:

1 *Married? It depends who I meet. I'll wait and see first. I'd like to have a*
   nice chap.
2 *If I get a good husband that's fine, but I'm not worried about it.*
3 *My father was on the railway at the station and then at different places.*
4 *He's not a porter, but he's good at his work. He's just that kind of man. He*
5 *took us out with him on a Sunday. He was always away walking.*
6 *We had a good mother too. We were well looked after. We had to go to*
7 *church on a Sunday. My mother didn't always manage to get, because*
8 *there was usually a wee one. After the baby was bit older my mother liked*
   to go.
9 *They're homely people, my folks.*
10 *There was a Mrs . . . I forget her married name. She died after I was there*
11 *a while, but she was awfully friendly.*

12 *There's some folks here you wouldn't want to be speaking to, but I can*
13 *speak to you. Some folks you're liking but you don't like speaking to. But*
14 *you feel you really like speaking to you.*

Judging from what we have here, everything for Maggie still revolves around relationships. There are those from her past to which she still seems very attached. The qualities of her parents are seen as admirable, and she sums up what they offered her with the word 'homely' (line 9). She applies a similar standard to any man she might marry (and here she may be talking as if from an earlier time in her life), and to the woman whose name she cannot remember (line 10). She measures some of the people in the home against it and is unable to endorse them (lines 12–13). Just as the dementia has left Maggie's language skills largely intact, it does not appear to have disturbed her adherence to the fundamental values that have informed her life.

Doris Adcock

Doris was a quiet, undemonstrative woman, who nevertheless conveyed quite an intensity once she began talking with John. These remarks were made on the fifth occasion they met:

1 *I think about it all. Everything. I pick up what I want, and what I don't*
2 *I leave. I sift it and the rest goes down.*
3 *There was a garden – there <u>is</u> a garden, and it's out. My mother*
4 *pushed me on the swing. Singing all the time. Singing and swinging on*
5 *the wing.*
6 *[scratching her nose] I've got an itchy coat.*
7 *[spreading her hands] My nails, my mother keeps me those. She's good*
8 *– she looks and tells me. I like her. Now she's going to be one of the*
9 *betime worlds.*
10 *When I was pushing up the stair, nobody stopped.*
11 *I had my whispers with Jim, my son. No secrets, not to me.*
12 *[pointing to notebook] These are lines from my crying book. It's all*
    wanting and waiting.

Like Maggie, Doris focuses on relationships that have meant a great deal to her, in this case these with her mother and her son. But there is a deeper, sadder air about these reflections than in Maggie's case. The references to 'sifting' (line 2) and 'crying book' (line 12) carry this quality of concentrated reminiscence and sorrow because they are in the past for her. She seems to express a lack of fulfilment: 'it's all wanting and waiting'. But Doris's recreation of her relationship with her mother in this passage also has a sensuous, poetic quality. The cameo is beautifully sketched in with the use of rhyming words 'swing', 'singing', 'swinging' and 'wing' (lines 4–5) The regret again comes in with the curious phrase 'one of the betime worlds' (lines 8–9). It is as if with Doris we are privileged to have access to a kind of internal meditation.

Relationships between people with dementia

When we think about relationships in the context of dementia, our minds spring most easily to those between individuals and their relatives and friends, and with staff carers. We have all been much slower to consider the subject of relationships between people with dementia.[6] This is a direct consequence of our longstanding failure to perceive and nurture the personhood of those with the condition, and the resultant assumption that meaningful relationships are not possible.

The neglect of this area in terms of research and attention in the practice context therefore leaves us quite ignorant about the whole subject. To what extent do people with dementia form relationships with each other? How much do they want to do so? When they do, what forms do these relationships take? For our own part, should we not be paying far more attention to this dimension of people's lives, and in practical terms what should we be doing to help to form supportive and satisfying friendships? We discuss this further in the implications for care section at the end of the chapter.

From John's work we have evidence that people with dementia living in care settings are interested in one another. In the words of Alice, whom we met in Chapter 1:

> How can we begin socially because people here don't want to understand my outlook and consequently have no desire to talk? I rather think that also because of my loss of memory people don't pay much attention to my conversation. And then there is my deafness. So I am left with very little social communication.

Here is someone, Pam Aders, showing her concern for her fellow residents:

> She's very rude to you, is Annie, but she's a poor thing. She was 92 recently. She fell and hurt the side of her head. I kissed her last night because she asked me to.
>
> I was here from near the beginning. I'd like to be more helpful to the others. I try to be helpful when it's all strange to them. After all, we're all strange here, you know.

And here is another lady, Meg Major, who on the surface accepts her situation but underneath is unhappy with the compromises that have to be made in living in the unit.

> I've nobody else, only myself. I do get upset but nobody notices.
>
> I don't like a grump of women with all their talking and taleing. I can't tell them nothing. Her over there that's talking, it's come and do this, and come and do that, but I never do. I don't like her. I thought she was my friend, but . . .
>
> There's good boys and bad boys in here. Him that's talking, he was sarky to me one day. He says 'What you coming in here for?' I just walked off. They sometimes tell tales of me, but I don't give a damn.
>
> It's not that I'm sulky or anything like that. I like everybody in a way, but not so as I can't manage without them.

Perhaps the last sentence sums up Meg's attitude to others, but it is a counsel of perfection she is unable to live up to. She seems to desire close relationships, yet she rejects the men and women alongside whom she lives as unsuitable companions. She appears to live in a state of anxiety, unable either to deny her need for friendship or commit herself to it.

Relationships and conversations between people with dementia can also involve much lightheartedness and playfulness. John overheard the following exchange between a woman and a man seated at a dining table, and studying a placemat. The man read out the title 'The Call of the Highlands'. 'Are <u>you</u> calling the Highlands?', she asked. 'Yes, I am.' 'In that case they could be very noisy', she replied.

Another form of humour is illustrated in this poem which John made from one woman's words, '*A Tour of the Menfolk*':

> *That man's supposed to be my father,*
> *but there's no more wrong with him than your boot.*
>
> *My mother would say that that man*
> *has a mouth like a chicken's arse.*
>
> *And that man's the biggest rogue in creation:*
> *the sooner he's under the dirt the better.*
>
> *That man, I tell you, he's absolute craft,*
> *and he tells lies like Tom Pepper.*
>
> *That one comes out with a string of swearings.*
> *If I catch him he'll get it across the kisser.*
>
> *That man's my brother-in-law. He's always trying*
> *to hitch it with me, but I'm not having any.*
>
> *And that man, his character goes before him.*
> *Like mine does. But I'm a Christian.*
>
> *I get on with all of these men all right.*
> *And if they want to do anything*
>
> *I tell them how: that the best way*
> *to get on in life is to agree with me.*[7]

In thinking about the subject of relationships between people with dementia, we must also give consideration to the matter of relationships which are sexual in nature. This is an uncomfortable subject for many people. It raises all sorts of difficult issues and dilemmas, and most prefer to avoid it altogether. However respect for personhood demands that these realities of people's lives be acknowledged, even celebrated.[8] We should also recognize that sexuality pervades many of our relationships even when there is no question of this being expressed in behaviour. As with anyone, people with dementia must retain a sense of their own and others' attractiveness, and the pleasure which can be found in talk and interaction which expresses mutual appreciation. To deny this reality and expression to people with dementia is to disregard deep and important facets of the human. As one woman put it:

I've got an eye for the men, but I didn't put it there.

We give further consideration to issues of sexuality in the section on ethical implications later in this chapter.

Pre-existing relationships which deepen in the context of dementia

It is our usual assumption that dementia has a negative influence on relationships, that there is inevitably great strain and ultimately loss. But what about the possibility that, in some cases, dementia in one party can actually bring about the deepening of a relationship? Only a few years ago this idea would have seemed unthinkable. But things have changed quickly, and happily we now have a growing number of accounts from the relatives and friends of these with the condition that new and positive developments in relationships can come about, not only despite, but actually through the experience of dementia.

Anthea McKinlay wrote:

Seventeen months before she died my mother told us that she felt her 'top layer' had been 'stripped'. I am her only child. After a lifetime of barriers and difference between us, we found one another. My mother used a new language to describe her experience. I was learning new ways of being and listening and to be unattached to assumptions.[9]

Another example comes from Beth Shirley Brough, who says:

In communion with Reg, my beloved soul-mate, I have grown in stature and spiritual independence. Our cherished interdependence has provided the companionship in which we can both increase the depth of our inner knowledge and experience.[10]

Also with a spiritual theme, Kim Zabbia, who produced paintings about her mother's dementia for an art thesis, quotes the following dialogue between herself and her supervisor (who speaks first):

'May I suggest that you refer to your relationship with your mother as a parallel journey, instead of a single journey?'
   'I can't call it a parallel journey. This may sound spooky, Bob, but it's like Mom and I are one person. It's difficult to explain. It's just that we are so much together in this adventure, this voyage, that we seem almost to be one.'
   'That's great, then,' he said sincerely 'You've apparently landed onto something spiritual and unique.'[11]

New relationships

Completely new relationships can also blossom in the context of dementia. Care assistant Laurel Rust writes in her piece about Amy:

> Amy and I have developed an intimacy that is hard to describe, an intimacy that makes me think of companionship differently because Amy does not know my name and has never asked. We sit and simply take up talking, wherever and whenever we are. Talking with Amy who 'exhibits no orientation to reality' is a wonderful experience in which we are always in the present, and the present could be anything we choose to create between us.[12]

This example highlights the need to challenge the value we attach to knowing names and classifying relationships, and the assumption that they must always have a conventional sequence in time. It stretches our understanding about what the idea of relationship actually means.

A woman John worked with on only one occasion, and with whom it was clear that a true relationship was developing, summed up her feelings about their time together in this way:

> *We're a nice little two-lot, you and I. I like us being with us.*

Issues arising

The subject of relationships is so rich and complex, we could easily fill a whole book discussing aspects of change, persistence, loss and gain. In the following sections we can highlight only a few.

What we bring to working with people with dementia

The word 'person' in 'person-centred care' refers not only to the person with dementia, but also to those caring for them. Providing high quality personalized care for people with dementia is emotionally and spiritually demanding work, and we are coming more to the realization that to understand what is needed and how things can work best, we must acknowledge workers as people too. As we have already mentioned, for those engaged in close caring work, understanding their own thoughts, feelings, beliefs and motivations which underpin their commitment is of great importance. But what does this actually mean?[13]

One question we can all usefully ask ourselves is how and why we have come into this kind of work. As we have already discussed, there are different routes we might have taken, but in many cases the decision will have been influenced by certain key experiences, for example, encountering older people and people with dementia during the early years of our lives. These could be people who were well known to us and knew us well – relatives, family friends, neighbours and so on. Others may have been an important part of our lives but in a limited way, for example as teachers, doctors or ministers. There could be others with whom we came into contact only fleetingly but in a highly significant way. There are some people who have influenced us in important ways but whom we do not remember at all. Even if we do not recall particular people or incidents, however, we learn from them, and carry these lessons with us. Of course many of us continue to have relationships with older people throughout our lives. Bonds with grandparents, aunts and uncles, neighbours, friends and, as we get older ourselves, our own parents. Contact with people of increasing age and those who are ill and dependent, shapes our attitudes and exerts pressures on us to develop ways of coping.

All of these experiences feed into the way we see and interact with the people in our care in the here and now, how we interpret their behaviour and how we construe our relationships with them and responsibilities to them. Sometimes a certain person appeals to us strongly. We may feel especially able to understand their experiences and feelings, and be attracted to spending time in their company. Interacting and communicating with that person may feel rewarding in a way that contact with other people is not. This can be a very positive experience, but as reflective practitioners it is important to think about why the person elicits such a powerful reaction in us. Is it that they remind us of someone from our past? Could there be a reawakening of the sorts of feelings generated by an important person from our own history? If so, it is necessary to ask ourselves to what extent we are trying to re-create a previous relationship rather than exploring the possibilities for building a new one.

Some people make us feel particularly protective. We might feel more than usually concerned about risk and want to act on this even to the extent of actually constraining and disempowering the person. Again, could it be that old feelings of being called upon to take responsibility and nurture are being activated? Of course, not all of our reactions are positive. Some people just turn us off. We may find ourselves unable to respond, to engage and to embark on developing caring relationships with some individuals. It is important to think about why this might be so. Perhaps the person reminds us of someone who hurt, offended or frightened us in the past, especially as a child.

Powerful responses to people touch on the issue of reciprocity in relationships which we explore in some depth in the ethical implications section at the end of this chapter.

Relationships and change in the self

Our conventional notions of relationship rely on there being a sense of basic consistency in the person to whom we are relating. Although we believe in the basic preservation of personhood, as we have seen, dementia is a condition which can bring about significant change in areas which impact on relationship. For those around the person, being a witness to change can not only be a distressing experience emotionally, but also can be highly threatening at an existential level as well. If our personhood derives from relationships with others, then when someone who is close undergoes radical change, this raises profound questions about the nature of our own selfhood. In her book about her relationship with her mother who has dementia, Linda Grant says:

> When a member of the family starts to lose their memory it turns every-thing up because not only are they losing their recall of you, your recall of them is challenged. It's almost a challenge to your own existence. If you live in the memory of someone else and their memory starts to fade, where are you?[14]

In *Scar Tissue*, Michael Ignatieff provides a historical perspective on a similar issue:

> She is the silent custodian of the shadow zone of my own life. She is the only one who can tell me what I was like before I began to remember, the only one who can decipher those first senseless scenes when memory begins.[15]

Sometimes those around the person with dementia find ways of coping with this kind of challenge by coming to the conclusion that the person they have known and loved has disappeared altogether, that although they are still physically present, in essence they have died. This way of dealing with the problem may facilitate the kind of grieving seen after actual death, and may assist practical coping by allowing the carer to distance themselves emotionally from the reality of loss. However, such a strategy will have consequences, probably very negative ones, for the individual with dementia who is still struggling to retain a sense of identity and integrity. We reiterate that we all depend on each other for keeping that precious spark of self alive, and never more so when it is under attack from something like dementia.

Others take a different view on the issue of selfhood and identity, insisting that despite the changes and losses which dementia has wrought in their loved one, their essence persists. Michael Ignatieff says:

> I want to say that my mother's true self remains intact, there at the sur-face of her being, like a feather resting on the surface tension of a glass of water.[16]

Beth Shirley Brough expresses a similar conviction:

> Although institutionalised and no longer rational, Reg's integrity remained intact. His strength of character was clear in the way he had stood his ground. The unchanged core of the man was disclosed.[17]

It is interesting to note that the character in *Scar Tissue* prefaces his statement with the words 'I want', which is perhaps a tacit acknowledgement of the fact that his desire to see his mother as being in some core sense the same as she ever was, is related to his own needs. Some would say that to adopt such a position is as much a coping strategy as the alternative, that it is about our own need to perceive continuity and to reject the idea that that which we love and believe in can be destroyed by a condition like dementia.

We do not know the answers to all of these questions. They are certainly deep and difficult. But it can only help to raise and explore them. And we do believe that if anything can help us to unravel their complexities, it is the effort to establish and maintain real communication between ourselves and people with dementia. They are not the only ones who stand to benefit – whenever we deny the personhood of others, we are all threatened, diminished and damaged. As the sociologist Peter Coleman puts it:

> Dementia care reveals clearly how much our personhood depends ultimately on each other. We hold each other up in conditions of dementia, distress and dying. To allow ourselves to be held requires trust.[18]

The expression of emotion

We have already said that emotion seems to play a heightened role in the lives of many people with dementia, and of course it is in the domain of relationships that we experience some of our deepest emotions. We should expect, then, in the course of communicating with people, to find powerful feelings regarding relationships coming to the fore. This has certainly been John's experience, and includes occasions when expressions of anger, bitterness, disappointment and confusion have occurred. One woman launched a mockingly scathing verbal onslaught on her son, in which he was criticized in a variety of stinging ways, but despite her dismissal of him what shone through was a powerful assertion of her own selfhood – *'The truth is mine, not yours!'* Once she had dealt with the acute anger, what was very apparent, and something John was able to help with, was the need for the woman to be affirmed as real and valuable in herself.

Memory

If relationships are about knowing others, and being known to them, the memory problems which are part of dementia could constitute a real threat. Remembering who someone is, and what kind of relationship you have with them, seems very basic, at least within our conventional notions of what form relatedness should take. So what happens when someone starts to forget these things? When they cannot hold the information and bring it to bear on the interaction?

Difficulties with recognition

It often seems, as the condition progresses, that people have increasing difficulties recognizing close relatives, friends and staff. In a situation where someone is being visited, there may be variability from day to day and week to week in the extent to which family members and friends are acknowledged, with one encounter going very well with warm recognition and positive inter-action, and others failing to connect at all. How and why this variability occurs is one of the many aspects of dementia we do not understand. But when it does start to happen it is understandably very distressing for those who are close, and is one of the problems which puts a very great strain on the ability of those around the person to cope with the condition.

In some instances apparent difficulties with recognition may reflect deeper aspects of a situation. Here Thomas Cassirer speaks about his wife, who has dementia:

> While her face lights up immediately when I show up at the assisted living residence, and she is always very happy and affectionate, she wavers in her identification of exactly who I am. At times I am one of a group of 'Thomases', and she tells me about another Thomas who visited her the previous week. At other times when we arrive back at the residence she acts as though we had been out on a very enjoyable date, hopes that I will come again soon to take her out, reminds me of her name, and adds, 'But I don't know your name'. It is evident that she feels there are at least two of me: The one who is with her and the other who is out somewhere, who is leading a life that she cannot imagine but who is likely to turn up at some other time. Again she is right, though her language is not what we who are 'on the outside' consider normal, because I do lead two lives, one together with her on Sundays, and the other on my own in another world, yet with her tucked away in my mind just as the 'other Thomases' are tucked away in her mind.[19]

Of course this does not always just occur in situations where the person with dementia is living separately from family and friends. It can also happen in circumstances where more constant contact is maintained. This can lead to very complicated and challenging situations. One person, Fran, whom John knew, had been married twice. She developed dementia while living with her second husband, and as things progressed it became clear that she often believed herself still to be married to her now-dead previous husband, and did not recognize her current partner at all. Fran was frightened and confused by his presence, and often told him to go away, even locking him out of the house on occasion. Greatly distressed, she would telephone her daughter and com-plain that there was a stranger in her home. Her daughter was usually unable to persuade Fran that the stranger was her husband of more than twenty years' standing. It was a highly upsetting situation for all concerned. This kind of confusion about people's identities was one of the main factors which led to her entering a nursing home.

Sometimes people with whom we consider ourselves to have only 'virtual' relationships can become intensely real to an individual with dementia. Tele-vision presenters or actors often figure in these scenarios. It is quite a common observation of staff and relatives that a person responds to something said by someone on TV, or addresses them as if they were actually there. The distinction between the two-dimensional reality of the world portrayed on TV and their physical surroundings and companions appears to break down, for brief or more sustained periods. However, it can go even further than this. We have heard about Eileen, who came to believe that people who appeared on TV at regular times (for example, newsreaders) were actually visiting her personally, and she would carefully get herself and her house ready when they were due to appear. She seemed to believe that anything which was said in the room while the person was on TV could be heard by them, and throwaway remarks made by real visitors about the style or appearance of the presenter would cause her great distress and embarrassment. On one occasion when she had been persuaded to turn off the television so that her grandson could talk to her properly, at the specific time a programme was due to start she rose out of her chair and went towards the window. When asked what she was looking for, Eileen replied that it was time for Michael Buerk to arrive. The virtual world of the television goings on had clearly become a very vivid part of her lived experience, and her family and friends had to adjust to this aspect of her reality.

A case of mistaken identity

As well as the failure to recognize individuals who are actually known, the opposite can occur, and someone who is new to the person may be mistaken for a familiar individual. It may be that a physical similarity or resemblance in personality and manner between, say, a new member of staff or a visitor and someone the person knows or has known gives rise to a conviction that the new person is actually the other. This can precipitate a positive, sometimes very emotional, reaction or, if the perceived similarity is to someone whom they disliked or resented, it may prompt coldness, withdrawal or even open hostility.

John had a very striking experience of this kind. One day he arrived in a unit for the first time, and was greeted loudly, warmly and emotionally by a man he had never met before. It quickly became clear that the man had mistaken John for his brother, whom he said he had not seen for many years and obviously loved and missed greatly. He expressed his joy at seeing him, and his gratefulness for the visit. It was a powerful experience which unfolded rapidly, and put John in an extremely delicate position. What was the best thing to have done? Should he have gone along with the misunderstanding, responded with respect and an appropriate level of warmth and attempted to steer the interaction on to more normal ground? Or should he have acted immediately to attempt to dispel the man's misapprehension? Had this happened before with other people? Was it that any new male visitor was mistaken in this way? And what was the reality of the situation with the man's actual brother? Had he been absent for many years? Was he dead? Or had he just left from his usual weekly visit? Lots of questions, and no immediate answers to hand.

Using names

We normally consider the knowing and using of someone's name to be an integral part of a relationship with them. Finding out a person's name is one of the first things we do on meeting them (even if we do often forget it almost instantly!). If the relationship goes on to become part of our close inter-personal sphere, then we are likely to use their name on many occasions, and perhaps even modify it to a more intimate version, denoting a special significance. In very close relationships we may develop private forms of address reserved only for use within that exclusive bond. Outside the sphere of the family, one's friends and colleagues may introduce nicknames which stick and become part of a person's identity. Although in many ways we take names for granted, their evolution and use is highly personal. If using a shortened or idiosyncratic version of someone's name denotes intimacy, then using it in full usually means someone is angry and has a bone to pick! Hearing someone call you by a version of your name which comes from another part or time in your life can be a powerfully evocative experience.

Using someone's name can be seen as a shortened way of respecting their personhood. Conversely abstaining from using a name can have the very opposite effect. Prisoners, or those being persecuted, are often addressed only by number, and this can act to undermine or even strip away the person's identity, leaving them feeling reduced to the status of an object.

The matter of people with dementia using names also carries considerable emotional significance. It is a common observation that over time many individuals use people's names less and less, and members of staff who have come into the person's life once their dementia is well established may not expect their name to be learned and used at all. However, we can be surprised by this. Many a practitioner has been astonished when under particular circumstances the individual demonstrates that they do know their name, and can use it. When relationships are more longstanding, the issue may be more emotionally charged. Beth Shirley Brough, who had been for some time increasingly needful to hear Reg use her name, said:

> So it is this day that, fired by sheer envy of anyone else who can evoke an animated response from him, I ask and ask again if he can just say my name. Then I will be satisfied that he really does remember me.
>
> With pained eyes he watches my face. At least I show enough insight to see that he is struggling, as up from the depths of him comes a gurgle and the words, 'You're *someone*!'
>
> Even though the statement is full of conviction, I fail to understand the import of his words. I have the audacity to be disappointed once again, and it is not until later, when a wise and knowing friend listens to my grieving tales, then gently repeats the phrase – changing the intonation ever so slightly – that the full impact of Reg's words finally strikes me.
>
> Consciousness comes through little shocks of awareness and humbles me. I have been so concerned with my desperate need for recognition that Reg's heartfelt reply has passed me by![20]

Altered subjective age

We introduced the subject of altered subjective age in the chapter on person-hood, and we return to it to now to consider this matter in the context of the discussion about how a person's dementia can affect their relationships. When an individual appears to have periods when they are convinced that they are much younger than they actually are, one of the consequences of this is that they may construe their relationships with others in different ways too. This could mean that a son or even a grandson is mistaken for a boyfriend or hus-band, while the actual spouse may appear to occupy the role of father or uncle, or else is not recognized at all.

Such misperceptions are likely to cause embarrassment or even real distress in relatives, and their discomfort can then be reflected back to the person, who may be unable to understand why people are upset. Whether it is best in such circumstances to attempt to re-orientate the person to current reality or accept and attempt to enter into and empathize with their own version of reality is a complex question. There are no simple answers. Some family members may be more able to deal with such situations than others, but staff can probably also have a positive role in helping to promote understanding of what is going on. Here is an example of someone with dementia, Catherine, being humorously challenged by her daughter, Anthea, about her view of her age. Catherine speaks first:

> Guess what!
> What?
> I'm 18!
> but how can you be 18 when I'm 39 and you're my mother?
> mmm . . .
> and you've got thick grey hair and I've got thick black hair, so how do we explain that?
> shhh – when you come, don't say anything to anyone and maybe they won't notice![21]

Here Anthea enters into what seems like a kind of game where her mother was clearly experiencing herself in an altered state, and needs to relate to her from where she is in her own mind.

Attachment

We have all met people with dementia who frequently call out someone's name, speak often of their parents, and others who play constantly with dolls or soft toys. According to a Dutch psychiatrist, Bere Miesen,[22] these are examples of people who display what he terms 'attachment behaviour'. He borrowed this term from the psychoanalyst John Bowlby,[23] who studied the attachment behaviour of young children to one or more persons, usually par-ents; Miesen sees these behaviours as responses by the person with dementia to the stresses and strangenesses of the condition they face. If dementia disrupts the normal patterns of relationship by interfering with recall of people and places, he argues, the person must first find security where they can. Some are seen to regress to the first and most comprehensive attachments of their lives, those formed in the first year of life. Some choose 'attachment figures' like members of staff whom the person will 'shadow'. Those who cling to soft toys seem to be embracing 'transitional objects' which are symbols of the human reassurance they crave. All these are responses to a world that has become unknowable and therefore fundamentally unsafe.

Those who have read thus far in the book will know that we are not driven by theory, nor do we attempt, even if we were able, to offer critiques of any of the major theories in the dementia world. Attachment theory is an attempt to explain aspects of relationship which are clearly present in some persons with the condition, and which we need to have cognizance of if we are to develop effective strategies for communication.

Experience of bereavement and grief during dementia

The subject of grief in people with dementia is beginning to be recognized as a major issue which requires special attention. After all, by the time most people have reached later life, they will have experienced a series of bereavements. Loss of parents is most likely to have occurred in middle age. Most older people are also likely to have experienced the death of a sibling or of a close friend. A proportion of those in later old age will have suffered the loss of a child or even a grandchild. These bereavements, which buck the expected order of loss, may be experienced as particularly severe or even traumatic. Looking further back, it used to be much more common for children to lose a sibling to illness at an early age or for parents to lose children in infancy or early childhood, so some bereavements will be of very long standing.

But for any bereavement, and whenever it occurred, we need to realize that resolution of these losses may or may not have been achieved,[24] and where grief is still an active, if buried, process its experience and expression may change in the context of dementia. To complicate matters further memory problems may interfere with the process. Linda Grant, writing about her mother, gives the following example:

> I tell her that I am going to Poland to track down the family's history, my search for roots.
> 'My parents came from Poland, you know,' she replies.
> 'No, they didn't. That was Dad's family.'
> 'Well, where did mine come from then?'
> 'From Russia, Kiev.'
> 'Did they? I don't remember. Your Auntie Millie will know. Ask her.'
> 'Mum, Auntie Millie died.'
> She begins to cry. 'When? Nobody told me.'

'It was years ago, even before Dad died.'
'I don't know, I don't remember.'[25]

Judy Griffiths, an Australian grief counsellor, tells a story of a woman who used to visit her husband in a nursing home at the same time every day.[26] After he died she ceased to go there. But three years later, after developing dementia, she turned up to visit him, and continued to do so every day despite repeated assurances that he was no longer there. Even after she was confined in a similar home and immobile, she continued to display agitation at that time of day until she died. It seems that since the grief was unaddressed and therefore unresolved, it could not be quelled.

Grief in the area of relationships need not apply only to people when the individual has been lost through death. Emotional rawness about relationships which were highly significant to the person, but ended through the break-up of romantic involvements, missed opportunities for intimacy or marriage, divorce and so on may also be salient. Such attachments may or may not be known to others.

John has had many conversations with people in which thoughts and feelings related to grief have been expressed. It may not always be clear exactly who is being talked about, or the circumstances of the death or loss, and in some cases people employ metaphorical language to talk about feelings of grief, perhaps accompanied by particular types of nonverbal expression such as crying and rocking. Such expressions can be very powerful, and if there is deep emotional pain being shared, there may be an instinct to try to distract the person, and move onto what seem like safer topics. This could be related to ways in which someone else's anguish can touch on our own. It is often said, however, that we should 'give grief words', and this must apply as much to people with dementia as to the rest of us. The force with which feelings of grief are felt may be linked to the person's awareness of their own impending death, something we discuss at more length in Chapter 13 on awareness.

When someone with dementia becomes newly bereaved, this raises a host of difficult issues. There may be questions about whether, when and how to tell them, and how to help them to come to terms with the loss. This will be complicated further if memory difficulties apparently interfere with the process of taking in the new information, and beginning the adjustment process. There are no hard and fast answers here, and this issue touches on one we discuss later in Chapter 15 on ethical implications, that of whether we have a responsibility to try to protect people with dementia from emotional pain.

We end this part of the chapter with another quotation from Beth Shirley Brough's book, *Alzheimer's with Love*. It embodies the expression of both love and awareness, combined with the pain of loss, and forms a bridge to Chapter 13 on awareness:

'It's going to go on forever.' He stiffens and raises his voice.
'Forever! Forever, I tell you!'

'Yes', I agree, 'but you are loved.'
'Am I?'
'Yes.'

This statement of self-realization and the heaviness of his slight body against mine, fill my heart with compassion. He knows! This once-so-rational man knows what he has lost.[27]

Implications for care

If relationships are the main way in which the personhood of people with dementia is maintained, then clearly the principal aim of care must be to help people to remain in the relationships they most value, and also to be open to the possibility of them developing new ones.

As regards existing relationships, there is obviously a major role for staff in supporting relatives and friends of the person with dementia. This aspect of their role is often overlooked and undervalued, but it is crucial. The member of staff is a provider of information and support to those around the person, helping them to make sense of their words and actions and cope with their feelings about the changes which occur. Similarly practitioners can function as a link between the individual with dementia and their relatives, encouraging them to talk about them, tell stories and generally helping them to be as real to them as possible even when they are not present. Objects, photographs and even recordings of the voices of friends and family members can play a part in this.

We have talked a great deal already about the importance of relationships between staff and the person with dementia, and we address the matter of the extent to which relationships can be reciprocal below. But there is scope in a practical sense for staff to capitalize on people's remaining memory capacity for developing relationships by attending to the way they present themselves (for example through clothes or jewellery) and being distinctive from one another in ways the person can link into and make sense of. Finding particular ways in which individual staff members can relate to people (for example through special activities or routines) are other possibilities in this regard.

The final area of concern here is that of the extent to which we promote the development of meaningful relationships between persons with dementia. It has often been John's experience that people living side by side in nursing homes and in other sorts of services have hardly even been properly introduced to one another, and even those with a great deal in common remain virtual strangers. This is a dreadful waste of really important potential sources of enjoyment and meaning in people's lives. We all need to give much more thought to how we can promote the development of genuine contact in these ways.

Ethical implications

It is probably in the area of relationships where the most complex and taxing ethical issues arise. There is certainly sufficient material on this topic to fill a whole chapter, so we have to be concise.

Reciprocity in relationships with people with dementia

The issue of reciprocity in relationships was first raised in the ethical implications section of Chapter 2 on personhood, and we return to it here. We have already acknowledged that in order for a relationship to exist there must be something given back by the person with dementia, however unconventional or minimal this is. To move to the other end of the scale, however, we must ask ourselves about how far the possibilities in terms of relationships can go. These questions are important not only from the point of view of practical issues, but also in the sense that they can be seen as a test of our commitment to the idea of personhood.

Could you, for example, ever enter into a friendship with a person with dementia, with all that that implies? If so, and since friendship is certainly a reciprocal relationship, what kinds of demands would it be appropriate to make? If not, if we would say that a person with dementia could never be a potential friend in the full sense, what does this imply that we think about dementia as a condition and those who have it?

The extent to which relationships can develop is influenced by external factors too. Most people reading this book will come into contact with people with dementia through a work role. This immediately places the possibilities within a framework which has values and rules about the limits of relationship, whether or not they are explicit. In most settings the dominant way of thinking about caring relationships is underpinned by ideas about maintaining a 'professional distance'. Within this the role of the recipient of a service is characterized by passivity and deference, while the professional is seen as having special knowledge and expertise, exercising control by not becoming over-involved. This is an idea which has come most strongly from traditional medical and nursing training, but it has permeated all sorts of other organizations. These values are now changing, and so there are now much greater possibilities for conflict. On the one hand, there is increasing pressure (not least from this book) to develop deeper and more genuine relationships with service users, getting to know them as people, and sharing aspects of ourselves with them too. On the other hand, there are these pervasive values about the importance of maintaining a professional distance.

We suspect that many members of staff struggle with this tension in an ongoing way, and it may contribute quite substantially to the stress generated by the job. Many members of staff do describe the development of close relationships with people with dementia – with some people more than others – and very much value this closeness. But they may or may not feel that this is supported by colleagues and managers, or the culture of an organization generally. In Chapter 14 we explore the practical implications of these realities, and in Chapter 15 there is discussion of the emotional and spiritual demands of the work, but for now we simply acknowledge that there are important questions here we need to address.

Alongside the larger issues about the possibilities for relationships, workers are sometimes faced with more specific situations in which values about the reciprocity of relationships are highlighted. An example is from the experience of a colleague, Jackie, who was spending time with Joan in a creative activity. After several minutes of intense occupation, Joan began to speak about personal matters. However, before doing so, she turned to Jackie and said in a very deliberate way, 'You're my friend'. It was clear from the manner of its utterance that this statement was significant, and it seemed that in the moment, the response that was called for was to reciprocate the message. Jackie did so by saying 'You're my friend too', and the conversation proceeded in an intimate way with Joan sharing a lot of feelings about her current and past life.

Although the encounter was very successful, this exchange raised many issues. Was it right for Jackie to respond to Joan's statement in this way? Was she being insincere in stating a commitment of friendship to Joan even though she probably did not truly see her in this role? On the other hand, how else could she have responded? It seemed in the moment as if this was what Joan needed to hear in order to proceed with the conversation, that somehow a statement of reciprocity was necessary for her to have the courage to share her story. If Jackie had not said what she did, would this not have seemed like a rejection of Joan's generosity and might it not have curtailed the positive potential of the encounter?

Such questions must in turn lead us to reflect on what was meant by the statement 'You're my friend'. In saying this had Joan been meaning to bestow on Jackie a status which included responsibilities and duties as well as benefits? Or could it have been a simple way of saying, 'I like and trust you, and want to spend time with you?' If so, then Jackie's response was entirely appropriate and truthful, since she had the very same feelings about Joan. However, there are other issues which need to be considered. For example, does the notion of being a friend necessarily carry the suggestion that one is going to remain a friend, that there is going to be an ongoing relationship, a commitment extending into the future? In many situations this is not an undertaking that one can honestly give. But again we are prompted to ask what might be the other person's understanding of such a situation, and whether such statements do have the same status of durability in time. These are philosophical questions which do not lend themselves to easy answers, but if we are to honour fully the seriousness of our work with people with dementia it is important for us to give them due reflection.

Self-disclosure

In the Ethical Implications section of Chapter 3 on nonverbal communication, we raised the issue of ourselves being emotionally exposed to people with dementia who may become experts in reading nonverbal cues. This leads us to give further consideration to that aspect of reciprocity in relationships which involves the sharing of ongoing feelings and mood states. We who care for people with dementia are not machines. We all have emotional ups and downs, days when it is harder to achieve an equanimity, and times when it is impossible to forget about personal worries. If we are arguing that we have to give more of ourselves in order to affirm and engage with the personhood of the other, then surely this suggests that we cannot always keep our own emotional lives out of the equation. Indeed might it not be that some of our most meaningful encounters with people could arise out of shared experiences of vulnerability? But this has a whole range of ethical implications, again touching on our attitudes regarding professional distance, the sharing of ourselves, and our perceptions of people with dementia as being inherently in need of protection.

Negative reactions to people

Is it possible to develop rapport with everyone? What about people you just do not like? Not all people are pleasant or act towards you out of the best of motives. People who hold antisocial or objectionable values develop dementia too, and we are bound to come across them from time to time. What are the best ways of handling such people and coping with your own reactions to them?

The reality is that it is impossible to like everyone, and there will be times when you encounter someone with whom you feel you cannot develop a positive relationship. Sometimes you will be aware of the reasons for your negative reactions, at others you may find they are harder to pinpoint. Where the reasons for your dislike are less clear, it may be that the person reminds you of someone with whom you have negative associations.

In any case when it is likely that you will have ongoing contact with the person, this will be a difficult situation. If we are right in thinking that people with dementia often develop heightened sensitivity to nonverbal communication, then the chances of your being able to hide your feelings are slim. But can it ever be right to admit to someone that you have negative feelings towards them?[28]

In a similar vein, sometimes people with dementia do or say things which are hurtful. We all have our vulnerabilities, and at times it may seem that the person can spot them and knows how to hurt or embarrass. The making of personal comments is a common example of this sort of behaviour, and sometimes the embarrassment or anxiety is not for yourself but for others, including other people with dementia. There is no getting away from the fact that these are challenging situations, and they should prompt us to consider our values. But we should try to find reasons for such behaviour. Most people are not deliberately unpleasant, and so such a tendency may be related to their own feelings of vulnerability or a need to wield what power does remain in any way which will get a response.

In terms of responding to this kind of thing, is it best to be straightforward about your feelings? Would a simple, non-accusatory statement about finding something hurtful be appropriate? These are questions which can only be answered with a specific situation in mind, but in the context of a commitment to honesty within relationships, the possibility should not be dismissed altogether.

Sexuality

In Chapter 2 on personhood we discussed the fact that, as people first and foremost, those with dementia have a sexual dimension to their being, and that this reality must be recognized and celebrated in our dealings with them. We also acknowledged that there is a very powerful taboo which operates in the area of sexuality in relation to older people, and when the facts of illness, disability and being near death are superimposed, the taboos multiply. This means that we have to make a conscious effort to recognize the ways in which our prejudices influence our thinking and behaviour, and try to maintain an open-minded stance. At the same time, it is crucial to appreciate that, whether or not we are aware of doing so, we ourselves bring our sexuality into any interpersonal situation, even at work; it cannot be 'left at the door'.

Clearly there are strict rules which forbid sexual involvement between individuals within professional care relationships; these are necessary and exist to protect all parties. Where communication is concerned, and specifically the approaches we have described in this book, it is, however, only responsible to recognize that there is the potential for sensitive situations to arise. Particular features of an interaction, for example intensity of gaze, proximity of positioning and the use of touch are all open to misinterpretation, either by the person with dementia or onlookers, as having sexual intent. Such perception may be interpreted positively or negatively by the other person. A negative response may lead to the person becoming angry or distressed. A positive response might be characterized by the reciprocation of apparent sexual signals. While it is entirely possible for such a misunderstanding to arise when the person has a normal appreciation of their own age, where they see themselves as being much younger the likelihood is perhaps increased.

On a number of occasions it has become clear to John, either through verbal or nonverbal means or both, that a person would like an encounter to proceed to a sexual level. In these circumstances it was necessary to make it clear – as respectfully and gently as possible – that this was not an option. One way of doing this has been to pay the person a compliment which is at once a sincere gift and affirmation, but also a clarification of the limits of the interaction. For example, a statement like 'Mary, you're a lovely person' said with the right tone and accompanying body language can be very effective. One of the uncertainties of letting someone down lightly in this way is the extent to which the other person appreciates what is happening and is able to modify their expectations. In trying to understand such a situation, we have to remember that not only do many people with dementia retain a strong awareness of their own and others' sexuality, but also they exist in a state of deprivation in this respect, as in many others. Opportunities for sexual activity in institutional settings are almost non-existent and any such expressions are likely to be discouraged.

Many others, while still living at home, will have lost their previous sexual partner through death and still miss this dimension of the relationship. Dealing with these situations calls upon great tact and self-awareness. And the feelings of discomfort they give rise to in ourselves are real and powerful, even if they do derive from ways of thinking we need to reassess.

At the same time we have fully to recognize the part sexuality plays in all interactions. There are conscious and unconscious elements of surprise and pleasure present in every human encounter. This is natural and integral and contributes immeasurably to the richness of our social lives. Surely a person with dementia has the same right to enjoy this aspect of their humanity as much as anyone else?

13 Awareness: 'I'm thinking . . . when I'm not saying anything'

The following passage comes from *The Atom of Delight*, the autobiography of the Scottish novelist, Neil Gunn. Here he is recalling a formative moment from his childhood:

> The shallow river flowed around and past with its variety of lulling monotonous sounds; a soft wind, warmed by the sun, came upstream and murmured in my ears as it continuously slipped from my face . . .
>
> Then the next thing happened, and happened, so far as I can remember, for the first time. I have tried hard but can find no simpler way of expressing what happened than by saying: *I came upon myself sitting there.*
>
> Within the mood of content, as I have tried to recreate it, was this self and the self was me.
>
> The state of content deepened wonderfully and everything around was embraced in it.
>
> There was no 'losing' of the self in the sense that there was a blank from which I awoke or came to. The self may have thinned away – it did – but so delightfully that it also remained at the centre in a continuous and perfectly natural way. And then within this amplitude the self as it were

became aware of seeing itself, not as an 'I' or an 'ego' but rather as a stranger it had come upon and was even a little shy of.

Transitory, evanescent – no doubt, but the scene comes back across half a century . . .[1]

The subject of awareness (also often referred to as 'insight') is the most diffi-cult one that we tackle in the book. It is difficult because the whole concept of awareness (dementia aside) is tricky to think about. It is hard to find solid start-ing points and build a lucid argument, and we are quickly led into highly abstract fields in the disciplines of philosophy and psychology, where even the experts have argued and disagreed with each other over the centuries. It is also a challenge because grappling with this subject in relation to dementia demands that we clarify our own ways of thinking about the condition, what it is and how its effects come about, and what the individual is left with at the end. These are questions we have all only recently begun to ask, and we simply do not have answers for them.

Nevertheless, we have to do our best because it is a crucially important sub-ject. The degree of knowledge and understanding the person has of their own situation must be central to any attempts to establish opportunities for real communication and genuine relationships. Our efforts to develop a grasp of the nature of dementia as a condition must include exploration of the person's subjective reality. In any case, the subject cannot be ignored since in John's experience, and that of many others, themes of awareness have emerged strik-ingly in encounters with individuals, and in examination of their words. It is a fascinating area, with the potential radically to alter our perception of dementia and its impact on the person.

A lot of what we discuss in this chapter is closely related to the ideas explored in Chapter 6 on interpretation, and much of the material presented in the chapters on personhood, memory and narrative has direct relevance. As usual we begin with a more general introduction to the subject, and then move on to consider it in relation to dementia.

Normal awareness

When we introduced the phenomenon of consciousness in Chapter 2, we identified as part of that not only to be able to do sophisticated things, but also to be able to know and think about, and almost mentally to observe ourselves doing them. In maintaining this kind of ongoing account or story of our experiences, we can exist at a level which is separate from the immediate moment and its physical realities. For our conscious awareness is linked with memory, imagination and forms part of the vast, largely unmapped domain which we call the mind, and out of its complexity arises the capacity to know what it is like to be oneself.

Obviously this kind of mental attention can range over any subject, but our interest here is in that aspect of awareness which is concerned with the self, and that which impinges directly on it, including, most importantly, other people. As we discussed in Chapter 6, we are continuously engaged in an effort of trying to make sense of our experiences, to develop an internal representation of pattern and meaning, and to find ways of living with this. The distinction between awareness of the self and knowledge about other matters is more than one of mere subject matter. It is about instinct, emotion and our deepest drives. In contrast with knowledge about the external world, which may or may not have any great personal importance, awareness of the self always does. The bottom line is that we matter greatly to ourselves. We care in a deep, visceral and relentless way about how we feel. It must be this way since millions of years of evolution have programmed us to do so. The subject of self-awareness (which we hereafter simply refer to as 'awareness'), is imbued with all of this significance.

The nature of awareness

What exactly do we mean by awareness? Definitions like this are always difficult, but we can offer some thoughts. Awareness is certainly not a simple all-or-nothing matter. There are many different levels at which we can be aware of personally important information. We may have vague hunches or notions, nothing well defined, just a nagging sense. These may, with time or effort, develop into a clearer picture. Sometimes we can know things in an intellectual way, but without there being any real emotional dimension to the awareness. The absence of the emotional component may be part of a more general way of coping with aspects of life, perhaps of very longstanding. The opposite can also be true. On occasion we may become aware of the presence of emotional feelings which call attention to themselves, but do not have any obvious cause or trigger. Again it may take time and effort to work out what is going on.

  Awareness is also something which is patchy and uneven. It would be impossible to have or develop awareness about everything pertaining to the self. We are simply too complicated, and the picture is constantly in flux as we move through life, collecting new experiences and reworking old ones. The extent to which our awareness of personally significant information is integrated or fragmented is also important. It is perfectly possible to 'know' or understand things but in a way in which they are somehow separate. Two 'items' of knowledge may remain apart until a new experience or piece of information causes them to come together, and merge in such a way as to make us wonder why we never previously saw them as being connected. Once this first phase of reorganization has taken place, this can pave the way for further realizations. This seems to be what the renowned psychotherapist, Carl Rogers, was thinking about when he wrote (referring to a passage of dialogue quoted prior to this):

  This excerpt indicates very clearly the letting of material come into awareness, without any attempt to own it as part of the self, or to relate it to other material held in consciousness. It is, to put it as accurately as possible, an awareness of a wide range of experiences, with, at the moment, no thought of their relation to self. Later it may be recognised that what was being experienced may all become part of the self.[2]

Generally speaking it requires the investment of considerable personal resources to achieve a high degree of personal awareness, and it can never be a project which is complete. For one thing the longer one lives, the more experience there is to work on, and also there is no limit to how aware one can be. Attaining a certain depth will always bring new degrees of complexity and subtlety into view, and so it goes on. It seems safe to say that one of the effects of pursuing this goal is to render one's experience of life ever more complex, and this may mean it seems like very hard work, but the alternative – the 'unexamined life' – seems far less acceptable.

Variation between individuals

Although a certain degree of awareness is necessary for successful general functioning, there is variation between individuals in the extent to which they place value on the effort to understand the things that happen in their lives, and those of the people they love. While for some this is an essential aspect of their approach to living, others seem not to have any particular drive to try to make sense of their experiences at a deep level. Others again may find the idea threatening, perhaps because of what they fear they might discover if they were to look too far.

Sometimes the level of our awareness of certain realities is affected by the perception of our ability to cope with whatever it is that is prodding us. If the potential realization is likely to be emotionally painful, then our minds are very well adapted to protect us from its impact. Such a strategy is not thought through in a conscious way (if it were the system could not work), but it is nevertheless a very important aspect of the workings of awareness. In such circumstances, it may be that the reality of the situation is clear to others, and they may be faced with a decision about whether or not they should intervene.

There is also the more general social context to consider. Since the 1950s or so, certainly since the 1960s, there has been a move towards the more 'feelings-orientated' society, the kind of culture where talking about emotions and relationships, reading self-help books, and going to a therapist is increasingly considered normal.

Developing awareness

There are lots of ways of developing awareness, including introspection, talking to others, writing things down, reading, and expressing ideas, images and feelings through a wide range of artistic or creative outlets. The amount of

time and energy we invest in such activities varies over time, and is related to the amount of resources available. There are times in our lives when we can hardly spare a moment to think things over because there are simply too many demands on our attention. Sometimes it is necessary to try to take time out of our routine specifically for this purpose, whether this means lying in a bath, going for a walk or something more drastic, such as seeking therapy or going on a retreat. Sensing that there is a backlog of impressions, feelings and events to process can be a source of stress.

Our level of awareness or understanding of an aspect of our experience is to an extent related to the availability of relevant information. When we wish to understand more, then obtaining information is an obvious way forward. As well as providing us with relevant facts, this helps us to learn new concepts and develop new ways of thinking about what we experience.

Escaping from awareness

As well as being something which we aspire to and need, the state of awareness can also act as an obstruction to well-being, or even give rise to psychological pain. In order to function effectively from day to day it is necessary for us to have times when we can escape from the experience of conscious awareness that accompanies normal functioning. Sleep is an example of this, and sometimes people seek it in order to enjoy the respite from aspects of consciousness that it provides. For thousands of years human beings have also used alcohol and other drugs in order to loosen the constraints of awareness. But there are other ways of achieving it. The psychologist Mihaly Csikzentmihalyi has explored this subject as part of developing a more general theory of human happiness.[3] His argument, and it is based on accounts from thousands of people of all ages, from all walks of life and from all over the world, is that a crucial element of what he calls 'flow' or 'optimal experience', is a form of absorption in an activity or challenge in which the usual sense of the separateness of the self diminishes, as the following quote describes:

> people become so involved in what they are doing that the activity becomes spontaneous, almost automatic; they stop being aware of themselves as separate from the actions they are performing.[4]

Dementia and awareness

The relationship between dementia and awareness has received little attention even in recent work on the person-centred approach to care. There are some enlightening studies of insight and periods of 'lucidity' from Scandinavia, which form part of the stream of work on 'intergrity-promoting care',[5] and we refer to one of these later. The studies which have been done in the UK and the United States (and these are mainly from the psychiatric literature) have very different starting points.[6] They tend to begin with an assumption of what insight is and how to measure it, and then look at the relationship between insight and other features, for example severity, language fluency or depression. Although some of these studies do grapple with the problem of how to define the concept, they fail to advance real understanding of this aspect of dementia, nor point directly to developments in care practice. A large part of the problem is that we do not yet have a sufficiently robust understanding of the nature of awareness to underpin studies of this sort, and exploratory work, which takes the experience of the person as its starting point, is required.

Insight or awareness?

As we mentioned above, another word which is commonly used to talk about this subject is 'insight', but the term 'awareness' also appears. We took a lot of time to decide which to use as we believe that they are not identical, and may lead us down different paths. Our decision was to continue using the term 'awareness'. The major disadvantage of 'insight' is that it has come to be regarded as a kind of technical term used by medical practitioners, and sometimes with the effect (intended or not) of maintaining a power differential (where, for example, someone is judged as being lacking in insight if they do not agree with the expert). This hinders the development of a more multifaceted understanding of the nature of awareness in dementia. The term 'awareness' is more associated with psychotherapy and personal development work and suggests a greater openness, including the quality of 'being with' knowledge without necessarily striving to shape it into an explanation. This latter state feels more consistent with our present purposes and current state of knowledge.

Assumptions about awareness

Old ways of understanding dementia assumed that any awareness the person had of their condition was progressively and irreversibly destroyed. The following comes from a book by the psychiatrist Alan Jacques (published in 1992):[7]

> The patient herself . . . is unlikely to be aware of or feel any of these changes in a coherent fashion. She will not recall all the things that she used to do and so she will not be able to recognise the change in herself. She will not be able to feel the humiliation of her dependent position. She will not sense the passage of time. Or she may experience the wrong feelings, or jumbled bits and pieces of feeling, some appropriate, some not.
> . . . At the final stages the patient may be assumed to have no real subjective awareness, no sense of self at all, and to be in this sense mentally 'dead'.[8]

It may be helpful at this point to try to make explicit the sorts of assumptions that have characterized traditional views about 'insight'.

- The progressive loss of insight is a core feature of dementia.[9]
- By the time a person has reached the moderate stage of the illness they can be assumed to have little or no awareness of their problems.
- Insight is an all or nothing entity – it is either present or absent.
- The presence or absence of insight can be established by questioning a person in a clinical situation.
- If a person does not express insight this means that it is not present.
- Insight can be expressed only in words.
- People who retain insight are at a greater risk of depression.[10]
- Those who do not have insight are likely to be less distressed by their condition than those who do.

Awareness of what?

Clearly dementia affects many areas of an individual's functioning. Until recently, however, thinking about awareness has emphasized cognitive change to the exclusion of other aspects. This bias reflects our hypercognitive conceptualization of the condition, and means that we have all proceeded with an overly narrow perspective. In order to move our understanding forward we need a more inclusive concept which recognizes the possibility that an individual could be aware of many different sorts of changes, not simply those in the intellectual sphere. For example:

- personality, including change in style of coping with difficulties, basic dispositions such as sociability and impulsivity
- emotional experiences such as an increase in feelings of anxiety, sadness, confusion; more difficulty in controlling emotions
- mental health, including onset of conditions like depression, anxiety and even psychotic features
- spiritual values and beliefs, including attitudes about death and what follows, alterations in values about what is important in life, changes in religious convictions
- ability to use language
- motor skills such as the ability to drive, dress oneself, to eat independently
- physical health, strength and capacity
- behaviour of other people, e.g. greater protectiveness by relatives/carers
- the feelings of others, including grief at the loss of aspects of the relationship with the affected person
- one's status in the eyes of other people, including lowered expectations, a sense of having been 'written off' by society
- living circumstances
- that life is coming to an end.

This list is surely incomplete, but the main point is that there are many sorts of changes encountered by the person, and we need to consider this diversity in our attempts to better understand the issue of awareness. For all we know the individual may be aware of all or only some of them at any one point in time, and certain phases of the condition may be characterized by greater awareness of some aspects of change over others.

Why it is important to think about awareness in dementia

As we have seen, we all have a need to try to make sense of the events in our lives, and this applies as much, if not more so, to people with dementia as for those without. In order for us to try to understand their inner reality, and to respond helpfully to their needs, it is clearly crucial that we consider what the person is aware of and how they use that information to explain to themselves what is happening.

There are also practical reasons for needing to understand more about the matter of awareness. For many people opportunities to take part in therapeutic activities such as counselling may hinge on judgements about their level of awareness. When perceptions are negative their chances of being offered an intervention which could be helpful are reduced.

Often when a person does not comply with a form of support or intervention, this is attributed to their lack of insight into the reasons for it. While this explanation may be correct in some cases, there is a risk of it becoming an easy way of explaining away the person's rejection of an intervention which is, in fact, inappropriate or unacceptable to them for entirely valid reasons. For example, medication may be resisted because the rationale for its prescription has never been explained or because it gives rise to unpleasant side-effects, and not because the person is unaware that they need help. Routine recourse to the 'lack of insight' argument is likely to forestall consideration of other reasons for treatment refusal.

Arguments about awareness can also appear when judgements about risk are being made. Again negative perceptions will lead to more conservative decision-making, and a greater likelihood that decisions will be taken on behalf of, rather than in agreement with, the individual. This extends to occasions when it is considered necessary to invoke legal powers to enforce certain arrangements. All this touches on the important matter of the power differential inherent in caring relationships.

In the last few years those concerned with planning and providing services have acknowledged the importance of making far more effort to consult with users about their needs and level of satisfaction with support.[11] However, arguments about developing expertise in user consultation can be met with the objection that people often do not know that they are ill and in receipt of services, and therefore cannot meaningfully be asked to provide feedback. This point of view is exemplified in the following passage, again from Alan Jacques, and written at a time when our attitudes were more pessimistic:

Our feelings about what is good or humane for a severely demented patient cannot come from an understanding of what she feels as an individual, or of what she 'wants'. These concepts are meaningless and so any real understanding is impossible.[12]

This demonstrates how certain perceptions of one aspect of a complex condition can be given overriding importance, and judgements made which can have a huge impact on the individual and people with dementia generally. In order to find good ways of asking people with dementia what they want and need from services we must be prepared to set aside our assumptions about what they can and cannot understand, and provide opportunities for them to express their views.

The interpretation of behaviour

In normal circumstances trying to get a sense of what another person is or is not aware of would be done by asking them about their understanding of the situation. There could be an open discussion where points of ignorance or disagreement are identified and addressed. Where people with dementia are concerned, we have all been quick to assume that the individual is unable to engage in this way on account of core features of the condition, and their behaviour is interpreted by us in accordance with this assumption.

The following is from a description by the neurologist Antonio Damasio of the actions of a longstanding philosopher friend who has Alzheimer's Disease:

Once, I saw him move close to the single, nearly empty bookcase in the room, reach for a shelf at about the level of the chair's armrest, and pick up a folded paper. It was a worn-out glossy print, 8 × 10, folded in four. He set it on his lap, slowly; he unfolded it, slowly; and stared for a long time at the beautiful face in it, that of his smiling wife. He looked but he did not see. There was no glimmer of reaction, at any time, no connection made between the portrait and its living model who was sitting across from him, only a few feet away; no connection made to me, either, who had actually made the photograph ten years before, at a time of shared joy. The folding and unfolding of the photograph had happened regularly, from earlier in the progress of the disease, when he still knew that something was amiss, perhaps as a desperate attempt to cling to the certainty of what once was. Now it had become an unconscious ritual, performed with the same slow pace, in the same silence, with the same lack of affective resonance. In the sadness of the moment I was happy that he no longer could know.[13]

What is most striking about this description is the readiness of Damasio to assume that he knows exactly what is and what is not happening in the mind of his friend. As a scientist Damasio is surely familiar with the maxim that absence of evidence should not be regarded as evidence of absence, but here the absence of an observable response to the photograph is confidently regarded as evidence of the absence of an inner one, and the certainty which with this assumption is expressed is all the more remarkable for the fact that it is embedded in a 350 page book exploring the highly complex nature of human consciousness.

Would we be so presumptious in the context of any other condition? If the man with the photograph had been suffering from a deep depression, his lack of outward response would have been interpreted in a different way, as it would if he had been known to be experiencing the muscular rigidity of the face which can accompany Parkinson's Disease. What is it about dementia which makes us so ready to form judgements of this sort?

Our own motives

The final point Damasio makes in the above quote is highly revealing. It touches on the fact that our way of thinking about awareness in dementia relates intimately to ourselves, and our own reasons for holding certain beliefs about conditions like dementia. These are also the primary reasons why the subject of awareness is so emotive.

It is crucial to recognize that assuming lack of awareness has a central function for ourselves as people *without* dementia. It helps us to believe that those with the condition are fundamentally different from us, and to hold at arm's length our worst fears for our loved ones, for people with dementia, and for ourselves. Believing in lack of awareness enables us to avoid confronting the whole truth of what being human may mean – that the mind, capable of amazing achievements and creativity, is also capable of suffering in sophisticated ways too.

On an interpersonal level, assumptions about lack of awareness enable us to deny, or at least minimize, the person's psychological and emotional needs. We can reassure ourselves that although from the outside their predicament is heart-breaking, the person is spared suffering because they do not know what is happening to them. These beliefs also help us to tolerate poor standards of care, both in terms of features of the physical environments in which people with dementia are often placed, and also standards of interpersonal care, both physical and psychosocial.

The following is from Michael Ignatieff's book *Scar Tissue*:

My wife once said, 'Don't be hard on yourself. She doesn't feel a thing. The illness takes care of everything. It's worse for you.' Nothing could be further from the truth. I know she has insight. I know she has counted up every one of her losses. She looks at herself and asks what kind of person she is becoming. The illness spares her nothing.[14]

Texts and interpretations

Andrew Manbridge

Andrew had spoken with John on two previous occasions. The text of this particular conversation is complete and chronological. John's role was confined to giving brief words of encouragement:

1 *How am I today? Well, generally speaking, standing up in a sitting*
2 *down situation! In short, I'm okay. Nobody's kicking my behind. Of*
3 *course, if it's too hard it's a matter for the police. But if it's only*
4 *tickle-wickle it's all right.*

5 *You'll be writing this down? Right, get the bloody thing back to me,*
6 *and I'll be your corrector.*
7 *What I say is not important, but it can be stated and looked at.*

8 *They were playing music, but it's gone now. When it came to both*
9 *sides, some would sing this and some would sing that. It was a nice*
10 *suite. We had a lot of Solomon. Having sung this, I said I'd never*
11 *sung that before. I don't care much for the ha-ha-ha-hee-hee-hee-*
12 *and-then-what-have-we-got-kind.*

13 *She spoke to me, that lady; she said 'Every time you speak you put*
14 *the word "what-d'ye-call-it" in the middle. Well, go and learn it for*
15 *next time!'*

16 *There was none of this in my young days. They wouldn't have*
17 *tolerated anything like this place, but it's a nice area, it's a sunny*
18 *day.*

19 *That chap who's doing what you're doing is original – he could be*
20 *on to quite a big thing.*

21 *I thought a lot of things would have gone by now. But they haven't,*
22 *they cling on. I go out and I make do, but it's difficult to make do.*

Andrew appears very self-aware. At the outset he interprets a question about his health as applying to his state of mind, a subject to which he returns at the end. He retains a good command of language, so it is not clear whether his use of the term 'tickle-wickle', or the extraordinary description of the kind of music he does not like, are the result of difficulty with language or examples of his wit. But he admits to struggling with vocabulary in lines 13–15 in the story he tells against himself. He also seems to understand about the kind of place in which he is living, hence his comments in lines 16–18. The view he puts across there seems a considered one, with pros and cons. He is also very conscious of John's role, on which he comments on two occasions, though his attribution of it to a third person in lines 19–20 is curious. The final sentence appears to be a clear statement of his awareness that he is undergoing losses, and that although his negative expectations have not been entirely borne out, he nevertheless struggles to cope.

There appears to be a great deal going on beneath the surface of this piece. On the one hand there is a bluffness, even belligerence ('get the bloody thing back to me'); on the other a sensitivity and reticence ('What I say is not important'). It may be that the former is adopted to cover up the latter, but the dementia has robbed him of the control which would have ensured that he presented a consistent face to the world. Andrew seems to be a complex person who is attempting to come to terms with the knowledge of his difficulties. The final paragraph could constitute an acknowledgement of that fact.

Some conversations are short because the person chooses that they should be so, or is unable to sustain a longer interaction. Some are close-packed with emotion because this is what the individual needs to express. Andrew's piece has both of these characteristics. It conveys little information about his life but a great deal about his state of mind.

Gladys Parr

Gladys also spoke with John on a number of occasions. The main body of this text is a slightly condensed version of a single conversation with some personal references removed. The final paragraph arose a few days later when John was helping another resident at the meal table:

1 *You hear many strange things in a hospital like this. It's God's blessing*
2 *that we have a sense of humour.*

3 *Do I detect a left-hander? They have all the brains. My husband was a*
4 *left-hander.*

5 *Are you a doctor? Oh I'd have liked to be one of those after my exams!*
6 *What do you write about? People? Well, you'll come across many*
7 *interesting side-lights on people's character.*

8 *Is this building in your parish? That's not tonight's sermon you are writing*
9 *by any chance?*

10 *It's old age that bothers me. I am a student of history and the loss of*
11 *memory irritates me.*

12 *That's beautiful writing. One of my brothers could write like that. All your*
13 *v's become w's if you write too fast.*

14 *When the place is silent like this I don't think it's helpful to the people.*
15 *It's the dead silence. Dead silence makes dead faces. There are no*
16 *smiles in this room. Except mine. And that is because I've got you to talk to.*

17 *There is no music here. Think of all the orchestras and choirs we could*
18 *have playing quietly.*

19 *I got my niece to sell my house. That was a mistake, it should have been*
20 *subdivided. When it goes through I may not stay here. I'll decide where*
21 *I want to end up.*

22 *Do you write under your own name? Between you and me, when I was*
23 *young I could never spell the word 'pseudonym'. I had to look it up in a*
24 *damned dictionary!*

25 *I'm one of the fortunate people of this world. I have relatives in Scotland,*
26 *England, France, America and Canada.*

27 *I'm very glad they did this place up. It was a very good idea. I've just*
28 *been here a week-and-a-half. It's a nice place, but I would rather go and*
29 *stay privately somewhere.*

      * * *

30 *Poor thing, there's something wrong with her mind. Do you think that's*
31 *what's happened to them? Is it something they were born with or does it*
32 *develop in later life? It's the lack of something in the brain that causes it,*
33 *they say. Are you a medical man? Well you've got the rapport and manner*
34 *to get through to them.*

Gladys is somewhat confused about where she is. The nearest she comes to identifying it is in the first line where she speaks of a hospital. She is perturbed, however, about what is wrong with her fellow 'patients'. At the outset she identifies 'strange things' that people say, and her most extended reflection about this occurs in lines 30–4 where she speculates on what 'they' may be suffering from. Her characterization of dementia as following from 'the lack of something in the brain' is quite accurate according to current medical thinking. Although she does not see herself as exhibiting these symptoms she admits that 'old age . . . bothers' her, and locates her concern in the area of memory loss. The paragraph in which she speaks of 'dead faces' (lines 14–16) indicates that she identifies with her fellow-residents. She states that it is only John's presence that gives animation to her features.

Gladys analyses her environment acutely. She says that the quality of the 'silence' is 'dead', and that it is the lack of activity which makes the place so sterile. Following on from this she remarks on the absence of music (lines 17–18), and seems to suggest that this would have a transforming quality. Despite a sense of helplessness in her text there is also a positive spirit shown in the references to how she might proceed in the future (lines 20–1, 28–9), and her enthusiasm for her extended family (lines 25–6).

As well as commenting on her surroundings, Gladys is actively attempting to discover what John's work is. She considers various options, but despite some confusion her reflections on his actual role are perceptive. She speculates on lefthandedness, on handwriting, on human foibles, and on using one's own name for published work. She also appreciates the value of the conversations that lead to the writing. Her own command of language is largely intact and she seems to find exercising her mind a rewarding activity.

Further reflections on awareness

Awareness and denial

A popular idea about the issue of awareness in dementia is that those with the condition use denial as a way of coping with its impact. Thus when a person talks of a possession having been stolen when in fact they have mislaid it, we may interpret this behaviour as being an expression of denial. Such an instance may be part of a much larger strategy of denying the nature and extent of difficulties, and maintaining the illusion that life is normal and usual activities ongoing. Some people engage in elaborate covering behaviour often with considerable plausibility that keeps others from realizing the true nature of the situation. Sometimes others can be drawn into these scenarios, and a complicated set of manoeuvres set in train.

From John's experience there was a man who lived in a nursing home, and who said:

Everyone here has Alzheimer's Disease – except me!

Social work researchers Victoria Cottrell and Laura Lein report an account of a man who refuted even the most blunt descriptions of his problems.[15] He continued to behave as if he was in his normal working routine, and demonstrated considerable ingenuity in reframing situations (that is, living in a nursing home) to be consistent with his previous lifestyle – by responding to other residents as if they were delegates at a conference.

Others show no such tendencies to conceal their difficulties. The difference may be a matter of personalities, but we suggest that rather than attempting to explain this entirely in terms of individual factors, the attitudes and behaviours of those around the person with dementia play their part.

As we mentioned in Chapter 2, it is important to recognize that dementia remains the subject of much stigma and shame in our society. The very language we use to describe it betrays this. Instead of talking about 'dementia' we often prefer to use terms such as 'memory problems' or 'confusion'. Many doctors continue to be reticent about diagnosing the condition, and little in the way of information or explanation is available to those undergoing investigation of their difficulties. We may tell ourselves that our behaviour is motivated by efforts to protect the affected individual, but at times it seems as if we are all involved in the perpetration of a kind of cover-up. When this is most clearly expressed by the person with dementia, we turn on them and point up their actions as yet another symptom which reinforces the need to maintain the illusion.

Relationship between the existence of awareness and its expression

So far we have talked about awareness and its expression without making any clear distinction between them, as if they always go together. Of course this need not be true. It is conceivable that an individual may have awareness of their condition (either continuously or episodically), without it being expressed. The absence of any expression may occur either because the individual is unable to do so or is unwilling for fear of the effect this could have on others. The following quote is from John Bayley's book about Iris Murdoch:[16]

> In old days she used to weep quite openly, as if it were a form of demonstrable and demonstrated warmth and kindness. Now I find her doing it as if ashamedly, stopping as soon as she sees I have noticed. This is so unlike the past; but disturbing too in another way. It makes me feel she is secretly but fully conscious of what has happened to her, and she wants to conceal it from me. Can she want to protect me from it?
>
> . . .
>
> Her tears sometimes seem to signify a whole inner world which Iris is determined to keep from me and shield me from. There is something ghastly in the feeling of relief that this can't be so: and yet the illusion of such an inner world still there – if it is an illusion – can't help haunting me from time to time.[17]

Bayley also hints here at the possibility that the rich inner life which Iris had – she was one of the most noted intellectuals of her generation – may still be operating, though hidden from him by the screen erected by the condition. It is speculation, but such speculations must, in many cases, be powered by a strong desire on the part of the relative or carer that it be so. This raises the further question of how much of the awareness we think we perceive in the person with dementia is a wish-fulfilment, and how much a genuine perception of what is occurring.

Another alternative is that the person may have awareness of their situation, and attempt to express it, but in a form which others do not recognize or understand. In turn, the individual may or may not be aware that others have not understood their message. Many, perhaps most, people with dementia sadly are still immersed in cultures which assume that their words and actions are meaningless, and therefore interpret their behaviour within this frame of reference.

The relationship between the existence of awareness and its expression is difficult to think about because it is so speculative, and we quickly have to start to talk about further levels of awareness – for example that of awareness about awareness. But it is an important example of a situation in which our lack of understanding of dementia demands that we maintain an open mind, and hope that by careful observation and greater sensitivity to the messages being offered, enhanced understanding will be achieved.

Different ways of expressing awareness

It is easy to identify a certain sort of response which conforms to our expectation of the expression of a heightened state of awareness – meaningful words and appropriate actions. However, although language is important, it is only one of many modes of expression which could be used to express awareness. Emotional behaviour such as rage or crying may be equally valid responses of someone who experiences awareness yet is unable to express it in language. Others include actions such as becoming withdrawn, or acting out in an aggressive way. The person may respond to awareness of loss of competence in practical matters by refusing to try to use a skill. Such behaviour, however, is likely to be regarded as evidence of the progression of the condition, wilful lack of cooperation or simply failure to recognize the appropriateness of a certain course of action. The woman whose words form part of the title was able to state in a direct way that words do not always accompany meaningful inner activity.

Some carers and members of staff have given accounts of when they thought episodes of awareness were occurring although outward signs were minimal or extremely subtle. The following comes from Margaret Forster's novel, *Have the Men had Enough?*:[18]

> And I am sitting in front of Grandma so she can see me and know she is not alone. I have my feet up too. I pretend to be reading a book. And I look up and stare at Grandma and for a moment she catches my eye and I hold my breath. It is there: sanity. If I move, if I speak, if there is an unexpected noise it will go. What can I do with it? It is so precious. I want to scream for Mum to come quickly and look, *look* . . . She is *there*, she really is, she knows, she communicates, what shall I do? I smile. Grandma raises her eyebrows. Then Mum drops something, there is a bang. Grandma blinks and she has gone.[19]

Alternatively the person may perform a task or demonstrate an ability which they have been assumed to have lost. Their nonverbal behaviour may suddenly revert to a previous style, and one which was especially characteristic of the person when well.

As we have emphasized throughout the book, humour has great power, both as a way of coping with reality and also in communication. An example of a humorous expression of awareness comes from Kim Zabbia's book about her mother:[20]

> Mom leaned over to her granddaughter and said jokingly,
> 'Don't listen to your Mama. She's the crazy one, not me. What're you playin'?'
> 'I was trying to play Solitaire,' Kate said, 'but I can't. There's only fifty cards. I don't have a full deck'
> 'That's okay, baby,' Mom grinned. 'I don't either.'[21]

We also suggest that given the right sort of support and opportunities people could tell us a great deal about their understanding of their circumstances through the use of the arts. Some may utilize chances to paint or draw in order to share their experiences, and mime, dance or drama may also be appropriate outlets. As an example of this kind of expression we heard a story about one man who, when encouraged to draw, produced a picture of a complicated machine, part of which was on fire. When invited to talk about his work, he indicated that although part of the machine was clearly damaged, other parts were intact. Could this have been a metaphor for his own mind or self?[22] This recognition of alternative modes of expression is crucial for us to develop our understanding of this aspect of dementia.

Fluctuations in awareness and 'lucid episodes'

As we have described elsewhere, it is a common observation that for many people the features of dementia seem to fluctuate. Some of these variations will be explicable in terms of tiredness, mood, effects of drugs or aspects of physical health unrelated to the condition. What goes on around the person in terms of the environment and the actions of others are also bound to influence how well the person fares from day to day.

But there sometimes seem to be other less obvious factors which affect how a person is able to function. Every so often individuals say or do something which has obvious meaning and unexpected clarity or purpose. For example, John encountered a woman in a nursing home who in the midst of many statements which were curiously phrased or difficult to interpret said 'I think it is a pity to have all these people together in here – they don't wear as well as they would outside.' Another woman, on previous occasions of their talking together, and prior to the quoted remark, had shown no recognition of him, awareness of the nursing home where the interactions took place, or of her condition. Yet she turned to him and commented in a seriously reproving tone 'I find your visits to us here demeaning.' Nothing which followed in the conversation was on that level.

Another example comes from work done by Astrid Norberg in Sweden in which video recordings of the behaviour of 'severely demented' patients living in a hospital ward were being analysed:[23]

> One woman had not said anything for a year and exhibited muscular rigidity . . . At the end of the study, after 12 days, the patient was drinking milk, swallowed the wrong way and coughed. The nurse said, 'It's OK.' 'Yes, I agree,' the patient answered. The nurse looked at the glass and said 'There's some milk left in the glass.' 'Yes, I can see that. But I can leave it, can't I?' the patient answered quite distinctly. After that occasion the patient did not say anything for another two years. Then she died and the autopsy confirmed Alzheimer's Disease.[24]

Some episodes of awareness are characterized not only by unusual facility with language, but also by other very marked modifications of bearing and expression. These can create a striking effect. They are often referred to as 'lucid episodes'.[25] John has written about these times as 'when the clouds part' (and the account of the clergyman who had been paragliding on pp. 102–3 is an example of this).[26] There is a dramatic, often sudden, change in the way the person presents. It may be that something is said which indicates clear recall of events which have taken place since the onset of dementia. A series of flashes of wit or humour may occur, or remarks may be made which show that the person has sized up a situation or seen through the pretensions of others. There may be a marked improvement in the ability to use language, with greater fluency or command of vocabulary than usual.

What allows someone who passes much of their time in a state of apparent unawareness and incapacity to behave in the ways described above? Perhaps a complex constellation of factors needs to coincide in order for them to express – in a comprehensible form – the extent of their awareness of their situation, and the changes which have come upon them. Some of these factors could be internal – for example their mood or what they dreamt the previous night. Some could be external – the effects of the physical environment, and behaviour of others, both those with dementia and without. Wherever our speculations lead, they must prompt us to question what is often taken for granted about the nature of dementia, and how it acts on the mind and brain.

The following example comes from Bernard Heywood's book about *Caring for Maria*.[27] It is difficult for us to supply an account of a lucid episode as it is necessary for someone to be in the company of a person for long periods in order to identify episodes which stand out particularly in terms of awareness. While John may well have encountered many individuals who were experiencing unusual lucidity, it would not be easy to judge this as there is often little other experience with which to compare it. In contrast, the following events occurred in the context of an ongoing caring relationship in which Maria's style and level of functioning were well known to those concerned.

Maria was an old friend of Bernard's, and he took a large part in caring for her when she developed dementia. She was German-born, although she had lived in Britain for many years. Anna was a nurse who helped with Maria's care. At the time of writing neither knew that Maria had only a week to live.

29 August: Anna took me in 10.30ish, and suddenly Maria was in the most touching and wonderful form with her. Coming round, she recognised her, smiled at her, touched and stroked her, and talked (in German) in her best old-time style, calling Anna 'Liebchen' (darling) and so on. It was quite remarkable.

The cherished mother–daughter feeling has now, I feel, got another dimension, with Maria regarding Anna as her mother as well. It was really most moving and Anna was wonderful at it. I only wish Maria could have died in that happy period, which went on remarkably for over an hour, till she began to be conscious of some pain and it was time for another injection.

This was an extraordinarily moving happening. Maria showed no signs of distress. She laughed and smiled so naturally, and she chattered alertly in German as she stroked Anna's cheek. Anna responded, stroking Maria's cheek and hand, and talking back as she always used to do. I just held Maria's other hand and watched with a sort of golden amazement.

As I wrote later, it had a 'sense of Lazarus emerging from his tomb' and it seemed to be a sort of ave atque vale, a 'hail and farewell'. But it was a hail and farewell imbued with triumph, as if saying: 'Thank you. All shall be well. We shall meet again.' It was so eloquent, and so remarkably out of keeping with Maria's present condition and situation that it was like sunshine suddenly bursting through a dark cloud. It was extraordinary, and extraordinarily moving and uplifting. Unforgettable and unforgotten.[28]

Emotional consequences of periods of awareness

As part of a discussion of awareness itself, we also need to consider the matter of its emotional consequences. There are bound to be emotional ramifications of both continuous and episodic awareness in the person with dementia, and for those around the individual who suspect it is present or actually witness its expression.

While recognizing that in considering this subject we are again forced to speculate, we should ask ourselves what might be the emotional impact of an episode of awareness for the person with dementia. Let us think of a someone who is normally not, or at least does not appear to be, aware of their condition. For whatever reasons this individual experiences a period of awareness. How might it feel? To 'come to' and find oneself in a situation, perhaps one that is not recognizable at all, and being treated by others in the way people with dementia often are? The person may realize that for most of the time, they are not in control of their daily life and decision-making, and that they have undergone a series of radical losses. Perhaps they are aware that the current period of lucidity is likely to give way at any time, returning them to a state (at least in the eyes of others) of partial or non-existent personhood.

This awareness and its accompanying feelings may or may not be expressed to others. If they are, and the significance of what is happening is recognized, the response may be supportive and comforting. This could help the person to cope with what is happening. However, given that many people spend long periods unattended, it is more likely that they will not be in a position to communicate their state of awareness to another. Even if an attempt is made, it may not be recognized as such, and therefore accompanying emotions stand little chance of being acknowledged.

Different people may respond emotionally in different ways to episodes of heightened awareness. Perhaps personality characteristics are a crucial factor. Some people may regard lucid moments as gifts. Others may see them as cruel reminders of how things used to be. It probably depends upon how adjusted the individual is to their present state, and to the quality of support available.

Emotional consequences for those around the person

It is also important to ask what happens to us, as people without dementia, when an individual unexpectedly expresses an awareness of their situation? What do we experience when the person seems to return from a state of deterioration and resumes their old self, even momentarily? It may be like having a sense of connecting properly with the other again, with all the resonances of the previous relationship. This could give rise to a wide range of different emotions for both parties.[29]

The person who was present at the moment of clarity may assume that it was something they did which triggered the response. They may examine their own behaviour and the situation in minute detail in an attempt to understand what happened. If they were the only one to witness the event they may question the accuracy of their perceptions, especially if others express scepticism about its veracity or significance. Such doubts may generalize to other aspects of how the condition is observed or understood.

Subsequent contact may be scrutinized more closely in an attempt to discern evidence of the lucid episode. If it is seen as a positive event, the situation and what led up to it may be reproduced in the hope that the occasion will be repeated. If there are no repetitions, or if the person demonstrates none of the characteristics of the previous episode and shows no awareness of it in subsequent hours and days, a deep sense of disappointment and renewed loss could follow. Feelings of helplessness and bewilderment may prevail, and also (whether or not this is felt to be rational) anger towards the person with dementia when it seems that they are making no effort to connect with others. Interaction with the affected person could feel more difficult than ever.

Alternatively, episodes such as these may act to renew a sense of commitment to help the person to get the most out of their remaining abilities and to enhance their capacity for enjoyment and intimacy. Faith that the essential person is 'still there' may be strengthened, and those around the individual could be motivated to try harder to find ways to be close to and supportive of them. These efforts may be rewarded with more satisfying contact, and a positive cycle would then be established.

Awareness and the self

Earlier in this chapter, in the excerpt from the writings of Carl Rogers, we touched on the relationship of the existence and experience of awareness to the self. It seems undeniable that at least some degree of consciousness (however that is defined or quantified) is basic to the idea of personhood, but what about awareness? It is certainly true that as part of our hypercognitive culture we tend towards the assumption that awareness, understanding and the ability to give a coherent account of oneself and one's actions are part of what a real person must be able to do. As with so many other things about being human, the existence and reality of dementia, and the way that it affects per-

sons, invite us to revisit and stretch conventional ways of seeing and understanding.

The following excerpt comes from Oliver Sacks' book about his experience
working as a neurologist with those who survived the great 'sleeping sickness'
epidemic of the 1920s.[30] Since their acute illness these people had existed in a
kind of limbo state in which, except for brief and infrequent intervals, they
appeared frozen – motionless, speechless and apparently unaware, but not in
a classic coma. The drug L-Dopa was been found to be effective for some, reviv-
ing them and bringing about a resumption of normal consciousness, events he
has called 'awakenings'. Reflecting on the nature of the transformation, Sacks
writes:

> The comparison of such awakenings to so-called *'lucid intervals'* will at
> once occur to many readers. At such times – despite the presence of mas-
> sive functional or structural disturbances to the brain – the patient is sud-
> denly and completely *restored to himself* . . . In patients with advanced
> senile dementias . . . where there is abundant evidence of all types regard-
> ing the massive loss of brain structure and function, one may also – very
> suddenly and movingly – see vivid, momentary recalls of the original, lost
> person.[31]

He goes on to describe similar phenomena in people with longstanding psychotic illness, and continues thus:

> But one need not look for such far-out examples. All of us have experi-
> enced sudden composures, at times of profound distraction and disor-
> ganisation: sudden sobriety, when intoxicated; and – especially as we
> grow older – sudden total recalls of our past or our childhood, recalls so
> complete as to be a re-being. All of these indicate that one's self, one's
> *style*, one's *persona* exists as such, in its infinitely complex and particular
> being, that it is not a question of this system or that, but of a total organis-
> ation which must be described as a self. Style, in short, is the deepest thing
> in one's being.

Expression of awareness before death

We finish this chapter with consideration of yet another facet of this subject:
the extent to which people with dementia show an awareness that they are
approaching the end of their lives. John's experience in talking to people has
been that the subject of death frequently arises, and may be referred to directly
or indirectly. One woman said:

> *All I'm interested in is my life's going!*

Another voiced a positive approach:

> *I've made a resolution to live till I die. You mustn't waste a moment. You
> mustn't let up.*

Some do not talk directly about the prospect of dying, but their awareness is implied by broaching the subject of things that need to be done before death. There may be a sense of unfinished business from much earlier in life which needs to be addressed. Alice, who features in Chapter 1, identified the death of her father, which occurred when she was a child, as falling into this category:

> *Nearly seventy years since that day and I got over the first shock, then on with my life. Now I feel the need to become reconciled with my father's death in some way. Afterwards my mother asked my sister 'Do you remember him?' To which she replied 'No, was he the poorly man in the bed?' But I think I have not done with grieving. I must see about it straightaway. I shall go to the place and buy a posy of flowers to place on his grave. Can you understand how I cannot rest until I have made this peace?'*

There are also those who seem to have completed some kind of life-review, and are able to look back at the past with a sense of fulfilment, and to face the future with calmness:

> *No bitterness or anguish, all loving-kindness. Now the evening is coming to its close for me. You can't barge it or dish it – all of it was everwell.*

Sometimes the person seems to be expressing an actual intimation of what is to come for them. Anthea McKinlay reports this conversation with her mother, Catherine, less than a month before her death. Anthea speaks first:

We're hoping you're coming home very soon to live near us.
Am I? We'll see.
Don't you believe it?
No, no. You see I have to go to a meeting upstairs to find out which way I'm going.
How do you mean?
You just go away and think about it.[32]

As well as evidence of awareness of approaching death, there are some remarkable reports of pre-death lucidity in people with the condition – extended periods of awareness and heightened functioning. We have no explanation of these to offer. They may be isolated examples, although it is possible that such phenomena are under-reported. But they are sometimes of such intensity and duration that they must be taken into account in considering the subject of awareness, and the nature of dementia itself.

The manager of a mental health unit in a nursing home supplied us with the following account:

> *'I used to be happy, I used to be sad,*
> *I used to be single before I was wed*
> *I used to have money – pounds, shillings and pence,*
> *I used to have claes,* and I used to have sense . . .'*

---

*'claes' is a Scottish dialect word for clothes.

Bill Morris would sing this song for anyone who stopped to speak to him – it was how he communicated. For the most part he was humorous and cheerful, even when he was in pain. I think he covered up his real feelings and his memory loss by this show of enthusiasm. Only when we tried to get him to do things to help us and to help himself would he sometimes get irritable.

Then one day about a fortnight ago he stopped eating. I tried to persuade him. I said 'Do you know what will happen if you don't eat?' 'I expect I'll not be here long' he answered. I was struck by his seriousness, as if he wanted his words to be noted. And also by his calm. His wife was amazed that he seemed so sure of what he wanted, that he was so quietly assertive.

Then he asked for his son to be brought over from America. This took a few days but eventually he arrived. During this time he ceased singing, except once, when he was shown a photograph of his son the night before he came.

Bill had no pain, and two days after his son's appearance he died peacefully with his family around him. The most extraordinary thing was that from the day of his announcing his decision not to eat, a resolve out of which he could not be shaken, he was consistently lucid in a way he had not been in the months preceding.

Implications for care

If we accept the possibility that many people with dementia are more aware of their situation than might be assumed, and that there is a need to express this awareness to others and have them appreciate its implications, then this means we have to think carefully about our responses.

If it is true the ability to express awareness fluctuates, then it is obviously important that we look out for times when the person may be more able to communicate their thoughts and feelings, whether this is done verbally or nonverbally. It means being alert to the subtlest of signs, and giving the fullest of attention to the person when something significant does seem to be happening.

As we have discussed previously, the act of talking aloud about experiences or reflections seems to be associated with the development of heightened awareness. Generaly this suggests that providing opportunities for people to talk, or otherwise express themselves, is extremely important. Being with someone who is trying to express their understanding of the deepest and more personal aspects of their condition is demanding, however. This is a subject we consider at greater length in Chapter 15 on ethical implications.

Another practical aspect of dealing with the subject of awareness is the availability of information about the condition for the person with dementia. Practice regarding sharing of information at the time of diagnosis is still very patchy, and there has been almost no work done looking at people's information needs subsequent to this phase. This is an area which requires much more work.

Ethical implications

If we are right in thinking that many people, at least some of the time, have much greater awareness of their situation than has been hitherto believed, then this has major implications for the way we understand the condition and think about the people who are affected by it. Would we talk to people differently? Would we treat them in a different way? Would we expect different things from them? A whole swathe of moral issues would demand consideration, in-depth treatment of which is beyond the scope of this book. For the present we can give thought only to those issues which we are faced with in the context of our current state of knowledge.

Awareness and hypercognitive values

It could be argued that by looking for evidence of awareness in dementia we are reinforcing the tendency to value people primarily for their intellect. This is not our intention. We agree with Stephen Post when he suggests that encountering people with dementia is an opportunity for society to challenge its hypercognitive values, and to find ways to nurture and celebrate alternative ways of being human.[33] But we should recognize the danger that, given the depth of our attachment to this way of thinking, we might be tempted to accord higher status to those people with dementia in our care who do demonstrate evidence of awareness than those who do not.

Encouraging the growth of awareness

We have presented the argument that, in common with everyone else, people with dementia need to feel that they understand what is happening to them, and to have a sense of meaning in their lives. We have also suggested that the development and expression of awareness may be encouraged or facilitated by certain styles of interpersonal behaviour – that the things we do or refrain from doing in this respect can make a difference. Are we then saying that it is desirable to set out to attempt to increase people's awareness of their situation? This is certainly a moral question.

   One aspect of this issue concerns the person's emotional reaction to experiences of heightened awareness. Some may say that people with dementia are in greatest distress when they demonstrate awareness of their condition. A corollary to this is that if the person can exist in a state of ignorance of the chasm between their former and present selves, then this is a mercy akin to being free from physical pain in the context of terminal physical illness. This assumes, however, that the distress occasioned by the experience of awareness is an inevitable and core part of the condition, and cannot be alleviated by others and their actions. Perhaps people with dementia, when they are so distressed, are not only expressing a pain which is inherent in their condition (surely this is so?) but also are giving voice to anguish at the behaviour and response of others to their predicament?

Further, if it is true that experiencing awareness in the context of dementia brings with it emotional, even existential, distress then what might be the compensating factors which lie on the other side of the balance? This question brings us back to the fundamental need for sense-making in our lives. Perhaps, despite pain stimulated by the realization of one's diminished capacities and situation, there is a deeply prized sense of mastery occasioned by episodes of awareness. If we accept this, then surely it must be our moral duty to do as much as we can to promote and sustain the experience of awareness in dementia.

The other important facet of this argument is the fact that the person's awareness and understanding of their situation has direct links with the ways they find to cope with it. We therefore need to tread carefully since there is potential for harm if these issues are approached in a careless manner. For example, if someone in the dementia unit of a nursing home expresses her view that she is there because she has trouble walking, is it right to intervene in such a way that she is confronted with the reality of her dementia and its consequences? Would the answer be different if it was clear to staff that at times she experiences real distress and confusion on account of her dementia-related difficulties? What about someone who states the view that his current situation is a punishment for past sins? We might feel it to be kinder to try to persuade him that his having dementia has nothing to do with previous behaviour (assuming that this is what we believe). It may seem the best thing to do, but the reality is that specific beliefs of this nature are only expressions of one part of a much larger system of beliefs.

As we discussed at length in Chapter 6 on interpretation, and again in this chapter, our efforts at sense-making do not occur in a vacuum. We seek meaning according to a unique and complex set of needs, desires and other biases which have evolved over a lifetime. The way that any one person interprets a situation will differ from that of the next person, as will the depth and quality of meaning sought. These individual differences must be borne in mind whenever we take action which could alter the way the person understands their particular circumstances.

Conflict with others' needs

Earlier in this chapter we raised the issue of our own investment in certain ways of thinking about awareness. The development of dementia in a loved one can be an excruciatingly painful experience for those around them, and the perception that they have no awareness of what is happening to them may offer some comfort. The idea, then, that the situation is so simple, that the person may in fact be much more aware, would be highly threatening to their ways of coping. And of course these ways of coping are much needed.

This is one example of how the promotion of a person-centred approach to care will inevitably disrupt previously stable balances of power, advantage and disadvantage between individuals with dementia and those connected with them. If we are to take seriously the possibility of awareness then this will have painful ramifications for the coping style and behaviour of others. But we would hope that the admission of the possibility of greater levels of awareness than was hitherto assumed could be part of a much more extensive and constructive reappraisal of what this condition is and how it affects persons. Then there could be great benefits for those around the individual as well as uncomfortable challenges. Surely if we are committed to the attempt to understand dementia we have to be prepared for what we find to change us as deeply (and positively) as we would wish for those directly involved?

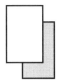 **Part 4:** Implications

14 **Implications for care:**
'I need help, yes.
But it's the way
that it's done'

We have already offered some ideas for more specific aspects of care practice within individual chapters, but in what follows we focus on some more general issues. We shall not go into any great depth with these, but they certainly form part of the bigger picture of improving practice as regards communication and deserve mention.

The need for a sense of meaning

Again, as already stated, if we are to make care which recognizes and supports the personhood of people with dementia a reality, then this must mean fully honouring the personhood of staff as well. The two cannot be separated. Poor systems of care pose a threat to their well-being, alongside those who are the recipients of that care. How, then, is this to be achieved? One major element in upholding the personhood of staff must be recognizing their need for a strong and positive sense of meaning, which embraces an appreciation of the deep importance and complexity of what they do. As we saw in Chapter 6 on interpretation this is of more than abstract significance, since the sense we make of our experiences has a direct relationship with how we feel about ourselves, other people and the world, and what we do. The Swedish researchers Britt Akerlund and Astrid Norberg highlight the issues of the mutuality of our need for meaning in the following:

> Just as the patient is dependent on the caregiver to survive, the caregiver is dependent on the patient to experience meaning in care-work and meaning with the patient's life. This could be regarded as an expression of their interdependence.[1]

The specific ways in which those who work with people with dementia make sense of their role depend on a number of factors. Some relate to influences beyond the individual, such as the way health and illness are constructed at a cultural level, how care is organized, and the attitudes of others. It is also affected by a range of personal factors. Let us consider those external to the person first.

At the most general level, our cultural inheritance in terms of thinking about issues of health and illness is that illness is something which is alien to the norm and should be eradicated. In line with this way of thinking, those whose conditions are not curable are stigmatized and excluded. We fear them and avoid them as examplars of what we most dread in our own lives and futures.

As a consequence of this, traditionally work with older people generally has been regarded as low in status, unskilled and inherently depressing. Involvement with older people with dementia is seen as an even more desperate domain. This view is part of the wider culture of ageism and finds expression in various ways including low rates of pay, poor conditions of employment, lack of training opportunities and almost nonexistent career structures.

There are also the reactions of others to learning that one is involved in such work: expressions of bewilderment ('Why would anyone want to do that?'), horror ('It must be dreadful!') or undue sympathy ('You poor thing!'). Being part of a culture which routinely enacts lack of respect for the status of the work must affect individual workers' understanding and experience of their jobs, and their day to day approach and behaviour.

Alongside external influences on an individual worker's sense of meaning in what they do there are internal factors which include:

- personality – general disposition, style and habits
- one's outlook at any one time, encompassing mood, self-esteem and confidence
- one's health – both mental and physical
- one's circumstances, including external demands on time and energy.

All of these factors will interact to influence the particular quality of the felt experience of a practitioner, and the way they make sense of it. For example, when we are feeling stressed by events in our lives outside of the sphere of work this may well have an impact on the way we feel about life in the workplace. However the precise form this takes will depend on the nature of the stressor, and also how we ourselves view it. If, say, the extra demands from one's personal life arise from the illness of an elderly relative then this is quite likely to have an effect on how time at work is experienced. If situations at work keep reminding one painfully of the personal scenario then the overall influence is likely to be negative. If, on the other hand, opportunities to make a positive contribution to the lives of people at work give one a sense of hope for the loved person then the effect will be different.

This is just one example of how personal factors influence one's sense of meaning at work. Like so many other things in this sphere, the situation is highly complex. In addition to more longstanding influences, one's personal sense of meaning is subject to much more short-term variations, depending on factors such as how a particular interaction went or how close one is to the end of an exhausting day!

The final set of influences on a sense of meaning that we discuss here relate to the response of others to one's efforts, and this includes responses both from people with dementia and those from peers and seniors. We all need to feel that our efforts are generally appreciated, and benefit from specific feedback about aspects of our performance. When forced to proceed without such affirmation, our sense of meaning is bound to dwindle and atrophy. On the other hand, a remark or gesture which demonstrates that the person with dementia welcomes and enjoys your attention, or praise from a colleague, can transform our feelings about what we are doing.

Clearly, then, many things need to be in place, or in place to a reasonable degree for enough of the time, for a positive sense of meaning to exist and play a full part in the work. But another point which needs to be emphasized here, though we hope it emerges from every page of this book, is that the quality of communication is a vital factor in creating and sustaining this much needed sense of meaning. The following comment by a staff carer, who took part in a Swedish research study,[2] provides a powerful description of what happens when it is lacking:

> When you cannot get into contact with the patient you feel insufficient, without hope, dissatisfied or burnt out. Care seems meaningless. You lose your commitment.[3]

An approach to care which is explicitly arranged around communication, with all its challenges and delights, will go a long way to helping staff members to establish and develop such a sense of meaning, but it needs to be supported and enhanced by the culture of the organization, and the attitudes, values and actions of senior staff.

Communication: taskless work

When the emotional and psychological lives of people with dementia went completely unrecognized, effort which was devoted to communication was clearly not seen as having a place in care. Thankfully we have now reached a point where the personhood of those with dementia is more widely acknowledged, and there is a recognition that communication plays a central part in nurturing well-being. But for some reason there is still a problem in seeing effort devoted to sustaining and enhancing communication as being legitimate work. This means that in circumstances where time and resources are limited (and that includes every care service there is), even staff, particularly direct care staff who are aware of the psychological and emotional needs of their users find themselves tending strongly in the direction of carrying out more conventional 'tasks', rather than devoting their energy to trying to communicate with people. In order to appreciate why this is so, we have to take a step back and think about the whole concept of work.

Again at a cultural level, our notions about the nature of work are still heavily influenced by the model of traditional manufacturing where a series of discrete tasks, that can be described in specific terms, are carried out and which result in a tangible outcome or product. This model conceptualizes the worker as a kind of unit in the process, depersonalized and entirely replaceable. Of course, this image, which derives from the days of the Industrial Revolution, no longer remotely fits the diversity of forms that work generally now takes, and it certainly has little or no utility in understanding the nature of work with people generally, or care work specifically. Nevertheless, it is deeply woven into our ways of thinking about it. Where work with people is made to fit this kind of template, it is easy to see that the result means giving primacy to tasks relating to say physical care over that of devoting energy to meeting people's psychological or emotional needs. And it is important to acknowledge that we all labour with a powerful pull towards the satisfaction generated by the feeling of having completed a task which has a clear outcome or product.

Some organizations that provide ongoing care are so geared towards meeting only physical needs that there is no opportunity for a decision to invest effort in communication work to arise. However, even in circumstances where there is recognition of personhood and its implications the situation is still complex. Where there are conflicting demands on time (meaning all the time), individual staff members have to make decisions as to how to invest their energy. How might this be done? To explore this further, it might be helpful to introduce the idea of the cost-benefit analysis. Whenever we are faced with conflicting demands, we perform a kind of quick calculation of how our limited energies should best be spent. In work settings, the kinds of factors which come into play in the reckoning include the following:

- *perceived* amount of effort involved
- *perceived* difficulty of the task
- *perceived* likelihood of success
- *perceived* tangibility of results of the effort
- *perceived* durability of benefits
- *perceived* likelihood that the effort will result in being accorded credit or reward by others.

In relation to work with people with dementia in residential settings, when a period of time has been invested in physical care, resulting in a set of clean, dressed and well-fed people, although this will have been hard work, the outcome is clear. The amount of work to complete the task is (reasonably well) known and quantifiable, the outcome is predictable, obvious and can be enjoyed by both the recipient of care and the worker. The effects of the work will not last for ever, but this is understood and accepted. Also the results of the work are salient to others and there is therefore a reasonable chance of the worker receiving credit for their effort. When the effects have dissipated the cycle of work can start again.

Effort devoted to communication work is very different. The same factors come into play in making a decision about whether to invest energy, but in these circumstances, unless the relationship is very well established and predictable, many of the answers to the above questions will be more difficult to ascertain. On entering into an interaction you will not know how hard you will have to work in order to establish rapport, whether this is likely to elicit a positive response, and whether (except in a most general and abstract sense) the approach is going to contribute to the person's well-being. Even if your effort *is* appreciated by the person, there are further doubts over whether they will be able to give you any clear signals to this effect, and even more over whether any signals will be sufficiently tangible to convince anyone else that something worthwhile is happening.

In addition to these considerations, there is another set of questions relating to the durability of positive effects. Getting a response from the person, and feeling that this has enhanced their sense of well-being in that moment is one thing, but if you think that because of their difficulties with memory the person may very quickly forget that anything has happened at all, might this not lead you to question whether your time and effort is justified? When there are so many other demands on your time, all of these uncertainties will often be sufficient to push you in the direction of doing something more concrete.

There are no easy answers to these dilemmas, but in an organization which is aware of the tensions and committed to trying to place genuine communication at the centre of care, there needs to be an openness to discussing issues around what constitutes work, and readiness to support staff in departing from the conventional model.

Lack of time

This is always the first and main response from staff to exhortations for greater commitment to enhancing communication with people with dementia. It is therefore necessary first to acknowledge that lack of time (caused primarily by low staff to service user ratios) is a very real and problematic issue. It should be obvious to anyone who spends time in services that the staff have a great deal to do. Part of the answer to this problem, therefore, is for forceful arguments to be made at all levels for greater resources to be devoted to the support of people with dementia. These representations need to emphasize the skilled and demanding nature of the work, and the complexity of the needs that staff are encountering.

The other part of the response to the issue of time pressures is for a reconsideration of the way that the time which is available is used. As part of our central message about the importance of communication as a primary activity, we are also keen to encourage people to seek out the many opportunities for meaningful connection which arise in the course of day-to-day contact and other activities. It is necessary to approach each and every interaction with a fresh attitude and openness to the possibilities. What already occurs in the way of communication may be heightened in quality by greater attention to the responses of the individual, and more readiness to modify one's own actions and words to be in tune with their mood or disposition. This may mean inhibiting talk which has a 'filler' quality, and engaging more fully at a nonverbal level.

In the case of residential services it is often said that the need to maintain an acceptable level of provision of basic care excludes the possibility of devoting more time to engaging with individuals at an emotional, social or spiritual level. While again acknowledging the importance of meeting people's physical needs, we would suggest that one type of activity need not preclude the other. Perhaps different skills are needed, and perhaps the way that personal care is provided has to be modified, but there must be ways of combining emotional connections with intimate physical care work. Indeed in order for the experience of physical interventions not to undermine the individual's dignity and personal integrity, it is vital for their psychological self to be touched and refreshed also. This has a positive spin-off for staff as well. In settings where the provision of physical care is seen as the only possible response to those with dementia, there is a high risk of exhaustion, alienation and depersonalization for staff. Greater efforts at connecting psychologically with the person transforms the experience of providing 'basic' care. We are reminded here of the words of the respondent in the Swedish study earlier in this chapter.

The perception that large amounts of time are required in order to connect properly with people with dementia is commonplace. When acts of communication are of a sufficient quality and specifically tailored to meet the needs of an individual, however, it may be that only fairly brief periods of time are required. The frequency of contacts is another factor in this. Spending a minute or two with someone every couple of hours may be much more beneficial, for reasons of energy expenditure for both parties, than struggling to allocate half an hour at a time.

Another aspect of the lack of time argument is the possibility that when people with dementia are regularly in an environment and partake of relationships where communication work is given its proper status and share of resources, there could be an ongoing and cumulative effect on the way that individuals are able to function and use their remaining abilities. This touches on the concept, described by Tom Kitwood, of 'rementia', whereby persons with dementia, in the context of optimal care and support, actually relearn skills and function at an heightened level.[4] As yet we know little about this phenomenon – we are not good enough at providing people with the kind of help they need – but the possibility that an ideal quality of communication may help an individual to increase their cognitive and practical skills, along with emotional and spiritual well-being, remains to be explored.

Another issue regarding the use of time is rethinking the pace at which we do things. Tom Kitwood identified the practice of 'outpacing' – habitually presenting information or moving at a speed which exceeds the capacity of the person with dementia – as being a feature of malignant social psychology.[5] It is so easy, though, to fall into the practice of doing everything at maximum speed when time and resources are tight. This not only has an exhausting effect on staff, but also may create an impassable barrier to communication since staff members are effectively operating in a different 'zone' from that occupied by people with dementia. This may well have been what one woman was talking about when she said to John:

> *You can't see people, or it's 'so and so and so' and they don't care. Yes, I do think so, I think they don't care. Nice to see someone who's . . . like you are. Others are dashing and dashing and dashing. If you ask them they say 'You this and you this and you that', but it doesn't help.*

The process of learning new skills

Since what we are advocating is that staff embark on learning and developing a new set of skills in communication, we need to give some consideration to the psychological aspects of the learning process, and how these affect the outcome.

Any learning process comprises a series of identifiable stages.[6] Prior to the start of learning about anything new the situation seems relatively simple. We know that there are new things to be learned, and presumably are motivated to invest effort in the enterprise, but at this point there is insufficient knowledge on which to base judgements for any real appreciation of what is involved.

Once the process of learning has begun, however, there is a rapid increase in knowledge and the development of skills. The excitement and enjoyment of learning creates its own sense of mastery and satisfaction, and these are useful in maintaining motivation to continue the hard work of learning. Once the skills are established, but have yet to be tested out in a variety of situations, there is often still a pleasure in the sense of being able to do something useful, and the first period of routine practice is characterized by enthusiasm, confidence, perhaps even a degree of cockiness.

This period is over when the novelty and conscious sense of using distinctive skills has passed: they have become automatic. At this point the scene is set for another phase to begin. The transition of skills from conscious to more habitual status brings with it the tendency to devalue them – 'I'm not doing anything special'. Once they have become more automatic and demand less thinking energy, this frees up cognitive space and facilitates an awareness of much greater complexity in the challenges facing one than was first appreciated. This is likely to be accompanied by a developing sense of the relative crudeness of one's tools to deal with these challenges.

Awareness of one's own limitations, and the reality of making mistakes or failing to achieve the desired objectives, combined with the awareness of layers of complexity hitherto unappreciated, can make this phase a testing time. Instead of feeling confident and competent, there is a sense of uncertainty, inadequacy and even anxiety. Some new practitioners will conclude at this time that the field is not for them and give up.

In fact all of these experiences are part of a healthy learning process. The world *is* difficult and complicated, and if we are to become sensitive and reflective, we need to be constantly aware of this. Much more alarming is the individual who is so convinced of the rightness of their own approach that ambiguity and subtlety are denied. With the right kind of support and perseverance, the uncomfortable phase can give way to a more mature and balanced perspective, where an appreciation of complexity and one's limitations can coexist with a realistic valuing of skills and a fair estimation of the chances of making a positive difference. The feeling of needing to know everything and how to cope with every eventuality diminishes, taking a good deal of the anxiety away with it.

In the longer run the exact balance of these thoughts and feelings will be affected by personal factors and the details of one's work at any one time, but ideally that a general stability will be maintained, and in time foster the growth of special areas of interest, expertise and professional development.

Although the qualities and skills required to work successfully with people with dementia have until very recently been totally undervalued, we believe that these same stages apply as much to work in this field as other areas. Setting out on developing communication skills is very likely to take this form. Armed with an understanding of the phases involved in learning and appropriate support from peers and seniors will go a long way to helping people to stick with the effort.

Support

There is no doubt in our minds that if staff are to achieve and maintain the level of work that we are describing then specific arrangements for supported reflection on a regular basis is essential. Staff need time when they are not actually calling on personal qualities and using skills to reflect on the nature of their experiences generally, specific situations or incidents that have arisen, and the factors in their own lives which may be influencing their practice. Just as we have been advocating the value of actually talking with another person in the process of enhancing understanding and achieving a sense of meaning, it is essential, we believe, that this kind of reflection takes the form of discussion with another person. If this can be supplemented by private reflection and even writing, its value will be further enhanced, but the interpersonal element is fundamental.

Admittedly allocating time regularly to activity which is not given over to direct practice has cost implications for an organization, but so does the failure to do so. When staff are encouraged to explore and express their thoughts and feelings about their work, one of the effects seems to be an enlarged sense of meaning and satisfaction in what they do, which is in turn likely to be associated with better performance, fewer absences from work and in the longer run reduced staff turnover of the kind which is so prevalent and costly in direct care work.

But this is merely the economic argument. The human aspects must point directly to finding ways of increasing practitioners' self-esteem and pride in the work they do. This subject is discussed at greater length in Chapter 15 on ethical implications.

Specific arrangements for support could take a variety of forms. Some regular one to one time with a manager or supervisor is necessary, but there are also great possibilities in bringing together small groups of peers, and encouraging them to share their experiences and reflect on their role. Ways to facilitate discussions could include having staff talk about an experience which had particular meaning for them, shared reflection on the possible significance of the words or actions of a person with dementia, looking at clips from films or TV programmes. Having some sessions include people from other similar organizations (with appropriate arrangements for confidentiality) could be very beneficial, enhancing sharing and learning.

Whatever specific form the arrangements take, it is very necessary, of course, for them to be continued and developed in a consistent way. Trust and confidence take time to develop. So often in the busy and complex world of services with all the complexities of shift systems, large numbers of staff, part-time working, staff illness and other absence, and the unpredictability of the health and well-being of service users, arrangements for supervision and support fall through at the last minute. We really do appreciate how much of a challenge it is to set up and maintain these sorts of arrangements, but if this is not successful then it is not realistic to expect staff to be doing new and difficult things by themselves. When staff feel overstretched, undervalued and are struggling to maintain a sense of meaning in what they are doing, the factors which gave rise to the problems maintaining arrangements will surely worsen.

Specialist nurses Tracy Packer and Jan Dewing are currently exploring the nature of support work in dementia care, and how it can be made more effective.[7] They stress the importance of finding a balance between offering support to staff and challenging them regarding their attitudes and practices. If there is too much support at the expense of challenge, then there is no impetus for development. If there is too much challenge relative to support, then staff will feel demoralized and under attack. It is only by achieving the right mix that staff will feel affirmed, be able to expand their understanding and acquire new skills, and find personal satisfaction in their work. They also emphasize that workers must be prepared to take an active role in clarifying and meeting their own needs in this respect.

Organizational factors

In what we have written so far we have tried to bear in mind the fact that the term 'services' covers an ever-widening range of different types of intervention and support, and similarly that the term 'staff' refers to a highly diverse set of people. Some reworking and adjustment on the part of the reader to the details of practical material will no doubt have been necessary, particularly in relation to the institutional bias which derives from the fact that John's experience has been predominantly in nursing homes.

But here we consider the effects of how we organize services in relation to their outcomes on communication practice.

Keyworker systems

We have talked previously about how it is impossible for any one member of staff to be able to develop rapport and deep communication with everyone they come into contact with. This is due in part to variations in personal style between individuals. Given that many services now operate keyworker systems in order that users relate particularly to one or two members of staff, we need to give more consideration to how we can make the most of its potential. For example, how are new people allocated? Is enough consideration given to the compatibility of the two individuals in terms of personality, outlook and communication style? There are obviously practical issues bearing on this, but if we are to uphold the importance of communication and relationships generally, then this is an area which needs to be looked at.

Shift working

The way that work is organized again clearly depends on many factors, but there is a need to recognize that sometimes systems act to undermine the chances of staff being able to build up regular supportive routines which nurture good communication. An example of this would be the rolling shift system, which means that a member of staff is able to bath a particular resident only once every six or eight weeks (if the resident always has a bath at the same time of day). Such a way of working clearly has negative impact on the chances of developing a familiar pattern which could enhance communication. As well as undermining opportunities for the person with dementia, such ways of working also have an impact on staff, who are deprived of the chance to develop a consistent approach, and have constantly to relearn ways of doing things. Even more radical than the challenges posed by rolling shift systems are those in care settings where entire staff groups swap over, for example in two wings of a nursing home. We must ask ourselves what purposes this sort of practice serves, and what kinds of messages it gives to people with dementia.

Staff absence

A heightened awareness and valuing of the quality of relationships between individual members of staff and people with dementia raises a number of practical and ethical issues. The matter of staff absence is one of these. It is an accepted part of working arrangements that people will have periods of absence from work. These may be brief or extended, anticipated or unexpected. Given that this kind of thing happens, what should we be thinking about in relation to the needs and experience of people with dementia?

The first thing to recognize is that the absence of a familiar member of staff with whom the individual has a positive relationship will be experienced as a loss, however mundane the event seems to us. This points us on to thinking about how the person with dementia might understand their absence. We need to consider the possibility that they might worry about the welfare of the person who is missing. It is also not uncommon for people to interpret events in such a way as to lead to worry that something they themselves have done might account for the absence of the other person. Similarly we need to think about how things are handled when staff leave their jobs altogether. At present we do not give enough consideration to the feelings of loss the person with dementia might have at such a time.

Just in case in discussing these issues in the abstract we forget about the reality 'on the ground', we conclude this chapter with examination of the following quotation.

An experience of care

The full paragraph from which the title quote for this chapter is taken goes as follows:

> I have felt completely cut off from everybody. I feel dumped. I have on occasion called out things but I don't get a response. I don't have that much private conversation or it gets advertised all round the place. I can't cope with all this silly nonsense that goes on. I need help, yes. But it's the way that it's done.

The woman, Nancy Adams, who said this seems to have been talking directly about her experience of receiving care, specifically nursing home care, and she says several very telling things. To examine them more closely, the first sentence is a strong statement about social isolation. Nancy may have been referring to feeling 'cut off' from people outside of the setting, or feeling distanced from those with whom she shares a physical space, or both. The second sentence gives an indication of how she views her situation more generally, perhaps implying that she is there against her will. The idea of being 'dumped' certainly suggests that Nancy feels that she has been rendered passive, treated as an object rather than a person. Alongside the notion of abandonment, there is the suggestion that she may see herself as being no longer useful or able to contribute. Or perhaps she retains a feeling of having something to give – hence her need for proper communication – but sees others as having negative views. As a further point, it may be that her sense of having been dumped has an important bearing on the feeling that she has been cut off from others. Even if there is contact, the fact that she is now marooned in a context she has not chosen may make her feel that the relationships she now has are less meaningful, somehow restricted and made artificial.

What Nancy says about 'calling out things' appears to be a very direct simple statement about being ignored. Following on from the messages about isolation and abandonment, this description of her attempts to reach out and being overlooked is all the more powerful. She continues with the theme of communication in the next sentence, identifying the fact that for her speaking on a one-to-one basis is a rare experience, and when it does happen its value is undermined by the fact that her privacy is violated. It seems as if she feels that what is shared through individual conversation becomes public property – clearly not a situation which respects her personhood and encourages genuine communication. We begin to get a picture of extremes here – either Nancy is ignored, no one pays any attention when she does try to establish contact, or when there is some meaningful interaction this is betrayed by a lack of confidentiality.

Her next statement is more mysterious. She does not explain what she means by 'silly nonsense', but it is clear that she disapproves of it and wishes to distance herself from it. The final two sentences sum up her situation. She makes it clear that she knows she cannot manage by herself, she acknowledges her dependent position. However, by referring to 'the way that it's done', she is expressing the view that the manner in which the help she needs is provided is of great importance. She does not state explicitly what difference it makes, but it seems likely that she is referring to what we would call personhood, and whether it is undermined or enhanced. And what it hinges on is communication. If we still needed any convincing that this is what lies at the heart of care, then Nancy provides us with it.

15 Ethical implications: 'What I want to know is, what is this doing for you?'

We begin this chapter with the words of Tom Kitwood:

> Dementia will always have a deeply tragic aspect, both for those who are affected and for those who are close to them. There is, however, a vast difference between a tragedy, in which persons are actively involved and morally committed, and a blind and hopeless submission to fate.[1]

We hope that by now there can be no question about any of us adopting a 'blind and hopeless submission to fate', but what might Kitwood have meant about being 'morally committed'?

Throughout this book we have raised ethical issues in relation to specific aspects of our subject; here we address some of the more general ones. We hope that this material will present itself not merely as an anthology of doubts. The challenge for us as the authors of this book has been to find the right balance between engendering enthusiasm and trust in the person's reality and robustness on the one hand, and on the other encouraging respect for their mystery and fragility and privacy.

Why we prefer to avoid tackling ethical issues

We appreciate that thinking about ethical issues can be uncomfortable and off-putting. This is especially so when the subjects under discussion have a direct bearing on the things we ourselves do from day to day, and the values which underpin our actions. None of us likes to confront the possibility that what we think, believe and do falls short of being ethically sound, and it is always difficult to try to change attitudes and behaviour. Nevertheless, we have to marshal our courage and proceed with resolve because, as we have seen throughout the book, caring work, and practice regarding communication in particular, is replete with moral questions and dilemmas, and it is far more hazardous to ignore them than to confront them. But before we continue, the following thoughts are offered by way of reassurance.

There are very few absolute rules in this sphere. Most issues and values are relative and have to be considered in context on an individual basis.

Nobody is perfect. We can all think of instances involving people with dementia where remembering our behaviour or words makes us cringe. We may feel ashamed of the way we responded to someone or feel guilty because we ignored something which should have been picked up. As well as the specific examples of poor practice, we all have ongoing blindspots and biases, things that we find hard to acknowledge and confront. Although it can be painful to do so, it is by acknowledging our shortcomings and mistakes, and talking about them with trusted others, that we can free ourselves of the habits or dispositions which gave rise to them. We should remind ourselves that those people we admire the most in terms of their personal qualities – their knowledge and understanding, skills and intuitive capacities – have not acquired these without cost.

Our understanding of the nature of dementia and the kinds of difficulties faced by people with the condition has changed so rapidly within the last few years that it would be surprising if we were not to find ourselves in the position of questioning our own practices and even sometimes being aghast at what was seen as normal in the not too distant past. In re-evaluating past actions, however, it is easy to forget the context which has such a powerful effect on our behaviour, and see what now seems so clearly unacceptable in an unduly isolated way. This kind of thing happens a lot, which is unfortunate as it can make people feel ashamed and demoralized, and tends to inhibit the very kind of reflection we so much need. As we discussed in Chapter 6, we interpret situations within the filter of our systems of belief, and it is only as these change that we see other possibilities. Setting out to gain more knowledge and develop one's practice is such an opportunity, and it brings with it excitement, pleasure and discomfort.

A final point here is that whenever we enter into an area which is new and has not been properly 'charted', there are great challenges in ethical respects. It is like this with communication work with people with dementia. Although we believe that it is right that we should do as much as we can to improve practice in this area, it can seem that by trying to do the right thing, we are often in the position of wondering whether we might be doing the wrong thing. At times like this we ask ourselves whether it would not be easier to give up altogether, and so avoid being in this uncomfortable position. The answer to this, of course, is that it would be far more wrong to give up, and that in commItting ourselves to exploring the subject, we have to muster our courage and proceed.

Before moving on to another account from John's experience, we pause to consider some general points.

General issues

A very basic moral issue is that of how we should regard people with dementia at all, specifically in respect of questions about how similar to or different from ourselves they are. While acknowledging that each individual is unique, where people are concerned there are certain generalities. There are a set of assumptions that we make about everyone – for example, that they want and need to be recognized as unique and irreplaceable, that they seek the acceptance of others, that they value opportunities to express themselves and be understood by others. Should we assume that people with dementia are similar to anyone else or should we think in terms of there being a more basic quality of differentness?

Unless we have a specific reason to think otherwise, our natural disposition is to assume that another person is similar to ourselves – that they like and pursue similar things, that they have more or less the same fears and preoccupations. While the presence of dementia has historically certainly been seen as sufficient reason to regard someone as 'different', this is now thankfully beginning to shift. But some, even those committed to improving the welfare of those affected, may argue that dementia brings about changes which mean that the person's ways of thinking, feeling and behaving should be understood differently, and that we owe them this recognition. However, as we know only too well, the traditional perception of differentness has had hugely negative consequences for both them and us. Any tendency to see people as being different in ways which are constructive rather than destructive would have to be based on a much more precise understanding of the nature of the condition than we have at present.

The alternative, which is what we have embraced in this book, is to assume that people with dementia are similar to other people in all respects unless experience suggests otherwise, in which case we explore ways of modifying our behaviour and expectations accordingly while leaving everything else the same.

This next point follows on from the above, although rather than being about individual people, it relates to how we should try to understand dementia as a condition. There exists a tension which revolves around whether we are committed to trying to find out and see it as it actually is – which could be called a scientific approach – or whether we adopt a more pragmatic approach and base our actions on certain 'positive' or 'helpful' assumptions. For example, we have been talking a great deal about the need to assume that people's actions and words are meaningful. This is crucially important, and, we believe, the right approach to adopt. However, it may be that for some people, and at some times, or at certain points in the progression of the condition, behaviour on the part of a person with dementia truly has no meaning, that it is in fact a manifestation of brain damage, and cannot properly be considered an expression of the person's wishes, needs or inner reality. In accepting this, we are faced with the choice of whether we act on this belief, or decide that it is more helpful to continue to regard the person's behaviour as meaningful. Since our primary interest in the subject is how we can best care for those affected by the condition, our response is more likely to be pragmatic than scientific; however, there are ethical ramifications of both positions.

If we were to pursue a strict scientific approach confining our beliefs and actions to what seems supported by evidence gathered in a controlled way, we would be at risk of overlooking the person within the dementia and failing to respond to their needs. If, on the other hand, we were to decide that the most fruitful approach is simply to choose what it seems most helpful or practical to believe and act accordingly, then we would be at risk of failing in our duty to attempt to increase our understanding of the nature of the condition. It could then become something we have created ourselves. This certainly would not be respectful of the person with dementia or their experience. This point leads on to the final of these general points.

Since dementia is such a common condition, and we all stand a significant risk either of developing it ourselves or being witness to its development in someone we love, we simply cannot be dispassionate about it. We all have a powerful personal motivation to understand it in certain ways while rejecting other less palatable points of view. While recognizing the tragedy, there is a great need to see dementia as being survivable, as having no real power to destroy that which we consider essential in a person. So much of what we believe about the nature of humankind rests on this foundation. We have been very conscious of this bias when writing this book, aware of all the objections that a 'hard-nosed' reader could raise in response to the points we make – the accusations of being whistlers in the dark. We hope that it is by now obvious that we are entirely sincere in our arguments, and are confident that the right kind of scientific inquiry will increasingly bear out our beliefs. But the disposition to see things in certain ways is one we must all be aware of in our encounters with people and our efforts to understand their experience.

John's experience: five years on

Throughout this book we have advocated that developing communication practice has great potential for good. But like anything else which has powerful positive effects, we must accept that there is another side to things. It is not simply a benign intervention which can be used freely without caution. What then might be the dangers inherent in the work? In order to begin to address this question we present an account from John which is in many ways a follow-up to that which appeared in Chapter 2:

> Over a period of five years I went on to work with hundreds of people with dementia. For some of this work there is an outcome in terms of a text, for the majority no such record exists. In fact I was involved in more than 1000 interactions over this time. I should add that I had no formal supervision or support to enable me to understand or cope with what I was experiencing.
>
> I have since spoken of the work involving 'communicating as if your life depended upon it'.[2] It can readily be imagined that such effort, and the accompanying setbacks and rebuffs, as well as attempting to come to terms with the pain I so frequently encountered in the people with dementia, must take its toll. Right from the first I approached this work with a degree of innocence which probably enabled me to find my way. It was the same innocence that concealed from me my growing distress. I eventually became aware of a weariness, and a tendency to feel strong emotions in a variety of situations where I would not have before. The former I dismissed as lack of staying power; the latter I welcomed as a deepening of my responses.
>
> At the end of this five year period I realized I had reached the point where I could not go on without help. I approached a counsellor who expressed her view that in doing this kind of work with people with dementia I had undertaken 'a crash course in spiritual development'. On being confronted with such a description, I began to cry, and found that this was a process which once begun was difficult to stop. I did more crying in the first week of that counselling relationship than I had done in the previous five years.
>
> I came across a poem by C.K. Williams which contains the following lines and seemed to sum up what I felt:
>
>> what pathways through pain, what junctures of vulnerability,
>> what crossings and counterings? Too many lives in our lives already,
>> too many chances for sorrow, too many unaccounted-for pasts.'[3]

It is important to examine in some detail what happened to John. When he began the work he displayed both innocence and ignorance in large measure. He had the vague hope that the approaches he had used with other elderly people would transfer to those with dementia. In fact it became clear early on that some adjustments had to be made, but the approaches which are described in this book developed through instinct and trial and error. When things went well this was satisfying and exciting, when they did not there were difficult feelings to cope with. Either way, there were no emotional safe-guards built into his work, and in any case at the time he had no sense that such measures were necessary.

Looking back on the five years, it became clear to John that as he had been learning how to come close to people with dementia he had also been incurring a cost to himself. As well as sharing positive feelings, he had also unwittingly taken on the burdens and griefs of those he encountered. He did this for one individual, and moved straight on to the next. In course of time an enormous backlog of unaddressed emotions was built up. Some people's thoughts and feelings had been written down, but even here he still 'owned' them because the texts had been given to him and therefore become his responsibility. In many instances, however, people's feeling-states remained unformed in linguistic terms; instead it seemed that he had absorbed them by other means and they were added to his existing emotional baggage.

Although on reflection it was possible to see that these emotions actually belonged to others, the perception was that they had in some way become his own, and the load was further increased by his emotional reactions to the sense of burden which had developed. Eventually all this forced itself upon his attention, and it was necessary to take some time to deal specifically with it.

In attempting to make sense of these experiences, John read work by the psychiatrist Patrick Casement, who discusses the kind of process he had been through within the context of a formal therapeutic relationship.[4] Casement emphasizes the importance for the therapist engaged in deep psychological work with clients of establishing 'what belongs to whom' in emotional terms. Apart from the fact that John had had no training as a therapist, and had not consciously been acting in this role, there are some important parallels. For one thing, his approach resembled that of a therapist who has the potential to become the repository for the client's intimate thoughts and feelings. But in another sense his situation was very different. The therapist could in most cases proceed to a stage where the emotions, once expressed and clarified, could be 'handed back' to the client, in order that they take responsibility for them and how to integrate them in their lives.

This seemed a less feasible strategy in relation to these people with dementia. How was John to assist them to process the material they had vouchsafed to him? Some of it related to traumas from the distant past, some of it revolved around existential terror occasioned by ongoing challenges to what we now think of as their personhood. Whatever the specific nature of the distress, however, it seemed doubtful in most cases whether the individual had the resources, either within themselves or in terms of external support, to assimilate what could be reflected back to them. Sharing any texts which had arisen from an encounter was a possibility, and this usually took place. But in most instances in itself this act seemed insufficient to reflect the depth of the actual exchanges which had given rise to them. Another important consideration in the attempted parallel between his role and that of a therapist was that many of those who seek out a therapeutic relationship presumably have a reasonable hope of alleviating their distress. In contrast John was watching many of those he had come to know experiencing seemingly inevitable deterioration.

However, despite these challenges John was able successfully to undertake a process of sorting out some of the emotional backlog. This took time. It was to be six months before he returned to working with people with dementia, and even then it was on a much reduced scale and with time built in for reflection after each interaction. Although the acute nature of that time is now past, it is his belief that the work itself and the process of reflection it prompted, has had many lasting effects. The best way of describing these is the sense of having 'lost' a layer of skin so that many things in life seem now to have a greater and deeper impact than they did previously. Living in this more open way brings both new joys and new griefs.

We have devoted quite a lot of space to telling this story, and offering reflections upon it. Not only does it bring the narrative we began in Chapter 2 to some kind of a resolution, but also it illustrates that fully acknowledging and engaging with people with dementia has consequences for the personhood of others. John's may be an extreme case, but many staff suffer from 'burn-out' which probably results from similar processes.

In previous chapters we raised various fairly specific ethical issues. We now proceed to a more detailed discussion of what could be considered rather more general ones. Some of what follows arises directly from consideration of John's experiences.

The moral status of care work

Caring work is inherently moral in nature. The most basic moral questions in life revolve around how we should behave towards one another, and this kind of reflection has kept moral philosophers in work for many centuries. When the complexities engendered by a condition like dementia are added in the situation becomes even more convoluted. Given that we have only recently woken up to the reality of continued personhood, the history of this type of thinking is very short. When people with dementia were treated merely as physical beings with physical needs, the process of caring for them was relatively straightforward. Broadening our view of the individual to encompass all the many aspects of personhood, including emotional and spiritual dimensions, renders the caring task very much more complex and demanding. For those caring for people with dementia making the shift from thinking about people predominantly in terms of physical needs to that which Kitwood called 'person-centred' is a huge task, and then translating this into care practice of various sorts another enormous step. This should not be underestimated. After several years of embracing and laying claim to the concept of person-centred care we are now beginning to acknowledge and explore its real complexity, and we have yet to consider properly the way that staff experience and cope with the many demands which it presents.[5]

Before looking at the nature of some of the challenges which can arise, however, we should pause to think about the moral status of the idea of 'care' itself. The very word 'care' is suggestive of an activity which is benevolent and appeals to the highest of human motives. But as we have seen, the idea is open to a variety of interpretations. What it means to care for any other person is complex enough, even when both parties have roughly equal status as regards power and influence. But when one party is radically disempowered, this complicates the situation immensely. The fact that it is dementia which has brought about the loss of power only adds to this since it is a condition we do not yet properly understand, and affects different people in such different ways. How we understand the idea of caring, and how we act on it, is closely tied up with how we see and make sense of the situation the other person finds themselves in.

In practical terms, those who care for people with dementia are regularly faced with decisions which have a moral dimension, whether these relate to practical matters or pertain to the person's psychological, emotional or spiritual well-being. Let us think first about the matter of autonomy – having the opportunity to have some control over the details of one's day to day life. We tend to take our capacity for making mundane choices for granted, but, as we have seen, such opportunities play an important part in maintaining our sense of being fully a person. In the last few years we have become better at recognizing that people with dementia retain this need, and can, if given the right kind of support, often express their preferences. Within the busy world of services, however, it can often be difficult to uphold the person's opportunities in this way. The ways in which we organize and deliver services are not geared to maintaining the person's capacity for making choices, and the result is that it often falls on individual members of staff to act on behalf of the individual. The following comment from a member of staff in a Swedish hospital ward illustrates the situation:

> More and more it becomes a routine to decide (for patients). In the end you forget the patient – it is dangerous – sometimes I wonder what on earth I am doing.[6]

Another type of situation which puts the member of staff in a difficult position ethically is that where the person with dementia expresses a strong wish to do something which the member of staff feels will put him or her at risk in some way. Another is that when a person makes a choice which runs contrary to the staff member's values. The following excerpt from Linda Grant's book about her mother illustrates this:

> Michelle and I are too taken in by the advice we had received from the experts: respect the rights of the elderly; consult them; do not force them to do what they do not want. My mother's rights are allowing her to spend twenty three hours alone, overdosed or under-medicated, and crying. Her nightmare goes on and on.[7]

Yet another kind of situation which places staff in acute moral dilemmas is that where they have to do things for people (for example, carry out intimate care tasks) when they know that this is an unpleasant, even frightening situation for the individual. There may be very powerful expressions of resistance or distress from the person, which they are forced by the nature of their responsibilities, to override. An example of such a scenario comes from a paper by the Swedish researchers Goran Holst and colleagues.[8] This is a nurse's description:

The patient screams and behaves aggressively when we try to get her clothes off. She does not understand what we intend to do. I guess it's her way of defending herself. It's difficult to know if I am doing the right thing.

When we approach the bed her eyes shine with fear. She clings tightly on to the bed when we lean over her, and I wonder what she has been exposed to in the past. It is a burden when she is frightened.[9]

As regards the same woman, this nurse said that she:

felt scared when she met the patient's eyes: 'her glance seems cold as ice'.

Apart from the fact that such distress on the part of a person with dementia must command our deepest compassion and moral concern, we all need to recognize just how much we are asking of staff who face such agonizing situations, often on a routine basis.

Could engaging with such people at a deep level be hazardous for them?

One day when John had been spending some time in a particular home, a member of staff remarked with a degree of exasperation, and a sweeping gesture around the room:

Everybody was quite happy till you came along, and now look at them!

It was certainly true that John's visit had occasioned what could be called disturbance and even distress, in the sense that during some conversations people had cried and otherwise expressed strong feelings. The implication of her words was that John's intervention had caused problems which were not present before. Was she right to say this?

In Chapter 8 on developing the interaction, we discussed the fact that some people with dementia respond to opportunities for genuine communication by very quickly revealing a great deal about themselves and expressing strong emotion. Here we go further and raise questions about whether it is possible that for some people the kind of approach we have been describing could actually be hazardous by leading them into areas of their minds and memories with which they are no longer able to cope.

We have said that one of the characteristics of people with dementia is that they may be more in touch with the emotional dimension of life than the rest of us. This may be a good thing in many ways, but we should also recognize that it could mean that these emotionally-attuned people will experience a great deal of pain. This raises issues for us, one of which is whether and how much we should intervene in the extent to which people experience emotion. It is sometimes felt that an individual with dementia should be spared painful feelings, for example by withholding news about some sad event or minimizing their exposure to cultural observances such as Remembrance Day. There may be an implicit perception that one of the indicators of good care is a degree of emotional blandness, with extremes pointing to deficiencies. It is important that we take time to examine what are the underlying values and assumptions which dispose us to think in such a way. Using the downward arrow method described in Chapter 6 may be of assistance, as will the following questions like:

- Do we not have a duty to help people who are vulnerable to contain their emotions and not become overwhelmed?
- Who are we to judge what a person should and should not feel?
- When we do try to 'protect' people, on whose behalf are we really acting?
- To what extent are we withholding the opportunity for the person to take part in their own life when we reduce the potential for someone to feel strong emotion?
- What else in the domain of personhood might be put at risk when we try to protect someone from their own feelings?

Our values about the role of emotions in life generally are of major significance here. It seems that much of our behaviour in this regard is motivated by a basic fear of emotion. We tend to see strong feelings like rage, fear and grief as being cataclysmic forces which are prone to go out of control and destroy people and relationships. Since emotions have a way of jumping from one person to another, perhaps we see the potential for strong feelings in another as being a threat to our own internal equanimity.

These scenarios raise the deepest of questions about the role of emotion in human existence and in relationships. We should certainly not fool ourselves that actions in this sphere are of only practical significance.

Does engaging in in-depth communication work with people with dementia pose hazards to our own mental and physical health?

One of the main messages from John's account earlier is that undertaking in-depth work with people in a sustained way eventually took a toll on his emotional state and mental health. It is of course relevant that he was working in an exploratory way without support, and we are not suggesting that such consequences are inevitable, but it is important to recognize that the risks are real. Staff spend long periods of time in situations where their very personhood is continuously called upon, stretched and even threatened by the constancy of contact with people who are *in extremis*. As Professor Faith Gibson puts it, person-centred communication:

> requires us to get close to people who may be very troubled and very troubling. Person-centred communication is not costless in terms of physical and emotional wear and tear.[10]

In Chapter 14 we discussed the need for realistic arrangements for support and supervision of those who work in this way, and later in this one we discuss the important issue of the limits of what we should expect ourselves to give and the consequences of doing so.

But for now we would like to focus on the importance of the need to value oneself in minimizing potential for harm. This is crucial but often tends to get overlooked. But it is obvious that we cannot properly care for others if we are neglecting the very means of doing this – our own personhood. Part of this demands that we recognize and nurture those aspects of our own personhood which are both one of our greatest resources – our vulnerabilities – and also our Achilles' heel. Those who are good at being with people with dementia are people who recognize need in others and try to respond, but who perhaps often do so at the expense of their own needs. Perhaps we all have something of the martyr in us, but in order to curb this tendency it might be useful to imagine how fearful we would be if the tables were turned and suddenly we were in the shoes of the person with dementia, aware of their own dependency on someone who seems bent on sacrificing themselves to the caring role.

It is crucial fully to acknowledge the complex and demanding nature of the work – the spiritual impact of confronting another's pain, and its potential to touch on one's own griefs and fears. According proper recognition to the personal skills, qualities and knowledge which are necessary to succeed is another facet of the same thing. So often practitioners themselves are disposed to denigrate what they bring to the work, dismissing it as commonsense or otherwise merely ordinary. The fact that in the world at large the status of care work is so lowly compounds this tendency, but this is unlikely to change while staff themselves are contributing to this damaging perception. If blowing one's own trumpet seems too difficult, might we be emboldened by thinking of it as championing the rights of people with dementia to the skilled support they deserve?

To what extent can one person really help another? What are the limits of helping?

We have argued strongly for the potential of communication work to affirm and develop the personhood of both parties. But what about its limitations? What about the people it cannot help and the situations it cannot alleviate?

These questions are ones that we can ask of people in any situation in life. Are there aspects of human experience that simply remain out of reach, that we cannot enter into, even with the intention of helping or comforting? Do we have to be, in a deep sense, alone with some of our experiences? And if so, does a condition such as dementia intensify these realities? These questions lie in the domain of spirituality, and some would answer them in religious terms. Surely most of us would have to accept that we simply do not know the answers.

It is important to discuss these issues here, however, because sooner or later, frequently or infrequently, we will be forced to confront the limits of our capacity to help. The exact nature of the situation will vary. The woman whose words describing her feelings about what seem to be spots appearing before her eyes (on p. 175) is an example. She presented John with a request that he take the problem away, something he was not able to do. This inability seemed to preclude the possibility of him even acting to alleviate the distress she was experiencing. If she had asked him for comfort or distraction, however, this is something he would have been able to provide.

Sometimes the nature of a situation will be less straightforward to pinpoint, indeed the core of the problem may be the person's apparent inability to give any kind of shape to the difficulty, either through words or actions. In some situations, it may be that the person with dementia seems to feel that they *are* giving a clear description, and the problem lies in our inability to understand what they are telling us. Sometimes the difficulty will consist not in the manner and clarity of its communication, but simply in itself, such as when a person is overtaken by feelings of grief, or is dreadfully frightened of something, or is profoundly and apparently unreachably depressed.

Whatever the details of such a scenario it will give rise to a range of challenges for us. The first we discuss here is how we make sense of the situation, which (as we have seen) will have consequences for how we feel and what we do about it. This is another example of where we have to look into ourselves, and consider our buried assumptions, this time around the nature of helping. Do we, deep down, believe that we should be able to 'fix' everything? If so, does it follow from this that if we cannot, we are somehow inadequate? Where this is the case, the feelings arising from the kind of situation described above are likely to be very painful. Feelings of guilt and anger may arise. Anger is an especially complex emotion. It may be directed towards ourselves, or towards the person with dementia for making unreasonable demands, or with Fate or God for creating such a situation. If, on the other hand, one is open to the idea that part of being human is the experience, at times, of not understanding, not knowing what to do and not being able to sort things out, then one's reaction will be very different, and probably much less self-punishing.

The idea of humility comes to mind here. Surely, when we think properly about it, the idea that any of us could be in a position to address, even to touch, the deepest and most complex aspects of being human is rather arrogant. The quality of humility invites us to confront and accept our essential powerlessness, and, perhaps, through this come to a point where resolution can be achieved through alternative means. Some forms of spirituality would suggest that although many of us spend our lives struggling to meet and solve individual problems, this is actually to fail to perceive that the real challenge is how to achieve a state of serenity, or at least acceptance, within the apparent messiness of things.

This leads us to a consideration of the problem of pain. We can form questions such as: What is the function and meaning of pain? How should we respond to it? Should we always try to do away with it? We devote so much of our energy to avoiding and suppressing it in ourselves, and perhaps many of our efforts to help others are attempts to 'rescue' them from their pain. There are many ways of thinking about these things; again considerations of this nature are usually part of spiritual or religious systems of thought. Kahlil Gibran offers one perspective in his writings from *The Prophet*:

> Your pain is the breaking of the shell that encloses your understanding.
> Even as the stone of the fruit must break, that its heart may stand in the sun, so must you know pain.
> And could you keep your heart in wonder at the daily miracles of your life, your pain would not seem less wondrous than your joy;
> And you would accept the seasons of your heart, even as you have always accepted the seasons that pass over your fields.
> And you would watch with serenity through the winters of your grief.[11]

The other challenge which we have to confront when unable to help is that of how to face the person whose situation is giving rise to such complex and profound thoughts and feelings in us. One reaction would be to avoid them, both because we think that minimizing exposure might serve to dampen down our difficult feelings, and also because we might perceive that they would feel negatively towards us for not being able to help. While the tendency towards such a reaction is understandable, avoidance is not generally a helpful strategy where feelings of guilt and fear are concerned. It tends rather to make those feelings grow and even become attached to more and more situations. Also, it would be extremely unfortunate for the other person to feel that one was avoiding them because of their difficulties. That may very well be experienced as a punishment.

Further, our natural disposition when people talk to us about problems is to assume that they are asking us to come up with a solution. But we know that when we ourselves have difficulties, it is often most helpful simply to have another person be aware that we are struggling – 'answers' are not what is being sought. Surely it might not be so different for a person with dementia?

How far should we expect ourselves to go?

We already know how much need there is out there in the world, particularly in terms of the numbers of people affected by dementia. We hope that we have by now convinced the reader that there are important things we can do to help people with dementia to live with their condition. Does this mean then that we should, without further delay, mentally roll up our sleeves and get to work, do as much as we can, and as energetically as possible? There is a problem here. In recognizing the scale of the need, we are also reminded of the extent of our own limitations. Is there not a danger of being swallowed up?

Tom Kitwood writes here of the fears which may underpin such a concern:

> Professionals and informal carers are vulnerable people too, bearing their own anxiety and dread concerning frailty, dependence, madness, ageing, dying and death. A supposed objectivity in a context that is, in fact, interpersonal, is one way of maintaining psychological defences, and so making involvement with conditions such as dementia bearable.[12]

An alternative and optimistic view of this is presented by Marie de Hennezel, a psychologist who works with people who are dying:

> Accompanying someone involves engaging with that person; it is a matter of the heart. Above all, it is about one's common humanity. One cannot retreat behind one's white coat, whether one is a doctor, a nurse or a psychologist. This does not mean, however, that there are no limits. And that everyone must remain aware of his or hers. One actually is less exhausted by a total involvement of the self – provided one knows how to replenish one's reserves – than by the attempt to barricade oneself behind one's defences. I have often seen for myself how the medical personnel who protect themselves the most are also those who complain the most of being exhausted. Those who give themselves, however, also recharge themselves at the same time. There's a phrase of Lou Andreas Salome, one of the first women to follow in Freud's footsteps in the practice of psychoanalysis: 'It is in giving oneself that one possesses oneself completely.' In all her exchanges with the master of psychoanalysis, which are so subtle and full of intelligence, she never ceased to preach the lesson that love, far from being a reservoir that begins to drain with use, refills the more it overflows.[13]

The phrase 'provided one knows how to replenish one's reserves' seems to be the key to this. And then, of course, there is the word 'love' . . .

The place of love

Love is a word that we have rarely used in this book, but we hope that it has been implicit in much of what we have said. One reason we have not used it is that it covers such a wide range, and we would have had to qualify it by excluding whole swathes of its application, including its romantic and sexual dimensions. It is also not a word which sits comfortably with our understanding of the nature of work and the boundaries which seem to need to be maintained. Again we are faced with the question, how far should we expect ourselves to go?

However, the idea of giving love, or at least loving care, is undoubtedly applicable to aspects of the caring role generally, and certainly communication work. What specifically might this mean?

Love is closely allied to the concept of acceptance. The Quakers have a phrase about 'seeking that of God in every man', and without necessarily subscribing to a fully religious philosophy, we can surely assert that in our day-to-day contact with people with dementia we should be actively searching for qualities to value and celebrate. People with dementia, who so often labour with feelings of stigma and the reality of rejection by others, have desperate need of acceptance. In this they are not really any different from the rest of us. We all have deep fears about being found unacceptable and being excluded. At its best, then, the practice of loving acceptance can be fully mutual – in celebrating the other we can enlarge our appreciation of ourselves.

Part of being loving is accepting that we do not, and perhaps cannot, always fully know and understand that of which we are part. We have to learn to live with the mystery of the human. Coming into close contact with people who are living through such a profound and poorly understood condition as dementia certainly demands that we tolerate uncertainty, practise the qualities of hopefulness and faith, and be open to possibilities for which we cannot always plan or prepare ourselves.

Then again there is the concept of mutuality – that love has the power to awaken love in return. As we hope we have demonstrated in this book, increasing numbers of people are learning, through direct experience, that people with dementia have a very great deal to teach and to give us, that relationships need not be characterized only by dependency and self-sacrifice, that both parties can grow through the experience. Perhaps part of what Kitwood meant when he used the phrase 'morally committed' was the idea of finding and giving the best of ourselves to the work. This surely is love.

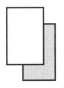 **Part 5:** Integration

16 Conversations with Jane: 'My mind, my whole sphere of life is full'

We began this book by introducing Alice as a person with dementia who was especially eloquent about her condition. We kept our commentary there to a minimum. We end by introducing Jane in her own words, and also provide a brief description of John's time with her the following day.

We believe this text to be very rich in terms of ideas, feelings and perspectives, and we offer it with only minimum pointers for your reflections. We suggest that you read the piece perhaps several times and observe and think about your reactions to it. We then provide some cues to assist in exploring the text further.

Jane Arnell

Jane was a quietly spoken woman who expressed herself slowly but intently. Sometimes she struggled to formulate what she wanted to say, and her words were accompanied by a real sense of strain and occasionally irritation with herself. She was quite tearful for much of the time:

I did notice you before. I've been here for quite a while. I have become very merciless or mercenary, I can never think of the word. Anyway, the person goes wandering off. I've become like that and it worries me [cries].

Walking is so difficult. I take about an hour to go down to the lav. I never thought that this would come to me. I'm becoming . . . I don't know what. That's your philharmonic isn't it? [indicating tape recorder] Or am I getting that way?

I'm forstering, I'm become more . . . well, put it this way, nothing would stop me talking if I could find something to talk about.

People haven't time to talk to me because it takes such a long time. I've never been an over-volulous person. I'm feeling I'm getting more silent. I feel that no one wants to bother with me any more [cries].

My mother is very old or more or less dying. I'm very fond of her and she of me. She was a very charming woman. I'd like to take after her. My life has been my mother's. When your home bolsters and unbolsters. I would do anything for her.

My mind, my whole sphere of life, is full. I was very fond of my life. It seems that I'm leaving it more and more. Oh dear, it isn't fair when your heart wants to remember! [cries]

I often wonder why people bother with people like us. I could have reeled it off for you what you are doing. It's a life story. It's the biography of the person you are writing about. It's me.

There's one thing about this world – they're very good to them, bringing them to the table. This is a mental home, you know. Most of the people living here need looking after. And if I were truthful I would say that includes me.

I really don't remember coming here. I never got a black book or anything like that. I don't care for black books anyway. I came here for the season and I'd only put my two feet on the flipping floor . . . it was a special sort of thing, and it was a nasty one. I said 'Coo, this would happen . . .' But she said 'It doesn't really matter.'

I've always had dogs. And puppies as well. They'll always tack into me. I prefer large dogs, but I don't mind what kind. I had up to two or three at a time. Spaniels I had for twenty years. I like every dog that will take to me. I have a photograph of Tess my Collie.

I was a keen gardener, but I didn't like getting my hands dirty. My brothers only minded it.

Tomorrow I'm nothing going to do. I'm doing things with my little . . . she'll be coming to greet me. She came yesterday, but she's studying quite a lot, and she's been off sick for quite a while. She doesn't run the home, it's she and I between us.

I'm tammering, stammering again. I've freed myself, but next week I'm having my conversation through breath.

He's a new gentleman. He's like a set of sentences: 'How do you settle? What do you do?'

Yesterday morning we thought she must have mistaken me for someone else. She goes around and around. I think she's a little confused. Everybody knows her. She's menace in a nice way.

I'm suffering from the same person. It is a sufferer. I don't like to hurt her. And I don't like to say anything. I haven't got the tongue for it.

I've known her since when. But even still I don't know her intimately. But she never insists on stressing me. It's very difficult to say no to people . . .

This lady who cries understands my voice. Some time during every conversation she goes into a grizzle.

When that chap leaps up I have to be careful.

That man, he's riding in a nice setting.

There are thirty people here, and they were settling in. . . .That was last week. Funny how people wanting to know you . . . and it's very difficult.

At the end of this interaction Jane expressed the wish to talk again the following day and invited John to look at her photographs with her in her room. However, when he arrived she was much more confused than on the previous occasion. Although he talked with her for over half-an-hour in the whole of that period she was unable to formulate a single sentence. She even had difficulty in finding the name of her daughter.

The variability between these two occasions illustrates the fluctuating process of the communication process in dementia. We do not know why Jane found it so difficult to express herself on the second day, but the contrast was so marked that had John encountered her then for the first time he would never have thought her capable of such profound and moving reflections.

Reflecting on Jane's words

The following are suggested starting points for interpreting the text:

- Language:
    creativity in expression
    difficulties with words
    comments on the process of speaking
    difficulties with formulating thoughts
- Memory:
    comments on the process of remembering
    feelings associated with it
    particular memories
    the meanings of particular memories to Jane
    gaps in memory
    objects which have memories attached to them
- Jane's life history:
    how she defines herself as a person
    things that were/are important to her
    interests and passions
    how she perceives herself and her life as a whole
- Emotion:
    the ways in which she expresses her feelings and her attitudes towards them

- Relationships:
    family relationships
    relationships with and perceptions of the other residents
- Jane's present situation:
    how she makes sense of it
    her understanding of her present circumstances
    her perceptions of care practice
- Awareness:
    of her current situation
    how it links with the past
- Communication:
    her attitude towards the place of communication generally
    concerns about the possibility of communication and its variability
    her awareness of problems with expressing herself
    her perceptions of others' attitudes towards those problems
- Ethics:
    her view of her worth as a person
    how people should treat one another
    to what extent we should intervene in her situation.

Postscript

At the start of working on this book we were not sure, other than in fairly general terms, what we were going to write. And now that we are in the position of needing to bring the book to a close, we find it hard to stop. We have begun to explore some ideas here, and are aware that they need further development. We also realize that there are important ideas we have hardly touched on, and no doubt many others not even yet thought of. In a sense this seems unsatisfactory, but then there is the feeling of a territory unfolding before us. This is exciting, so the ending of our task seems more like a beginning, just a stage on a journey.

It is now open to us all to carry on the exploration. We hope that ideas we have expressed will provoke fresh thoughts in you. In this way a dialogue is opened up. It is mirrored by the dialogues we are entering into with people with dementia. All communication is a partnership, and we would like to think of those with the condition as essential partners in this enterprise. That is why their words and actions have figured so prominently in these pages. Without their contributions and insights we could not proceed. There is a real mutuality here, and it must be cherished.

We leave you with the words of Oliver Sacks, which seem to capture the nature of the opportunity with which we are presented:

A Who has a What – Will the What overcome the Who? Will the Who emerge through the What? Or will the two combine in a way that embraces and transcends the Condition?[1]

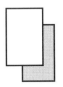

References and notes

Introduction

1 For further reading (and particularly the chapter by John) see S. Cox and John Keady (eds) (1999) *Younger People with Dementia: Planning, Practice and Development*. London: Jessica Kingsley.

2 Personhood

1 Alzheimer's Disease Society (ADS) (1996) *Opening the Mind*. London: ADS, p. 1.
2 See B. Bytheway (1995) *Ageism*. Buckingham: Open University Press.
3 J. Miller (1990) Goodbye to all this, *Independent on Sunday* (Sunday Review section), 15 April: 3–5.
4 For example, B. Reisberg, S.M. Ferris, M. deLeon and T. Crook (1982) The Global Deterioration Scale for assessment of primary degenerative dementia, *American Journal of Psychiatry*, 139: 1136–9.
5 T. Kitwood (1997) *Dementia Reconsidered*. Buckingham: Open University Press, pp. 46–7.
6 For example, D.C. Dennett (1976) Conditions of personhood. In A. Rorty (ed.) *The Identities of Persons*. Berkeley, CA: University of California Press.
7 Kitwood op. cit., p. 8.
8 For a review of research on the concept of personhood in dementia see M. Downs (1997) The emergence of the person in dementia research, *Ageing and Society*, 17: 597–607.

9 S. Post (1995) *The Moral Challenge of Alzheimer's Disease.* Baltimore, MD: Johns Hopkins University Press, p. 3.

10 Kitwood op. cit., p. 7.

11 For a discussion of these ideas see N. Harding and C. Palfrey (1997) *The Social Construction of Dementia: Confused Professionals?* London: Jessica Kingsley.

12 For a fuller exploration of the psychosocial model of dementia care see R. Cheston and M. Bender (1999) *Understanding Dementia: The Man with the Worried Eyes.* London: Jessica Kingsley.

13 T. Kitwood (1997) The uniqueness of persons in dementia. In M. Marshall (ed.) *State of the Art in Dementia Care.* London: Centre for Policy on Ageing, p. 39.

14 T. Packer (2000) Does person-centred care exist? *Journal of Dementia Care*, 8(3): 19–21.

15 I. Morton (1999) *Person-centred Approaches to Dementia Care.* Bicester: Winslow Press.

16 See C.R. Rogers (1951) *Client-Centered Therapy.* London: Constable.

17 N. Feil (1982) *V/F Validation: The Feil Method.* Cleveland, OH: Edward Feil Productions.

18 F. Goudie and G. Stokes (eds) (1989) *Working with Dementia.* Bicester: Winslow Press.

19 G. Prouty (1994) *Theoretical Evolutions in Person-Centred/Experiential Therapy: Applications to Schizophrenic and Retarded Psychoses.* Westport, CT: Praeger.

20 R.B. Adler and N. Towne (1993) *Looking Out/Looking In.* Orlando, FL: Harcourt Brace Jovanovich, p. 4.

21 J. Killick (1998) Learning a new language, *Alzheimer's Society Newsletter*, July: 4.

22 E. Goffman (1968) *Stigma: Notes on the Management of Spoiled Identity.* Harmondsworth: Penguin.

23 M. Goldsmith (1996) Slow down and listen to their voice, *Journal of Dementia Care*, 4(4): 24–5. See also M. Goldsmith (1996) *Hearing the Voice of People with Dementia: Opportunities and Obstacles.* London: Jessica Kingsley.

24 F. Gibson (1999) Can we risk person-centred communication? *Journal of Dementia Care*, 7(5): 20–4 (p. 24).

25 A. Damasio (1999) *The Feeling of What Happens: Body, Emotion and the Making of Consciousness.* London: Heineman, p. 5.

26 R. Harré (1998) *The Singular Self: An Introduction to the Psychology of Personhood.* London: Sage, p. 3.

27 S.G. Post (1992) To care but never to prolong? *Caring Magazine*, June, 40–3 (pp. 42–3).

28 For a full discussion of these ideas see E. Goffman (1969) *The Presentation of Self in Everyday Life.* Harmondsworth: Penguin.

29 S.R. Sabat and R. Harré (1992) The construction and deconstruction of self in Alzheimer's Disease, *Ageing and Society*, 12: 443–61 (p. 460).

30 J. Miller (2000) *The Body in Question.* London: Pimlico, p. 1.

31 For a review of this work see E. Aronson (1994) *The Social Animal.* New York: W.H. Freeman.

32 B. Macdonald (1984) *Look Me in the Eye: Old Women, Aging and Ageism.* London: The Women's Press, p. 14.

33 J.M. Hull (1990) *Touching the Rock: An Experience of Blindness.* London: Society for Promoting Christian Knowledge, p. 19.

34 S. Post (1995) *The Moral Challenge of Alzheimer's Disease.* Baltimore, MD: Johns Hopkins University Press, p. 3.

35 P. Ferrucci (1982) *What We May Be.* Wellingborough: Turnstone Press, p. 96.

36 F.G. Davidson (1995) *Alzheimer's: A Practical Guide for Carers to Help You Through the Day.* London: Piatkus, p. 7.

37 R. Gibson (1998) *Unmasking dementia, Community Care Inside Dementia*, 29 October–4 November: 6–7 (p. 6).

38 A. Storr (1994) *Solitude*. London: HarperCollins, p. 48.

39 J. Croft (2000) Communication day by day, *Pathways*, 6: 1.

40 See work by E. Barnett (2000) *Involving the Person with Dementia in Designing and Delivering Care: 'I Need to be Me!'*. London: Jessica Kingsley, and K. Allan (2001) *Communication and Consultation: Exploring Ways for Staff to Involve People with Dementia in Developing Services*. Bristol: Policy Press.

41 See M. Czikszentmihalyi (1992) *Flow: The Psychology of Happiness*. London: Rider.

42 O. Sacks (1984) *A Leg to Stand On*. London: Picador, p. 79, original emphasis.

43 P. Adams (1993) *Gesundheit!* Rochester, VT: Healing Arts Press, p. 66.

44 K.H. Zabbia (1996) *Painted Diaries: A Mother and Daughter's Experience through Alzheimer's*. Minneapolis, MN: Fairview Press, p. 60.

45 See C. Archibald (1997) Sexuality and dementia? In M. Marshall (ed.) *State of the Art in Dementia Care*. London: Centre for Policy on Ageing.

46 See E. Shamy (1997) *More than Body, Brain and Breath: A Guide to Spiritual Care of People with Alzheimer's Disease*. Orewa, NZ: ColCom Press.

47 O. Sacks (1985) *The Man Who Mistook his Wife for a Hat*. London: Picador, p. 36.

48 D. Everett (1996) *Forget Me Not: The Spiritual Care of People with Alzheimer's*. Edmonton, Alta: Inkwell Press, p. 167.

49 See T. Packer (2001) 'Everyone wants something': recognising your own needs, *Journal of Dementia Care*, 9(1): 26–8.

50 L. Rust (1986) Another part of the country. In J. Alexander (eds) *Women and Aging: An Anthology by Women*. Corvallis, OR: Calyx.

51 Ibid., p. 145.

3 Nonverbal communication

1 D. Wright (1990) *Deafness: A Personal Account*. London: Faber and Faber. p. 112

2 S. Post (1995) *The Moral Challenge of Alzheimer's Disease*. Baltimore, MD: Johns Hopkins University Press, p. vii.

3 M. Nind and D. Hewett (1994) *Access to Communication: Developing the Basics of Communication with People with Severe Learning Difficulties through Intensive Interaction*. London: David Fulton, p. 97.

4 For a full discussion of aspects of nonverbal communication see M. Argyle (1988) *Bodily Communication*. London: Routledge.

5 A.M. Lindbergh (1991) *Gift from the Sea*. New York: Vintage, p. 116.

6 For example, A. Pease (1997) *Body Language: How to Read Others' Thoughts by their Gestures*. London: Sheldon Press.

7 An exception to this is work from Scandinavia, for example, K. Asplund, A. Norberg, R. Adolfsson *et al.* (1991) Facial expressions in severely demented patients – a stimulus-response study of four patients with dementia of the Alzheimer's type, *International Journal of Geriatric Psychiatry*, 6(8): 599–606. Also, an older work from the US: S.B. Hoffman, C.A. Platt, K.E. Barry *et al.* (1985) When language fails: nonverbal communication abilities of the demented. In J.T. Hutton and A.D. Kenny (eds) *Senile Dementia of the Alzheimer Type*. New York: Alan R. Liss Inc.

8 T. Kitwood (1993) Towards a theory of dementia care: the interpersonal process, *Ageing and Society*, 13: 51–67 (p. 64).

9 O. Sacks (1986) *The Man Who Mistook his Wife for a Hat*. London: Picador, p. 79.

10 Ibid., original emphasis.
11 A. McKinlay (1998) *Inner→Out: A Journey with Dementia*. Rothesay, Isle of Bute: Charcoal Press.
12 T. Harrison (1993) *Black Daisies for the Bride*. London: Faber and Faber, p. 11.
13 See J. Rée (1999) *I See a Voice: Language, Deafness and the Senses – A Philosophical History*. London: Harper Collins.
14 M. Ignatieff (1993) *Scar Tissue*. London: Vintage.
15 M. Ignatieff (1994) *All in the Mind*. BBC Radio 4.
16 S. Mootoo (1999) *Cereus Blooms at Night*. London: Granta, pp. 126–7.
17 For a full discussion of this see R. Cheston and M. Bender (1999) *Understanding Dementia: The Man with the Worried Eyes*. London: Jessica Kingsley.
18 Nind and Hewett op. cit., p. 98.
19 For example, Nind and Hewett op. cit.
20 RCN video *When your Heart wants to Remember*.
21 B.L. Miller, K. Boone, J.L. Cummings *et al.* (2000) Functional correlates of musical and visual ability in frontotemporal dementia, *British Journal of Psychiatry*, 176: 458–63.
22 For a review of this work see: J. Killick and K. Allan (1999) The arts in dementia care: tapping a rich resource, *Journal of Dementia Care*, 7(4): 35–8; J. Killick and K. Allan (1999) The arts in dementia care: touching the human spirit, *Journal of Dementia Care*, 7(5): 33–7; K. Allan and J. Killick (2000) Undiminished possibility: the arts in dementia care, *Journal of Dementia Care*, 8(3): 16–18. Also, a new range of resources for encouraging communication through the arts is being developed by Dementia Services Development Centre, University of Sterling.
23 S. Jenny and M. Oropeza (1993) *Memories in the Making: A Program of Creative Art Expression for Alzheimer's Patients*. Orange County, CA: Alzheimer's Association.
24 For a review of this work see: J. Killick and K. Allan (1999) The arts in dementia care: tapping a rich resource, *Journal of Dementia Care*, 7(4): 35–8.
25 H. Finch (2000) Musical keys to communication, *Pathways*, 2: 1.
26 B. Heywood (1994) *Caring for Maria: An Experience of Coping Successfully with Alzheimer's Disease*. Shaftesbury: Element, p. 116.
27 J. Ellis and T. Thorn (2000) Sensory stimulation: where do we go from here? *Journal of Dementia Care*, 8(1): 33–7 (p. 36).
28 B.S. Brough (1998) *Alzheimer's with Love*. Lismore, NSW: Southern Cross Press, p. 19.
29 For further information on this topic, see G. Stokes (2000) *Challenging Behaviour in Dementia: A Person-centred Approach*. Bicester: Winslow Press.
30 F.G. Davidson (1995) *Alzheimer's: A Practical Guide for Carers to Help You Through the Day*. London: Piatkus, pp. 84–5.
31 See A. Grimes (1995) Auditory changes. In R. Lubinski (ed.) *Dementia and Communication*. San Diego, CA: Singular.
32 M. Downs (2000) A world without dementia? What do we need to do? *Dementia in Scotland:* Newsletter of Alzheimers Scotland – Action on Dementia, March, 6.
33 For example: D. Brandes and H. Phillips (1977) *Gamesters' Handbook*. Cheltenham: Stanley Thornes; T. Bond (1986) *Games for Social and Life Skills*. Cheltenham: Stanley Thornes.
34 P. Crimmens (1995) Beyond words: to the core of the human need for contact, *Journal of Dementia Care*, 3(6): 12–14 (p. 14).
35 Ibid.

4 Language

1 P. Lively (1988) *Moon Tiger*. Harmondsworth: Penguin, p. 41.
2 P. Newham (1999) *Using Voice and Song in Therapy: The Practical Application of Voice Movement Therapy*. London: Jessica Kingsley, p. 14.
3 J. Rée (1999) *I See a Voice: Language, Deafness and the Senses – a Philosophical History*. London: HarperCollins, p. 16.
4 S. Pinker (1995) *The Language Instinct*. Harmondsworth: Penguin, p. 21.
5 J-D. Bauby (1997) *The Diving Bell and the Butterfly*. London: Fourth Estate, pp. 48–9.
6 Lively op. cit., pp. 41–2.
7 An illuminating discussion of these matters is J. Aitchison (1994) *Words in the Mind*. Oxford: Blackwell.
8 Pinker op. cit., p. 19.
9 O. Sacks (1995) *An Anthropologist on Mars*. London: Picador, pp. 245–7.
10 O. Sacks (1991) *Seeing Voices*. London: Picador, pp. 38–9.
11 Ibid., pp. 39–40.
12 Ibid., pp. 56–7.
13 C. Antaki (2000) Why I study . . . talk in interaction, *The Psychologist*, 13(5): 242–43 (p. 242).
14 D.C. Dennett (1996) *Kinds of Minds: Towards an Understanding of Consciousness*. London: Phoenix, pp. 12–13.
15 T. Zeldin (1998) *Conversation: How Talk Can Change Your Life*. London: Harvill Press, p. 14.
16 See R. Lubinski (1995) *Dementia and Communication*. San Diego, CA: Singular.
17 D.N. Ripich and B.Y. Terrell (1988) Cohesion and coherence in Alzheimer's Disease, *Journal of Speech and Hearing Disorders*, 53: 8–14.
18 J. Appell, A. Kertesz and M. Fisman (1982) A study of language functioning in Alzheimer's patients, *Brain and Language*, 17: 73–91.
19 H.E. Hamilton (1994) *Conversations with an Alzheimer's Patient: An Interactional Socio-linguistic Study*. Cambridge: Cambridge University Press.
20 P. Becker (1988) Language in particular: a lecture. In D. Tannen (ed.) *Linguistics in Context*. Norwood, NJ: Ablex.
21 Hamilton op cit., p. 172.
22 M. Ignatieff (1993) *Scar Tissue*. London: Vintage, pp. 140–1.
23 Quoted in L. Grant (1997) *Remind Me Who I Am, Again*. London: Granta, p. 42.
24 B.S. Brough (1998) *Alzheimer's with Love*. Lismore, NSW: Southern Cross University Press, p. 2.
25 T. Kotai-Ewers (1999) Going into the middle: the search for meaning in the words of people with Alzheimer's. Unpublished paper presented at Australian National Alzheimer's Conference, Perth, September.
26 J. Aitchison (1994) *Words in the Mind*. Oxford: Blackwell, p. 154.
27 O. Sacks (1995) *An Anthropologist on Mars*. London: Picador, p. xiv.
28 C. Keegan (1998) *Talking with Jean*. Stirling: DSDC (Dementia Services Development Centre).
29 J. Crisp (1995) Communication. In S. Garrett and E. Hamilton-Smith (eds) *Rethinking Dementia: An Australian Approach*. Melbourne: Ausmed.
30 K.H. Zabbia (1996) *Painted Diaries*. Minneapolis, MN: Fairview Press.
31 Ibid., pp. 143–4.
32 Brough op. cit., pp. 52–3.
33 R. Watt and J. Anderson (2000) Fa yaav's you? Dialect and dementia, *Pathways*, 6: 20.

34 N. Patel and N. Mirza (2000) Care for ethnic minorities: the professional view, *Journal of Dementia Care*, 8(1): 26–8.
35 L. Rust (1986) Another part of the country. In J. Alexander, D. Berrow, L. Domitro-vitch *et al.* (eds) *Women and Aging*. Corvallis, OR: Calyx, p. 140.
36 M. Forster (1990) *Have the Men Had Enough?* Harmondsworth: Penguin.
37 Ibid., p. 98, emphasis as original.
38 Ibid., p. 72.

5 Memory

1 S. Rose (1993) *The Making of Memory: From Molecules to Mind*. London: Bantam, p. 1.
2 For an overview of this work see G. Cohen (1996) *Memory in the Real World*. Hove: Psychology Press.
3 For a general guide to the study of memory see A. Baddeley (1992) *Your Memory: A User's Guide*. Harmondsworth: Penguin.
4 For discussion of work on this, again see A. Baddeley, op cit.
5 See G. Bower (1981) Mood and memory, *American Psychologist*, 36: 129–48.
6 F. Bartlett (1932) *Remembering: A Study of Experimental and Social Psychology*. Cambridge: Cambridge University Press, p. 203.
7 L. Grant (1998) *Remind Me Who I Am, Again*. London: Granta, p. 29.
8 M. Mills (1997) Narrative identity and dementia: a study of emotion and narrative in older people with dementia, *Ageing and Society*, 17: 673–98. With reference to W.F. Brewer (1986) What is autobiographical memory? In D.C. Rubin (ed.) *Autobiographical Memory*. Cambridge: Cambridge University Press. A.J. Parkin (1987) *Memory and Amnesia: An Introduction*. Oxford: Blackwell. A.J. Parkin (1993) *Memory: Phenomenon, Experiment and Theory*. Oxford: Blackwell.
9 See U.P. Holden and R.T. Woods (1988) *Reality Orientation: Psychological Approaches to the 'Confused' Elderly*, 2nd edn. Edinburgh: Churchill Livingstone.
10 For an overview of this work see F. Gibson (1999) *Reminiscence and Recall*. London: Age Concern. A good practical guide is E. Bruce, S. Hidgson and P. Schweitzer (2000) *Reminiscing with People with Dementia: A Handbook for Carers*. London: Age Exchange.
11 For an overview of this work see U.P. Holden and R.T. Woods (1995) *Positive Approaches to Dementia Care*. Edinburgh: Churchill Livingstone.
12 A. Crump (1997) Room to remember, *Nursing Practice*, 9(3): 8–10.
13 Mills op. cit., pp. 695–6.
14 O. Sacks (1985) *The Man Who Mistook his Wife for a Hat*. London: Picador, p.105, original emphasis.
15 L. Slater (2000) *Spasm: A Memoir with Lies*. London: Methuen, pp. 219–20.
16 M. de Hennezel (1997) *Intimate Death: How the Dying Teach us to Live*. London: Little, Brown, p. 146, original emphasis.
17 M. Ikeda, E. Mori, N. Hirono *et al.* (1998) Amnestic people with Alzheimer's Disease who remembered the Kobe earthquake, *British Journal of Psychiatry*, 172: 425–8.
18 For an overview of this work see L. Hunt, C. Rowlings and M. Marshall (1997) *Past Trauma in Late Life: European Perspectives on Therapeutic Work with Older People*. London: Jessica Kingsley.
19 For discussion of the concept of identity in the context of a psychological model of dementia and the practice of psychotherapeutic work, see R. Chester and M. Bender (1999) *Understanding Dementia: The Man with the Worried Eyes*. London: Jessica Kingsley.

20 M. Ignatieff (1994) *Scar Tissue*. London: Vintage, p. 53, original emphasis.
21 D. Everett (1996) *Forget Me Not*. Edmonton, Alta: Inkwell Press, p. 85.
22 M. Ignatieff (1992) A taste of ice cream is all you know, *Observer*, 4 July.
23 S.G. Post (1995) *The Moral Challenge of Alzheimer's Disease*. Baltimore, MD: Johns Hopkins University Press, p. 37.
24 P. Coleman (1986) *Ageing and Reminiscence Processes: Social and Clinical Implications*. Chichester: Wiley.

6 Interpretation

1 R. Fulghum (1990) *It Was on Fire When I Lay Down on It*. London: HarperCollins, pp. 5–7, original emphasis.
2 N. Humphrey (1993) *The Inner Eye*. London: Vintage, pp. 36–7.
3 The ideas in the following sections come from the application of cognitive psychology to clinical problems such as depression and anxiety. Further information can be found in D. Burns (1990) *The Feeling Good Handbook*. New York: Penguin.
4 For a full discussion of these ideas see E. Aronson (1994) *The Social Animal*. New York: W.H. Freeman.
5 For a full discussion of this see N. Thompson (1995) *Age and Dignity: Working with Older People*. Aldershot: Arena.
6 D. Burns (1992) *Feeling Good: The New Mood Therapy*. New York: Avon.
7 T.M. Häggström, L. Jansson and A. Norberg (1998) Skilled carers' ways of understanding people with Alzheimer's Disease, *Scholarly Inquiry for Nursing Practice: An International Journal*, 12(3): 239–66; with reference to E. Athlin, A. Norberg and K. Asplund (1990) Caregivers' perceptions and interpretations of severely demented patients during feeding in a task assignment care system, *Scandinavian Journal of Caring Sciences*, 4(4): 147–56; and S.J. Pawlby (1977) Imitative interaction. In H.R. Scaffer (ed.) *Studies in Mother–Infant Interaction*. London: Academic Press, pp. 203–24.
8 Häggström *et al*. op cit., p. 240.
9 Ibid.
10 Humphrey op. cit., p. 57.
11 T. Kitwood (1993) Discover the person, not the disease, *Journal of Dementia Care*, 1(6): 16–17.
12 C. Keegan (1998) *Talking with Jean*. Stirling: DSDC, p. 1, original emphasis.
13 B.M. Hellner and A. Norberg (1994) Intuition: two caregivers' descriptions of how they provide severely demented patients with loving care, *International Journal of Aging and Human Development*, 38(4): 327–38.
14 P. Benner, (1984) *From Novice to Expert, Excellence and Power in Clinical Nursing Practise*. Menlo Park, CA: Addison-Wesley.
15 See G. Claxton (1998) Investigating human intuition: knowing without knowing why, *The Psychologist*, 11(5): 217–20.
16 For a useful discussion of these issues, see J. Crisp (2000) *Keeping in Touch with Someone who has Alzheimer's*. Melbourne: Ausmed.
17 S. Knocker (2000) 'A meeting of worlds – play and metaphor in dementia care and dramatherapy'. Unpublished manuscript, p. 7.
18 A. McKinlay (1998) *Inner→Out: A Journey with Dementia*. Rothesay, Isle of Bute: Charcoal Press.
19 A. McKinlay (2000) personal communication.
20 Keegan op. cit., p. 1.

21 J. Bayley (1998) *Iris: A Memoir of Iris Murdoch*. London: Duckworth, p. 44.
22 A. Norberg (1996) Caring for demented patients, *Acta Neurologica Scandinavica*, 165: 105–8, p. 106.

7 Making contact

1 L. Rust (1986) Another part of the country. In J. Alexander, D. Berrow, L. Domitrovitch *et al.* (eds) *Women and Aging*. Corvallis, OR: Calyx, p. 140.
2 J. Nussbaum, J. Robinson and D. Grew (1985) Communicative behaviour of the long-term health care employee: Implications for the elderly resident, *Communication Research Reports*, 2: 16–22.
3 The skills described in the following chapters can be explored in more depth in texts such as R. Nelson-Jones (2000) *Introduction to Counselling Skills*. London: Sage.
4 From T. Kotai-Ewers (1999) Falling apart: an in-depth view of one man's progress through early onset Alzheimer's. Disease paper given at International Alzheimer's Conference, Johannesburg, September.
5 Ibid.
6 T. Perrin and H. May (2000) *Wellbeing in Dementia*. London: Churchill Livingstone.

8 Developing the interaction

1 E.M. Starkman (1993) *Learning to Sit in the Silence: A Journal of Caretaking*. Watsonville, CA: Papier-Mache Press.
2 D.W. Lipinska (2000) Listening between the lines: counselling people with dementia, *Pathways*, 3: 1–2, (p. 2).
3 J.M. Hull (1990) *Touching the Rock: An Experience of Blindness*. London: SPCK, p. 17.
4 J. Crisp (1995) Dementia and communication. In S. Garrett and E. Hamilton-Smith (eds) *Rethinking Dementia*. Melbourne: Ausmed, p. 59.

10 Writing

1 G. Wallas (1926) *The Art of Thought*. London: Jonathan Cape, p. 106.
2 See P. Elbow (1981) *Writing with Power*. Oxford: Oxford University Press; M. Schneider and J. Killick (1998) *Writing for Self-Discovery: A Personal Approach to Creative Writing*. Shaftesbury: Element.
3 H. Hesse (1970) *Gesammelte Werke*, vol. 11. Hamburg: Suhrkamp Verlag, p. 80.
4 K. Allan (2001) *Communication and Consultation: Exploring Ways for Staff to Involve People with Dementia in Developing Services*. Bristol: Policy Press.
5 C. Keegan (1998) personal communication. See also C. Keegan (1998) *Talking with Jean*. Stirling: DSDC.
6 T. Kotai-Ewers (1999) Going into the middle: the search for meaning in the words of people with Alzheimer's. Unpublished paper presented at Australian National Alzheimer's Conference, Perth, September.
7 See J. Killick (1997) *You are Words: Dementia Poems*. London: Hawker; J. Killick and C. Cordonnier (2000) *Openings: Dementia Poems and Photographs*. London: Hawker.
8 K.H. Zabbia (1996) *Painted Diaries*. Minneapolis, MN: Fairview Press.

9 Ibid., p. 102.
10 R. Davis (1993) *My Journey into Alzheimer's Disease*. Amersham-on-the-Hill: Scripture Press.
11 Ibid., pp. 18–19.
12 B.S. Brough (1998) *Alzheimer's with Love*. Lismore, NSW: Southern Cross University Press, original emphasis.
13 Ibid., p. 6.

11 Narrative

1 I. Allende (1995) *Paula*. London: HarperCollins, p. 8.
2 O. Sacks (1986) *The Man Who Mistook his Wife for a Hat*. London: Picador, p. 105, original emphasis.
3 A. MacIntyre (1981) *After Virtue: A Study in Moral Theory*. London: Duckworth, p. 216.
4 A. Damasio (1999) *The Feeling of What Happens: Body, Emotion and the Making of Consciousness*. London: Heinemann, p. 188.
5 M. de Hennezel (1997) *Intimate Death: How the Dying Teach us to Live*. London: Little, Brown, pp. 111–12.
6 See E. Bruce (1999) Holding on to the story: older people, narrative and dementia. In G. Roberts and J. Holmes (eds) *Healing Stories: Narrative in Psychiatry and Psychotherapy*. Oxford: Oxford University Press.
7 D.P. Spence (1982) Narrative persuasion, *Psychoanalysis and Contemporary Thought*, 6: 457–81 (p. 458).
8 J. Crisp (1995) Making sense of the stories that people with Alzheimer's tell: a journey with my mother, *Nursing Inquiry*, 2: 133–40, (p. 137).
9 J. Bayley (1998) *Iris: A Memoir of Iris Murdoch*. London: Duckworth.
10 B.S. Brough (1998) *Alzheimer's with Love*. Lismore, NSW: Southern Cross University Press, p. 39.
11 Ibid., p. 68.
12 L. Grant (1998) *Remind Me Who I Am, Again*. London: Granta, p. 37.
13 P. Crimmens (no date) Drama therapy in the care of people with dementia. Unpublished paper.
14 For example P. Batson (1998) Drama as therapy: bringing memories to life, *Journal of Dementia Care*, 6(4): 19–21.
15 G. Holst, A.K. Edberg and I.R. Hallberg (1999) Nurses' narrations and reflections about caring for patients with severe dementia as revealed in systematic clinical supervision sessions, *Journal of Aging Studies*, 13(1): 89–107. See also G.M. Kenyon and W.L. Randall (1997) *Restorying Our Lives: Personal Growth Through Autobiographical Reflection*. Westport, CN: Praeger.
16 Holst *et al.* (1999), p. 90.
17 Ibid., p. 104.

12 Relationships

1 Aristotle (1926) *The Nicomachean Ethics*, translated H. Rackham. London: Heinemann, pp. 573–4. (This quote is an adapted version from this translation.)
2 M.S. Peck (1978) *The Road Less Travelled*. New York: Simon and Schuster.

3 For an overview of this work, see E. Aronson (1994) *The Social Animal*. New York: W.H. Freeman.

4 See E. Goffman (1969) *The Presentation of Self in Everyday Life*. Harmondsworth: Penguin.

5 See for example, R.G. Adams and R. Blieszner (eds) (1989) *Older Adult Friendship*. Newbury Park, CA: Sage.

6 An exception to this is J. Reed (1999) Keeping a distance: the reactions of older people in care homes to confused fellow residents. In T. Adams and C.L. Clarke (eds) *Dementia Care: Developing Partnerships in Practice*. London: Ballière Tindall.

7 J. Killick (1997) *You are Words*. London: Hawker, p. 38.

8 C. Archibald (1997) Sexuality and dementia? In M. Marshall (ed.) *State of the Art in Dementia Care*. London: Centre for Policy on Ageing.

9 A. McKinlay (1998) *Inner→Out: A Journey with Dementia*. Rothesay, Isle of Bute: Charcoal Press.

10 B.S. Brough (1998) *Alzheimer's with Love*. Lismore, NSW: Southern Cross University Press, p. 23.

11 K.H. Zabbia (1996) *Painted Diaries*. Minneapolis, MN: Fairview Press, pp. 171–2.

12 L. Rust (1986) Another part of the country. In J. Alexander, D. Berrow, L. Domitrovitch *et al.* (eds) *Women and Aging*. Corvallis, OR: Calyx, p. 140.

13 T. Packer and J. Dewing (2000) 'Crossed lines: crossed words – is the support in your team as helpful as you'd like?' Workshop presented at *Journal of Dementia Care* conference, Bournemouth, 17 May. See also T. Kitwood (1997) *Dementia Reconsidered*. Buckingham: Open University Press, for exploration of the idea of 'scripts' in Chapter 8.

14 L. Grant (1997) *Remind Me Who I Am, Again*. London: Granta, p. 268.

15 M. Ignatieff (1993) *Scar Tissue*. London: Vintage, p. 50.

16 Ignatieff op cit., p. 58.

17 Brough op. cit., p. 15.

18 P.G. Coleman (1996) Last scene of all. Inaugural lecture delivered at the University of Southampton, April.

19 T. Cassirer (1999) Separate and yet together: living with a spouse suffering from Alzheimer's Disease, *Last Acts: Innovations in End of Life Care*. 1(4): 1–4, (pp. 3–4).

20 Brough op. cit., pp. 63–4, original emphasis.

21 McKinlay op. cit.

22 See B. Miesen (1999) *Dementia in Close–up*. London: Routledge.

23 J. Bowlby (1969) *Attachment and Loss*, vol. 1. London: Hogarth Press.

24 See J.W. Worden (1991) *Grief Counselling and Grief Therapy: A Handbook for the Mental Health Practitioner*. London: Routledge.

25 Grant op. cit., p. 14.

26 J. Griffiths (1994) Addressing the need for mourning in bereaved people with dementia. Unpublished paper.

27 Brough op. cit., p. 37.

28 See T. Packer (2000) Facing up to the Bills, *Journal of Dementia Care*, 8(4): 30–3.

13 Awareness

1 N.M. Gunn (1986) *The Atom of Delight*. London: Polygon, p. 20, original emphasis.

2 C. Rogers (1967) *On Becoming a Person*. London: Constable, p. 78.

3 M. Csikszentmihalyi (1992) *Flow: The Psychology of Happiness*. London: Rider.

4 Ibid., p. 53.

5 For example, M. Kihlgren, A. Hallgren, A. Norberg *et al.* (1990) Effects of training in integrity – promoting care on the interaction at a long-term ward, *Scandinavian Journal of Caring Sciences*, 4(1): 21–8.

6 See work by S.M. McGlynn and D.L. Schachter (1989) Unawareness of deficits in neuropsychological syndromes, *Journal of Experimental Neuropsychology*, 1: 143–205; A. David (1990) Insight and psychosis, *British Journal of Psychiatry*, 156: 798–808; M.B. Markova and G.E. Berrios (1995) Insight in clinical psychiatry: a new model, *Journal of Nervous and Mental Disease*, 183(12): 743–51; R. Mullen, R. Howard, A. David *et al.* (1996) Insight in Alzheimer's disease, *International Journal of Geriatric Psychiatry*, 11: 645–51.

7 A. Jacques (1992) *Understanding Dementia*. Edinburgh: Churchill Livingstone.

8 Ibid., p. 172.

9 K.D. McDaniel, S.D. Edland, A. Heyman *et al.* (1995) Relationship between level of insight and severity of dementia in Alzheimer's Disease, *Alzheimer's Disease and Associated Disorders*, 9(2): 101–4.

10 F.R.J. Verhey, N. Rozendaal, R.W.H.M. Ponds *et al.* (1994) Dementia, awareness and depression, *International Journal of Geriatric Psychiatry*, 8: 851–6.

11 K.M. Allan (2001) *Communication and Consultation: Exploring Ways for Staff to Involve People with Dementia in Developing Services*. Bristol: Policy Press.

12 Jacques op cit., p. 172.

13 A. Damasio (2000) *The Feeling of What Happens: Body, Emotion and the Making of Consciousness*. London: Heinemann, pp. 104–5.

14 M. Ignatieff (1994) *Scar Tissue*. London: Vintage, pp. 49–50.

15 V. Cotrell and L. Lein (1993) Awareness and denial in the Alzheimer's Disease victim. *Journal of Gerontological Social Work*, 19(3/4): 115–32.

16 J. Bayley (1998) *Iris: A Memoir of Iris Murdoch*. London: Duckworth, p. 178.

17 Ibid., p. 178.

18 M. Forster (1990) *Have the Men Had Enough?* Harmondsworth: Penguin.

19 Ibid., p. 42, original emphasis.

20 K.H. Zabbia (1996) *Painted Diaries*. Minneapolis, MN: Fairview Press.

21 Ibid., p. 143.

22 We are grateful to the Psychology Deparment of Hull and East Riding Community Health Trust for permission to quote the example.

23 A. Norberg (1996) Caring for demented patients. *Acta Neurologica Scandinavica*, 165: 105–8.

24 Ibid., p. 105.

25 Also termed 'spontaneous intermittent remissions' by S. Thorpe (1996) Language changes in Alzheimer's Disease, *Alzheimer's Disease Society Newsletter*, July.

26 J. Killick (1997) When the clouds part, *Journal of Dementia Care*, 5(1): 24.

27 B. Heywood (1994) *Caring for Maria*. London: Element.

28 Ibid., pp. 203–4.

29 See work by H.K. Normann, K. Asplund and A. Norberg (1998) Episodes of lucidity in people with severe dementia as narrated by formal carers, *Journal of Advanced Nursing*, 28(6): 1295–300.

30 O. Sacks (1982) *Awakenings*. London: Picador.

31 Ibid., p. 312, original emphasis.

32 A. McKinlay (1998) *Inner→Out: A Journey with Dementia*. Rothesay, Isle of Bute: Charcoal Press.

33 S. Post (1995) *The Moral Challenge of Alzheimer's Disease*. Baltimore, MD: Johns Hopkins University Press.

14 Implications for care

1 B.M. Akerlund and A. Norberg (1990) Powerlessness in the terminal care of demented patients: an exploratory study, *Omega*, 21(1): 15–19 (p. 18).
2 S.L. Ekman, A. Norberg, M. Viitanen and B. Winblad (1991) Care of demented patients with severe communication problems, *Scandinavian Journal of Caring Sciences*, 5(3): 163–70.
3 Ibid., p. 168.
4 T. Kitwood (1995) Positive long-term changes in dementia: some preliminary observations, *Journal of Mental Health*, 4: 133–44.
5 T. Kitwood (1997) *Dementia Reconsidered.* Buckingham: Open University Press, p. 47.
6 Discussion of the stages of learning can also be found in F. Strandgaard (1981) *NLP Made Visual.* Copenhagen: Connector.
7 T. Packer (2000) A person-centred approach to the people who care, *Journal of Dementia Care*, 8(6): 28–30.

15 Ethical implications

1 T. Kitwood (1997) *Dementia Reconsidered.* Buckingham: Open University Press, p. 69.
2 J. Killick (1997) Communication: a matter of the life and death of the mind, *Journal of Dementia Care*, 5(5): 14–16 (p. 14).
3 C.K. Williams (1997) *The Vigil.* Newcastle-upon-Tyne: Bloodaxe, pp. 4–5.
4 P. Casement (1985) *On Learning from the Patient.* London: Routledge.
5 See T. Packer (2000) A person-centred approach to people who care? *Journal of Dementia Care*, 8(6): 28–30.
6 S.L. Ekman and A. Norberg (1988) The autonomy of demented patients: interviews with caregivers, *Journal of Medical Ethics*, 14: 184–7 (p. 185).
7 L. Grant (1997) *Remind Me Who I am, Again.* London: Granta, p. 159.
8 G. Holst *et al.* (1999) Nurses' narrations and reflections about caring for patients with severe dementia as revealed in systematic clinical supervision sessions. *Journal of Aging Studies*, 13(1): 89–107.
9 Ibid., p. 99.
10 F. Gibson (1999) Can we risk person-centred communication? *Journal of Dementia Care*, 7(5): 20–4 (p. 21).
11 K. Gibran ([1926] 1994) *The Prophet.* London: Bracken, pp. 61–2.
12 T. Kitwood and K. Bredin (1992) Towards a theory of dementia care: Personhood and wellbeing. *Ageing and Society*, 12: 269–87, p. 270.
13 M. de Hennezel (1997) *Intimate Death: How the Dying Teach Us to Live.* London: Little, Brown, pp. 130–1.

16 Conversations with Jane

1 Quoted with permission, O. Sacks (1994).

Index

DEMENTIA RECONSIDERED
THE PERSON COMES FIRST

Tom Kitwood

Over the last ten years or so Tom Kitwood has made a truly remarkable contribution to our understanding of dementia, and to raising expectations of what can be achieved with empathy and skill. This lucid account of his thinking and work will communicate his approach to a yet wider audience. It is to be warmly welcomed.

> Mary Marshall, Director of the Dementia Services
> Development Centre, University of Stirling

This is a very radical book; it could be called revolutionary . . . (it) is relevant to all professionals engaged in direct practice with people with dementia as well as policy makers, service planners, managers and resource holders . . . I believe that it will profoundly influence the development of dementia care in the years ahead.

> *Journal of Dementia Care*

Kitwood's book is an eloquent reminder of the importance of relationships in caring.

> *Mental Health Care*

Tom Kitwood breaks new ground in this book. Many of the older ideas about dementia are subjected to critical scrutiny and reappraisal, drawing on research evidence, logical analysis and the author's own experience. The unifying theme is the personhood of men and women who have dementia – an issue that was grossly neglected for many years both in psychiatry and care practice. Each chapter provides a definitive statement on a major topic related to dementia, for example: the nature of 'organic mental impairment', the experience of dementia, the agenda of care practice, and the transformation of the culture of care.

While recognizing the enormous difficulties of the present day, the book clearly demonstrates the possibility of a better life for people who have dementia, and comes to a cautiously optimistic conclusion. It will be of interest to all professionals involved in dementia care or provision, students on courses involving psychogeriatrics or social work with older people, and family carers of people with dementia.

Contents

Introduction – On being a person – Dementia as a psychiatric category – How personhood is undermined – Personhood maintained – The experience of dementia – Improving care: the next step forward – The caring organization – Requirements of a caregiver – The task of cultural transformation – References – Name index – Subject index.

176pp   0 335 19855 4 (Paperback)   0 335 19856 2 (Hardback)